VERTIGO, NAUSEA, TINNITUS AND HYPOACUSIA DUE TO HEAD AND NECK TRAUMA

VERTIGO, NAUSEA, TINNITUS AND HYPOACUSIA DUE TO HEAD AND NECK TRAUMA

Proceedings of the XVIIth Scientific Meeting of the Neurootological and Equilibriometric Society: Vertigo, Nausea, Tinnitus and Hypoacusia due to Head and Neck Trauma, Bad Kissingen, 22–25 March, 1990

Editors:

Claus-Frenz Claussen
Bad Kissingen, F.R.G.

Milind V. Kirtane
Bombay, India

 1991

EXCERPTA MEDICA, AMSTERDAM – LONDON – NEW YORK – TOKYO

© 1991 Elsevier Science Publishers B.V. All rights reserved.

No part of this publication may be reproduced, stored in a retrieval system or transmitted in any form or by any means, electronic, mechanical, photocopying, recording or otherwise without the prior written permission of the publisher, Elsevier Science Publishers B.V., Permissions Department, P.O. Box 521, 1000 AM Amsterdam, The Netherlands.

No responsibility is assumed by the Publisher for any injury and/or damage to persons or property as a matter of products liability, negligence or otherwise, or from any use or operation of any methods, products, instructions or ideas contained in the material herein. Because of rapid advances in the medical sciences, the Publisher recommends that independent verification of diagnoses and drug dosages should be made.

Special regulations for readers in the USA – This publication has been registered with the Copyright Clearance Center Inc. (CCC), 27 Congress Street, Salem, MA 01970, USA. Information can be obtained from the CCC about conditions under which photocopies of parts of this publication may be made in the USA. All other copyright questions, including photocopying outside the USA, should be referred to the copyright owner, Elsevier Science Publishers B.V., unless otherwise specified.

International Congress Series No. 929
ISBN 0-444-81150-8

This book is printed on acid-free paper.

Published by:
Elsevier Science Publishers B.V.
P.O. Box 211
1000 AE Amsterdam
The Netherlands

Sole distributors for the USA and Canada:
Elsevier Science Publishing Company Inc.
655 Avenue of the Americas
New York, NY 10010
USA

Library of Congress Cataloging-in-Publication Data

Neurootological and Equilibriometric Society. Scientific Meeting (17th : 1990 : Bad Kissingen, Germany)
  Vertigo, nausea, tinnitus, and hypoacusia due to head and neck trauma : Proceedings of the XVIIth Scientific Meeting of the Neurootological and Equilibriometric Society : vertigo, nausea, tinnitus, and hypoacusia due to head and neck trauma, Bad Kissingen, 22-25 March 1990 / editors, Claus-Frenz Claussen, Milind V. Kirtane.
    p. cm. -- (International congress series ; no. 929)
  Includes index.
  ISBN 0-444-81150-8 (alk. paper)
  1. Head--Wounds and injuries--Complications and sequelae--Congresses. 2. Neck--Wounds and injuries--Complications and sequelae--Congresses. 3. Vestibular apparatus--Diseases--Congresses. 4. Hearing disorders--Congresses. I. Claussen, Claus-Frenz. II. Kirtane, Milind V. III. Title. IV. Series.
  [DNLM: 1. Head Injuries--complications--congresses. 2. Hearing Disorders--etiology--congresses. 3. Labyrinth Diseases--etiology--congresses. 4. Neck--injuries--congresses. 5. Ocular Motility Disorders--etiology--congresses.   W3 EX89 no. 929 / WE 706 N494 1990v]
RD521.N46 1990
617.5'1044--dc20
DNLM/DLC
for Library of Congress   91-34650
                                                                  CIP

Printed in The Netherlands

FOREWORD

From March 22nd till 25th, 1990, the XVIIth international congress of the Neurootological and Equilibriometric Society Reg. was held at Bad Kissingen, West Germany. The meeting was attended by participants from 30 nations.

Most of the contributions are dealing with the 2 main themes of this congress, of which the first is related to investigation methods: Objective and Quantitative Equilibrium Tests, and the second to an outstanding clinical problem: Vertigo, Nausea, Tinnitus and Hypoacusia due to Head and Neck Trauma.

The symposium on objective and quantitative equilibrium tests was especially organized in honour of Prof. Dr. Pedro Luiz Mangabeira Albernaz from São Paulo, Brazil, who has introduced a special method of triangular electronystagmographic derivation. He has also created a deep interest in objective and quantitative equilibriometry not only in the countries of Latin America, but also in the English speaking world.

The XVIIth scientific NES congress was convened under the patronage of the president of the Bavarian Senate, Dr. Hans Weiß. Clinically it dealt with the mechanisms and the sequalae of head and neck trauma. Besides the general aspects of head and neck truama, the epidemiology of neurootological findings resulting from head and neck trauma was also discussed from a more basic and morphological point of view. Then special functional clinical aspects were analyzed like inner ear trauma, pathological nystagmus findings after head trauma, audiovestibular disturbances because of head trauma, posttraumatic neurootological disturbances resulting from cervical lesions, posttraumatic vascular problems with respect to neurootology, and vestibular spinal disturbances due to head trauma. Attention was also paid to changes in evoked potentials and EEG due to concussional trauma, and also to fractures of the skull.

In addition, audiovestibular and taste and smell disturbances were elucidated including psychological features in head and neck trauma. Finally, the various aspects of the treatment of posttraumatic vertigo, nausea, tinnitus and hearing loss have been presented and debated, including surgical, rehabilitative and drug treatment.

Thus, the XVIIth NES congress, as shown by the results printed in this volume, fulfills the aims of the Neurootological and Equilibriometric Society to promote clinical neurootology in practice and in the field of clinical research, to standardize clinical methods, to create functional standards, as well as to develop diagnostic and therapeutic modalities in neurootology.

We thank all contributors and participants, who have helped us to bring these results together and especially Dr. Dieter Schneider, who took care of the indices. We are also very much obliged to Elsevier Science Publishers BV, Amsterdam, for their close cooperation and kind support in the completion of this volume. Finally, we thankfully acknowledge the help and support of the city of Bad Kissingen, the Bavarian government and the DAAD, who have supported the meeting. We are also grateful for the help of our industrial sponsors, especially the laboratories Intersan, Ettlingen, West Germany, who substantially support the publication of this volume.

Bad Kissingen, June 1990   Claus-F. Claussen *Editor*
M.V. Kirtane *Editor*

CONTENTS

NYSTAGMOGRAPHY

The many faces of Pedro Luiz Mangabiera Albernaz
   W. Rubin   3
4- Generations of automatic nystagmus analysators
   G.O. Bertora, J.M. Bergmann, C.-F. Claussen and E. Claussen   5
The possibility of adequate stimulation of the phasic canal in the vestibular system
   P. Schwartze, K. Mukherjee and F. Thoss   9
Physiological nystagmic and non-nystagmic ocular movements recorded by means of the Peng-method by H.R. Gestewitz
   B. Gestewitz   13
On the diagnostic importance of saccadic ocular movements (waves and square waves) in the nystagmogram
   D. Gestewitz   17
The Peng-apparatus with computer-aided evaluation made by VEB Kombinant Carl-Zeiss Jena – First clinical experiences
   H.R. Gestewitz   21
Visual suppression in the caloric and rotatory tests
   J. Deblen, T. Ledin, L. Noaksson and L.M. Ödkvist   25
Oculomotor disturbances in normal children learning to read
   V. Gabersek   31
Electrical vestibular stimulation of cochlear implanted patients
   B. Frachet, V. Gabersek, T. van den Abbeele and P. Tison   37
Influence of the head-body position on optokinetic afternystagmus
   H.J. Scholtz, A.W. Scholtz and U. Sievert   41
Brain electrical activity mapping – A new frontier in neurootology
   A. Hahn, C.-F. Claussen, D. Schneider, U. Fraass and B. Büki   45
Experiences gathered so far with the investigation of the direction changing somato-autokinesis
   E. Černý   49
Auditory blink reflex in children with cerebral palsy
   M. Uzunova and L. Stamatova   53
Head shaking nystagmus and right/left vestibular asymmetry
   S. Takahashi   57
Oculomotor stimulations in a patient with an ocular epileptic equivalent
   V. Gabersek   63

Vergence nystagmus physiopathological considerations about five cases
  D. Caputo, A. Cesarani, D. Alpini and M. Mini   67
A new concept of Meniere's syndrome
  L.H. Hiranandani   71
Influence of asymmetric peripheral vestibular activity on optokinetic
after-nystagmus in man
  K. Brantberg and M. Magnusson   75
$GABA_A$ receptors induce hyperpolarization in outer hair cells of the guinea
pig cochlea
  A.H. Gitter, P.K. Plinkert and H.P. Zenner   79
α-Bungarotoxin binding to nicotinic acetylcholine receptors in the
mammalian cochlea
  P.K. Plinkert, A.H. Gitter and H.P. Zenner   83

GENERAL ASPECTS OF HEAD AND NECK TRAUMA

Posttraumatic dysequilibrium
  C.F. Claussen and E. Claussen   89
Neuroradiological aspects of posttraumatic brain lesions
  H. Gräfin von Einsiedel   97
Sequelae of injuries of the temporal region
  R.P. Firsching and A. Karimi-Nejad   103
Head trauma with associated vertigo
  W. Ruben   107

FRACTURES OF THE SKULL BASE

Functional complications after the otobasal fracture
  L. Kessler   113
Behaviour of the speech analysis after fronto-basal skull fractures
  H.G. Dieroff and G. Schuhmann   119
The function of the vestibular system after cranial injury – A critical review
  P. Christ, M. Meichelböck, W. Goertzen, S. Wolf and C.T. Haid   123
Otoneurological profile of patients examined for posttraumatic sequellae
  M.E. Norré   129
The neurootological findings following mild head injury
  A. Casani, P. Ghilardi, B. Fattori and R. Vannucchi   133
Vertigo as a cause of acute admission to a neurologic and ENT department
  H. Krejcova, R. Cerny, J. Jerabek and J. Tomas   137
Disbarism and oto-baro traumatism: Classification, clinical picture and
mechanisms
  C. Kolchev and N. Uzunov   141
Prognosis of vertigo in temporal bone fractures
  C. Wennmo   149

INNER EAR TRAUMA

Vectornystagmographic study of patients with Meniere's disease
C.A. Anadão, M.M. Ganaça, H.H. Caovilla and
P.L. Mangabeira Albernaz ... 155
The different types of perilymphatic fistule
G. Bodo and L. Heid ... 159
Does delayed labyrinthine hydrops develop in consequence of head trauma?
J. Czigner and É. Szabados ... 161
Traumatic perilymph fistula
W.G. Hemenway, F. Owen Black, R. Grimm and S. Pesznecker ... 167
Vestibular traumatic action of the different loadings
K.F. Trinus, V.S. Oleinik, V.I. Cherniuk, V.B. Lastovchenko,
G.V. Meshcheriakov and V.Y. Nikolenko ... 171
Multivariate statistical procedures for the differentiation of cochlear and retrocochlear hearing impairments
J. Kluba, S. Kropf and H. Deike ... 175

PATHOLOGICAL NYSTAGMUS FINDINGS AFTER HEAD TRAUMA

Oblique pursuit eye movements in normal adults and in cases with vestibular disturbances
A.W. Scholtz, H.J. Scholtz and U. Sievert ... 181
Detection and localization of vestibular lesion due to head and neck trauma. A vector-nystagmographic study
H.H. Caovilla, Y.I. Ito, T.T. Costa Neto, F.A. Suzuki, C.A. Anadão,
F.F. Ganança and M.M. Ganança ... 185
The influence of postcontusional ocular disturbances upon the ENG
W.D. Schäfer and C.-F. Claussen ... 189
Rationale for routine evaluation of provoked NY in CNS diseases
D. Alpini, A. Cesarani, D. Caputo, A. Ghezzi, M. Zaffaroni and
M. Mini ... 193
Late electronystagmographic findings in patients with head trauma
J.C.R. Fernandes, A.C. Cedin and V.H. Guimarães ... 197
Visual-vestibular interaction and optokinetic modifications in the post concussional syndrome
J.L. Cárdenas N. ... 201
Computerized caloric responses in chronic otitis media
C. Wennmo ... 205

VESTIBULO-SPINAL DISTURBANCES DUE TO HEAD TRAUMA

Posturographic findings in posttraumatic patients
M.E. Norré ... 213

Cranial trauma and posturography performed without and with caloric tests
   A.M.T. Hadj-Djilani   217
Motor control after head trauma
   M. Gospodinov   221
Scoliosis: A model to evaluate spino-vestibular interactions
   P. Sibilla, A. Cesarani, S. Barozzi, D. Alpini and G. Rainero   225
Dynamic posturography and aging
   T. Ledin, C. Möller, M. Möller and L.M. Ödkvist   229
Square wave perturbed posturography – Effects of vision, direction and amplitude
   T. Ledin and L.M. Ödkvist   233
Perturbed posturography – An experimental setup and simple applications
   T. Ledin, J. Hedbrant and L.M. Ödkvist   241
Lesions in the vestibular-spinal system in children and their determination by cranio-corpo-graphy and posturography
   G. Aust   247
Dynamic posturography
   W. Rubin   251

POSTTRAUMATIC NEUROOTOLOGICAL DISTURBANCES DUE TO CERVICAL LESIONS

Vertigo due to whiplash injury
   M. Sagnelli, L. Pollastrini, F. Baretti and M. Patrizi   255
Cervical syndrome due to trauma
   R. Becker and E.D. Meyer   259
Dynamic posturography in cervical vertigo
   M. Ålund, T. Ledin, L.M. Ödkvist, C. Möller and S.E. Larsson   265

AUDIOVESTIBULAR DISTURBANCES DUE TO HEAD TRAUMA

Causes of sensorineural hearing loss in Bulgaria
   D. Dimov and I. Spiridonova   269
Vertigo, nausea, tinnitus and hypoacusia after iatrogenic traumata
   O. Ribári and B. Büki   273
Impedance audiometric findings in patients with head trauma
   D. Scheidhauer and O. Schwetschke   279
Bilateral hearing loss and vestibular loss due to a triffling trauma of the head – A case demonstration
   K. Hamann   283
Differential diagnostics in patients suffering from sudden sensorineural hearing loss
   I. Šejna   287

New impedance measurements of the ear
  H. Eube — 291
ABR in high-risk neonates
  G. Katona, T. Timár and Z. Farkas — 295

POSTTRAUMATIC AUDIOVESTIBULAR SYMPTOMS IN NEUROOTOLOGY

Middle- and inner ear hearing disorders due to trauma
  G. Gavalias, J. Vathilakis, S. Sfetsos and L. Pastidis — 301
Diagnosis of central vestibular lesions after head injury
  S. Spellenberg and J. Láng — 307
Tinnitus and hearing reduction as a result of acoustic trauma in the Federal German Armed Forces
  M. Pilgramm — 311

POSTTRAUMATIC VASCULAR PROBLEMS WITH RESPECT TO NEUROOTOLOGY

Vestibulo-motor reactions during the free fall and in the landing phase of normal and perinatally hypoxic rabbits
  T. Schwartze, H. Tegetmeyer and H. Schwartze — 319
Audio-vestibular disturbances due to acute and chronic traumas of the carotid and vertebral arteries
  H. Haralanov, P. Shotekov and L. Haralanov — 323
Baro-trauma of the inner ear and its determination with neurootological tests
  G. Aust — 327
Vertigo and tinnitus in traumatic cervical vascular lesions
  I. Decker, A. Omlor, K. Schimrigk, G. Huber and H. Jäger — 333
Clinical and instrumented investigations into vertebrobasilar insufficiency
  B. Fischer and H. Von Specht — 339
Vertigo and nausea in patients with diabetic autonomic neuropathy
  W. Bossnev, M. Daskalov, N. Nikolova, S. Ghikova and Z. Stoyneva — 343
Doppler sonographical functional tests and otoneurological investigations in patients with cerebral trauma
  P. Shotekov, V. Raicheva, G. Poptodorov, J. Petrova and N. Popova — 347

PSYCHOLOGICAL FEATURES IN HEAD AND NECK TRAUMA

Vegetative responses due to posttraumatic nausea reactions
  C. Popivanova and L. Nakova — 355

The subjective symptoms compared with electronystagmographic findings
in vestibular neuronitis
    P. Silvoniemi and E. Aantaa   359
Vertigo, tinnitus and hallucinations due to head trauma
    S. Haralanov and L. Haralanov   363
Dynamic posturography in psycho-organic syndrome
    T. Ledin, E. Jansson, C. Möller, and L.M. Ödkvist   367

CHANGES IN EVOKED POTENTIALS AND EEG DUE TO TRAUMA

Auditory evoked responses in patients suffering from diabetes mellitus
    I. Chromej and J. Javorkova   373
Brainstem auditory evoked potentials in patients with subdural haematoma
    L. Haralanov and S. Haralanov   377
Brainstem audiometry in patients with head trauma
    Y.I. Ito, T.T. Costa Neto, F.A. Suzuki, R.G. Felipe, H.H. Caovilla
    and M.M. Gananca   381

TREATMENT

Infusion therapy in posttraumatic hearing defects and disorders of balance
    S. Spitzer, H.-J. Wilhelm, H. Kiesewetter, F. Jung and H.-J. Schieffer   387
Trans-ethmoid decompression of the optic nerve for post-traumatic
blindness
    M.V. Kirtane, S.R. Nayak and M.V. Ingle   391
Selective chemical vestibulectomy for the surgical treatment of intractable
Meniere's disease
    C.H. Norris and R.G. Amedee   395
Post-operative vertigo in chronic ear surgery
    G. Gavalas, M. Papamichalopoulos, G. Dokianakis and A. Pavlopoulos   399
Therapeutical concepts in posttraumatic vestibular lesions
    D. Futschik   405
New concepts in the treatment of positional vertigo
    A. Cesarani, D. Alpini, S. Barozzi and M. Mini   409
Central mechanisms of vestibular function compensation, following an
experimental unilateral delabyrinthization
    V. Chalmanov, H. Haralanov and C. Kolchev   413
Clamedex − Diagnostic neurootological expert system with a network
structure
    C.-F. Claussen and E. Claussen   419

POSTTRAUMATIC DISTURBANCES IN TASTE AND SMELL

On eventual changes of living habits due to posttraumtic dysosmias
    H. Gudziol and E. Beleites   427
Posttraumatic dysosmias
    U.E. Fraass and C.-F. Claussen   431

Index of authors   435
Subject index   439

NYSTAGMOGRAPHY

THE MANY FACES OF PEDRO LUIZ MANGABIERA ALBERNAZ

Wallace Rubin, M.D.

Otorhinolaryngology and Biocommunication Louisiana State University School of Medicine New Orleans, Louisiana

Pedro Luiz Mangabiera Albernaz was born in Campinas on June 20, 1932, where he attended public schools. He entered Escola Paulista de Medicina in 1949, and received an MD degree in 1955.

After working ten months in Rio with Professor de Lima, he obtained a Rotary Foundation Fellowship in 1958, and was accepted as a Clinical research fellow of the Department of Otolaryngology at Washington University School of Medicine in St. Louis, Missouri. There he worked with Dr. Walsh two days a week. The rest of the time he worked in research with Dr. Riesco McLure, Dr. Stroud, Dr. Hirsch, Dr. Davis, Dr. Eldredge and Dr. Silverman.

In 1959, Pedro entered Washington University Graduate School and obtained a Master of Arts in Otolaryngology in 1960. From July 1960 to July 1961, he was a research assistant on the staff of the Department of Oto at Washington University School of Medicine.

Pedro returned to Brazil in 1961 as an assistant professor at the Escola Paulista de Medicina. In 1965, he was promoted to associate professor. He became a Privat Dozent in 1966. In March of 1967, he was nominated Professor and Head of the Department of Otolaryngology, which position he presently holds.

In addition to his professional pursuits, Pedro was active in numerous medical societies. He also continued to research and publish, amassing some 443 publications in the field of OTO, and 69 non-ear contributions.

Here we have the scientist, and the professor as seen in the professional man. But the other sides are equally fascinating. He is a doting father to his Andrea, an established rancher and entrepreneur in his own right, and last, but not least, the eternal playboy to his beloved Marlene.

The faces of Pedro are many, and all reflect the great strength and character of a truly outstanding man.

4- GENERATIONS OF AUTOMATIC NYSTAGMUS ANALYSATORS

BERTORA GUILLERMO OSCAR
BERGMANN JULIA MATILDE
CLAUSSEN CLAUS FRENZ
CLAUSSEN ERIKA

INTRODUCTION

In the last, the neurootological studies were reduced to subjective observations such as walking and standing tests or looking at the eyes with Frenzel glasses. Nowadays, with the advantages of equilibriometrie an objective, measurable and quantitative evaluation can be obtained.

The modern methods of the Neurootologie allow a more exact differential diagnostic for vertigo patients. Owing to the improved as well as its evaluations through computer programs to obtain a fast and objective clinic diagnostic.

MATERIAL AND METHOD

Since 1972 our work team has developed 4 computers generations referred to the ocular movement diagnostic. In the first phase during 1972 an IBM 1800 Computer Main Frame was used.

Since 1976 microprocessors were developed having the advantage of being much smaller. This feature made computer devices portable.
Between 1976 and 1980 we worked with the INTEL 8080 system.
Between 1981 and 1985 the "NYDIAC" system was developed for the Z80 processor.
The fourth release, developed in the last years, called "CNG" (ComputerNystagmoGraphie) was based on the use of an IBM PC system an eliminating the register paper.

The CNG makes scrolling on a VEGA high resolution screen, as if it were a digital oscilloscope. The bioelectrical analogical signals are digitalized and appear on the screen, in a similar way as it is observed in the register paper with the advantage that all the data is stored in the computer disk for its subsequent analysis.

The CNG is menu driven, in this way the operator interactively controls the functions of the computer. These are hierarchically arranged, so that the first choice is referred to general operations, for example:

    1.- Patients data.
    2.- Record and evaluation.
    3.- Printing.
    4.- Manual correction of the evaluation.
    5.- Returning to the operating system.

When the record and evaluation option is chosen, the following menu allows you to choose the position of the electrodes, according to the operator's necessities. Besides you may add the recording of the electrocardiogram or other used stimulus.

The following step is the biological calibration of the device. Once this has been done the system is ready to do the following tests:

    1.- Caloric tests.
    2.- Rotatory tests.
    3.- Tracking tests.
    4.- Optokinetic nystagmus.
    5.- Saccadic tests.

The visual and rotatory tests are done under the watch of the computer, which automatically controls the periferic stimulators.

All these developments are based on the Electronistagmography introduced by Schott in 1922. The electrical registration of the movements of the human eyes is possible thanks to the fact that the eye behaves like an electric dipole. If derivation electrodes are placed around the eyes, variations of electrical potential are obtained according to the movements they make.

During the last 18 years, dedicated to the automatic analysis of the ocular movements, we have insisted on the recognition of the nystagmus signal form and its difference from noise. The nystagmus beat shows a typical triangular shape with unequal sides. One corresponding to a fast ascending side, called slow phase, and the other one, to a fast descending side, called fast phase of the nystagmus.

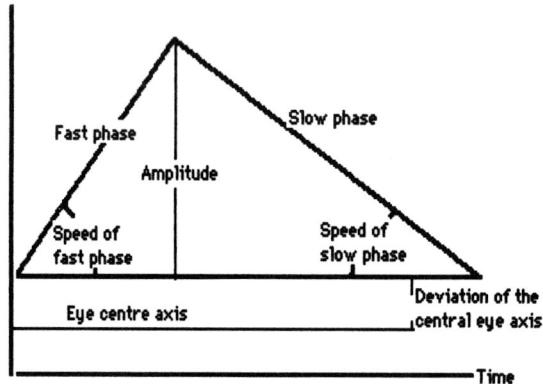

There are 9 main parameters studied in the recognition of the nystagmus signal by means of the evaluation with CNG:
  1.- Fast nystagmus phase.
  2.- Slow nystagmus phase.
  3.- Speed of fast phase.
  4.- Duration of fast phase.
  5.- Speed of slow phase.
  6.- Duration of slow phase.
  7.- Nystagmus amplitude in uVolts or grades.
  8.- Nystagmus speed.
  9.- Deviation position of the eye with reference to the midline of the gaze.

From the former parameters there are 3 which are the most important for the computerized evaluation: No. 3, 5 and 7.

From an algorithm point of view the nystagmus recognition is done by the evaluation of digitalized triads points. That is, as if it were a window that moves over the curve considering the following elements:

  1.- Components of analyzed current point.
    a.- Time in 1/50 seconds.
It is recognized and marked in the case that the point is a relative extreme and in the case it satisfies with nystagmus criteria.

b.- Measurement of that point related to the calibration.
This is the deviation of the point with respect to the isoelectric obtained from the calibration.

2.- Components of the previous point.
a.- Time in 1/50 seconds.
b.- Measurement of that point related to the calibration.

3.- Components of the following point.
a.- Time in 1/50 seconds.
b.- Measurement of that point related to the calibration.

Others measurements on the points:
a.- Amplitude of the ascendant side and descendant side in uVolts and grades.
b.- Speed of the ascendant and descendant side in grades/sec.

In order to recognize a nystagmus the main criteria is:
1.- Minimum amplitude: 20 uVolts or 1 grade.
2.- Minimum difference of 15% between the slow and fast phase.
3.- Roundness of the edges of the nystagmus.

To distinguish a rigt nystagmus signal from a left one, the phases are compared by searching for the corresponding alfa and ßeta angles.
In practice, the program has to recognize pathological shapes of the nystagmus, such as undulations, nystagmoids, etc.
A frequent obstacle observed in the recognition of the nystagmus signal is the presence of intermediate points in the curve before an extreme. These points modify the slope of the slow or fast phase of the nystagmus and are ignored if they do not exceed 15%.
The results of the analysis are printed with a printer device in a tabular form or in a graphical form such as the butterfly chart and the RIDT, in a cumulative distribution of the speed of the slow and amplitude. In order to compare the manual evaluation with the automatic one, it is possible to print the original curves where the recognized nystagmus are marked with a point.
In the tricky cases, the operator may make the nystagmus manually by means of the keyboard scanning the curves with the cursor.

CONCLUSIONS

The vertigo patients diagnostic has acquired a great importance from the beginning of century. Simultaneously, the nystagmus analysis of the ocular movements has improved. The analysis of sensomotors vias based on nystagmus analysis has a central place in the Neurootologie.
The nystagmus beat must be watched carefully and must have a great experience in its diagnostic. The nystagmus signals must be studied with the help of a pencil, and a ruler in order to get the exact parameters.
With the launching of computers during recent years we wonder: Is there any possibility of analyzing these phenomenons with the microprocessors?.
We have chosen the way of recognition of nystagmus form.During these 4 periods we have polished this process. At this time we have the CNG without paper, it gives us safety in the evaluation and fastness in the daily consultation.

REFERENCES

1. BERGMANN de BERTORA J.M., BERTORA G., CLAUSSEN C.F.: "Computarisierte Nystagmographie - CNG - Neue objetive Analysenmethode ".Verlag "Otoophtalmologische Neurophysiologie". Buenos Aires. Argentinien. August 1988.
2. BERTORA G., BERGMANN de BERTORA J.M.: "The optokinetic saccadic test evaluation by means of a digital computer". Elsevier Science Publishers B.V. (Biomedical Division). Vertigo, nausea, tinnitus and hypoacusia in metabolic disorders, 27-30 , 1988.
3. CLAUSSEN C.F., BERGMANN DE BERTORA J.M., BERTORA G.:"Otoneurooftalmologia. Modernas técnicas topodiagnósticas y terapéuticas" Springer Verlag Berlin - Heidelberg, 1988.

THE POSSIBILITY OF ADEQUATE STIMULATION OF THE PHASIC CANAL IN THE VESTIBULAR SYSTEM

PETER SCHWARTZE, KAKOLI MUKHERJEE and FRANZ THOSS
Carl Ludwig Institute of Physiology, Karl Marx University,
Liebigstrasse 27, Leipzig 7010, Germany

INTRODUCTION

In the vestibular nerve of adult mammals thick and thin axons with different discharge characteristics were found (1,2). The thick vestibular afferents have a irregular and the thin afferents a regular discharge pattern. After onset of adequate vestibular stimulation the thick afferents discharge phasic and the thin tonic. The thick fibres innervate as calyces in the central zone of the ampullary sensory epithelium and envelopes the nighboring type 1 hair cells (HC1). Thin fibres innervate predominantly the peripheral parts of the epithelium and furnish the bouton type endings which belongs solely to type 2 hair cells (HC2). Most of the normally executed head movements stimulate the HC2; these movements are too slow to reach the higher threshold of HC1. The usual clinical vestibular tests stimulate the HC2 too. To reach the threshold of the phasic reacting HC1 it needs a sudden intensive semicircular canal acceleration which can be produced experimentally if by means of a rigid coupling of the head and the stimulation device a steep acceleration impulse is transduced to the labyrinth.

MATERIAL AND METHODS

After implantation of chronic EOG-electrodes horizontal eye movements were recorded during acceleration steps, using 20 rabbits between the 20th and 30th postnatal day. The stimulus, produced by a computer steared step motor, had an amplitude of 0.6 deg., the maximum rotational velocity was reached 20 ms after start and the acceleration was approximately $1,5 \cdot 10^3$ deg $\cdot$ s^{-2}. The stimulation procedure was a sequence of 0.6 deg acceleration steps: the time between the steps were 1000, 500, 100, 50 and 25 ms. The eye movements were recorded during a sequence of 150 stimulating steps in each direction. The recordings were analyzed by hand.

The endolymph hydrodynamics was during the stimulation computer modelled using the general equation of motion

$$M\ddot{x} + W\dot{x} + Fx = f(t); \quad T_1 \approx \frac{M}{W}; \quad T_2 \approx \frac{W}{F}$$

The acceleration pressure is opposed mainly by the friction pressure $W\dot{x}$ of the streaming fluid in the narrow part of the semicircular canal and also by the inertial pressure Mẍ of the endolymph and the directive pressure Fx delivered by the elastic cupula (3). An acceleration step deforms the cupula with the short time constant T_1 after which the initial position of the cupula is reached with the long time constant T_2. These time constants in rabbits between 20th and 30th day are 0.01 s and 3.3 s respectively (3). The computersketch of the cupuladeviation 5 s after stimulus onset using a stimulation step sequence of $2 \cdot s^{-1}$, $4 \cdot s^{-1}$ and $10 \cdot s^{-1}$ showed an increase of the cupuladeviation angle with increasing stimulation frequency; the permanent deviated cupula oscillates in the frequency of the step stimuli (Fig. 1).

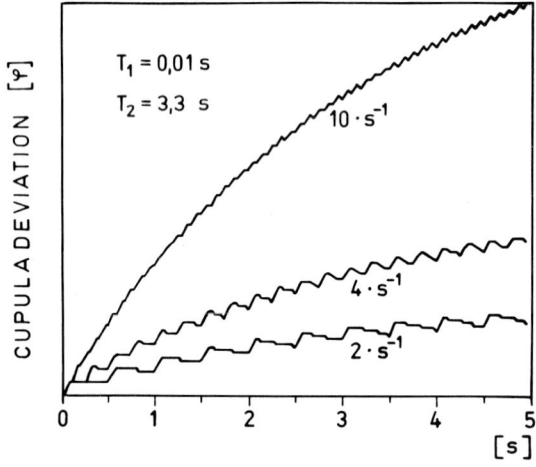

Fig. 1. The cupula deviation in relative units during the application of step stimuli of a tact frequency of 2,4 and 10 Hz. The stimulation duration was 5 s, time constants of the cupula deviation 0.01 s and 3.3. s respectively.

RESULTS

Already a step stimulus sequence of $1.0 \cdot s^{-1}$ induced horizontal eye movements. With the increase of the stimulus frequency from $2 \cdot s^{-1}$ to $15 \cdot s^{-1}$ an eye oscillation movement pattern was generated, the frequency of which was between 2 and 3 Hz and was independent of the stimulus frequency. Higher stimulation step frequencies up to $40 \cdot s^{-1}$ changed the eye movement pattern: now a 2-3 Hz regular nystagmus with slow and quick phase was generated (Fig. 2)

DISCUSSION

Stimulation step impulses of an amplitude of 0.6 deg induce 2-3 eye movements per s, if the time delay between the impulse is in the range of 500 to 75 ms. The application of the 150 stimulating steps lead to a 90 deg horizontal rotation of the turning table together with the animal in 45 s and 4.5 s respectively. The mean velocity of the turning table increases tenfold in this stimulation

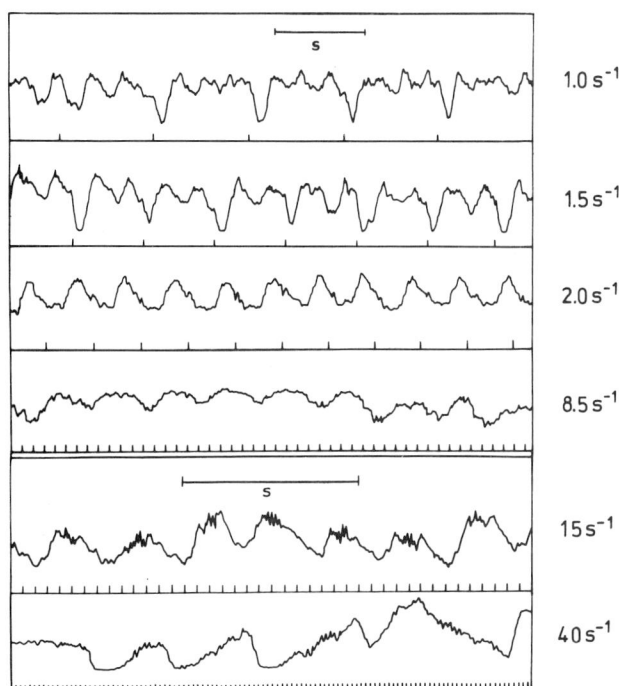

Fig. 2. Horizontal eye movements during step stimulation between 1 and 40 Hz; stimulus amplitude 0.6 deg, rabbits, 20-30 days of postnatal age.

range, but the number of oscillating eye movements is nearly constant. The impulse stimulation procedure induces a functional state in the vestibulo-ocular reflex system which is also observed during sinusoidal stimulation of 2 to 3 Hz. Stimulation step impulses under 50 ms changes the functional state of the system: instead of oscillating eye movements now nystagms are generated. To decide whether these phenomena are caused mainly by stimulating the HC1, that is the phasic vestibular canal, a study is in preparation, in which the eye movement parameters shall be tested using the same stimulation procedure as in this study, but using animals of which the HC1 are destroyed.

REFERENCES

1. Fernández C, Baird RA, Goldberg JM (1988) J Neurophysiol 60: 167-181
2. Baird RA, Desmadryl G, Fernández C, Goldberg JM (1988) J Neurophysiol 60:182-203
3. Schwartze P, Schönfelder J, Thoss F (1975) In: Drischel H, Dettmar P (eds) Biokybernetics V, Jena, pp 181-188

PHYSIOLOGICAL NYSTAGMIC AND NON-NYSTAGMIC OCULAR MOVEMENTS RECORDED BY MEANS OF THE PENG-METHOD BY H.R. GESTEWITZ

Dr. med. B. GESTEWITZ
Militärmedizinische Akademie Bad Saarow, DDR

Many studies on ocular movements aimed and aim at detecting oculomotor phenomena with vestibular, cerebellar and spinal reflex circuits.

In the literature only little attention was paid to eye movements or defined oculomotor phenomena occurring while looking into a dark field with eyes open (elimination of any fixation of a target).

Therefore, we carried out examinations on these problems.

MATERIAL AND METHODS

Examinations were carried out with PENG-apparatus by H.R. Gestewitz (Kombinat Carl-Zeiss Jena). This apparatus allows the continuous and simultaneous registration of both eyes in any position of the head and the body with the organism being in the condition of rest and in motion, respectively.

We tested 123 healthy subjects with normal balance (97 men, 25 women, mean age: 21,6 years) in order to examine spontaneous ocular movements when looking into a dark field. During the examination the probands were lying in supine position on a couch with head slightly raised.

Movements of both eyes were recorded simultaneously in vertical and horizontal directions with a registration sensitivity of 0,3 degrees/mm of eye movement when the probands looked into a dark field with eyes open.

To reveal possible relations between ocular movements and cerebellar coordination requirements subjects additionally performed the finger-nose, finger-finger as well as the heel-knee tests.

RESULTS

Figure 1 shows eye movements (while looking into a dark field with eyes open) both at rest and during the finger-nose test. While lying, the healthy subject exhibited small-amplitude, low-frequency nystagmic eye movements to the rigth upper side. Nystagmic movements of both eyes were horizontally interrupted by waves and square waves. Small-amplitude nystagmic ocular movements to the right with a rotatory component were found during the right finger-nose test.

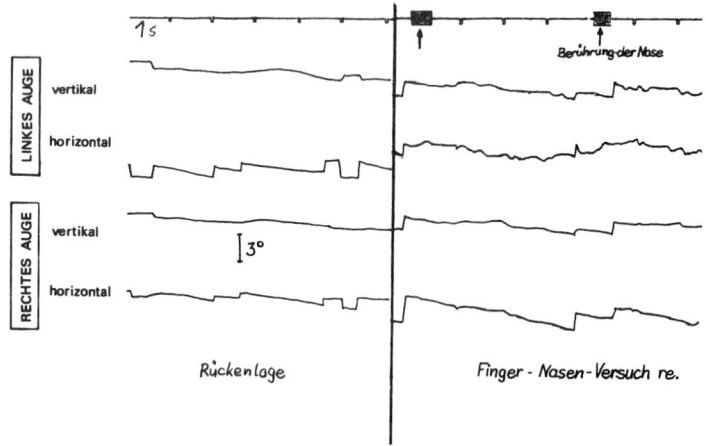

Fig. 1

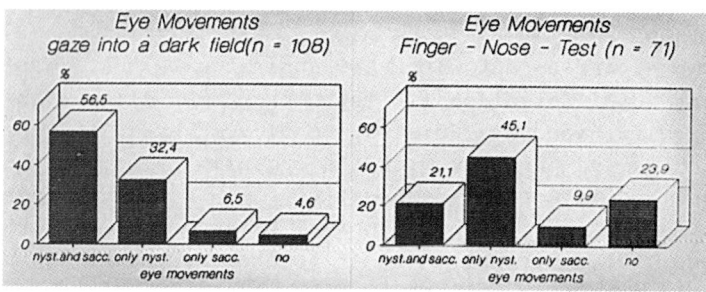

Fig. 2

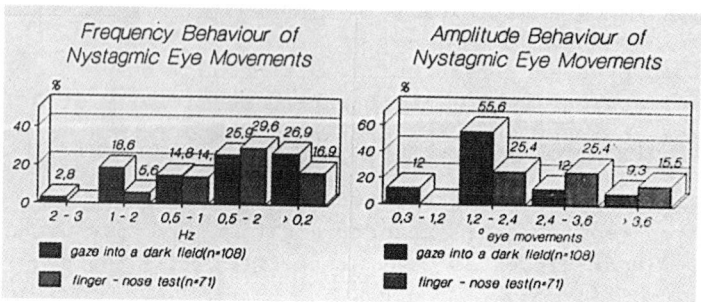

Fig. 3

The systematic interpretation of the PENG-curves recorded continuously with subjects in supine position and looking into a dark field revealed nystagmic and/or non-nystagmic saccadic ocular movements in 94.5 per cent of the cases (figure 2).

No classifiable eye movements were found only in 5 probands (4.6%). Fifteen curve could not be interpreted.

During the finger-nose test (figure 3) 71.6% of the subjects exhibited nystagmic and/or non-nystagmic saccadic eye movements.

The number of probands (23.9 %) without any eye movement was significantly higher than during the examination at rest. The frequency of nystgmic ocular movements was predominantly smaller than 1 Hz both during the examination at rest and during the finger-nose test.

Comparing both test groups, no significant differences could be found (figure 4).

A significant increase in the amplitude of nystagmic ocular movements was observed during the finger-nose test, as compared to the examinations at rest (figure 5).

Both tests showed no considerable differences in the direction of nystagmic ocular movements.

It was, however, obvious that there were no nystagmic ocular movements downwards.

In both test groups the frequency of non-nystagmic ocular movements was mainly in a range of 1.0 - 2.5 Hz (86.7% and 95,8% respectively).There were no significant differences.

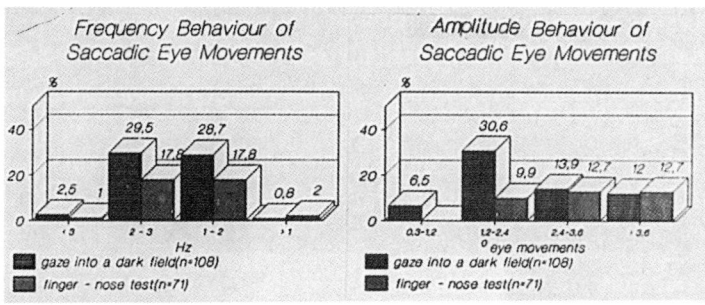

Fig. 4

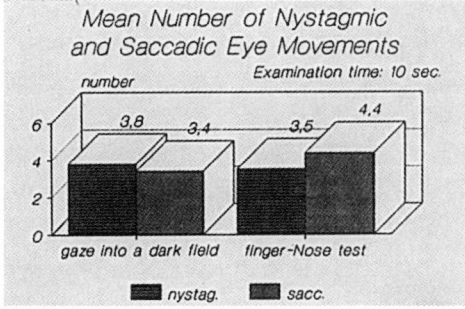

Fig. 5

A significant increase in the amplitude of non-nystagmic ocular movements was observed in cerebellar coordination requirements.

Non-nystagmic ocular movements were found in both test groups only in the horizontal recording channels.

No distinction in the direction to the right and left sides was made.

Related to an examination time of 10 s, the mean number of nystagmic and non-nystagmic saccadic ocular movements was 3.3 and 4.4 respectively.

Similar results were obtained during the finger-finger and heel-knee test.

SUMMARY

An optomotor spontaneous activity was recorded in a large number of healthy subjects when they were lying in supine position and looking into a dark field. This probably physiological optomotor spontaneous activity can be divided into nystagmic and non-nystagmic saccadic ocular movements.

An increase in these spontaneous ocular movements, especialy in their amplitude, was observed during the finger-nose, finger-finger and heel-knee tests.

ON THE DIAGNOSTIC IMPORTANCE OF SACCADIC OCULAR MOVEMENTS (WAVES AND SQUARE WAVES) IN THE NYSTAGMOGRAM

Dr. med. D. GESTEWITZ
Militärmedizinische Akademie Bad Saarow, GDR

Photoelectronystagmography allows to record the real movements of both eyes simultaneously.

Eye movements with a very small amplitude of less than 1.0 degrees can be recorded.

During the continuous registration of eye movements using this method an increased number of saccadic ocular movements is observed, especially in pathological processes in the CNS. Presenting the results obtained in a larger study the question should be answered, to what extent these saccadic ocular movements are of pathological charakter in neurootologic diagnostics.

We exemained 120 predominantly male patients with different central pathological processes or peripheral vestibular disorders.

The patients were divided into groups according to clinical aspects. They were compared with 50 healthy probands. The following groups were selected:
* 20 patients with supratentorial tumours
* 15 patients with infratentorial tumours
* 10 patients with acoustic neurinoma
* 30 patients with cerebrovascular disorders
  - of them 4 patients with occlusion of the A. carotis interna and
  - 3 patients with occlusion of the A. vertebralis
* 15 patients with multiple sclerosis and
* 30 patients with peripheral vestibular disoders, showing an unilateral disturbed labyrinthine function.

Diagnoses were established by clinical and X-ray examinations, including computerized tomography, cerebral angiography as well as neurootologic and neurologic special examinations.

The continuous registration of spontaneous eye movements was used to settle the question raised.

The examination ran as follows:
Patients were lying in supine position on a tilting couch. Then they were tilted 45 degrees to the right and to the left, respectively. Finally, they were in supine position again.

Each position of the body has been maintained for 60 s. Movements of both eyes were recorded simultaneously with a sensitivity of the registration of 0.5 degrees by means of the PENG-apperatus.

The amplitude, the number of the saccadic eye movements as well as the time between waves and square waves (retention time) were evaluated.

Nystagmic eye movements were evalueted only qualitatively.

RESULTS

It was ascertained that patients suffering from a disease of the CNS exhibited significantly more saccadic ocular movements than healthy subjekts.

Only single saccadic ocular movements occured in healthy subjects both in the supine and in the other positions of the body.

There was an average number of the ocular movements of 5 beats/minute in healthy probands. The mean amplitude of saccadic eye movements was 1.4 degrees and the mean time between wave and square waves (retention time) was 0.7 s.

Patients with a supratentorial tumour showed mainly saccdic eye movements with a mean amplitude of 2 degrees and a mean retention time of 1 s. The total beat rate was 14 beats/minute on an average.

Predominantly nystagmic ocular movemens with a high ampliude and low frequency were found in patients with infratentorial tumours. Saccadic ocular movements with mean amplitude values of 2.5 degrees occured inisolated cases. The mean retention time was 0.8 s in these cases.

Small saccades with amplitude values of 1 -2 degrees and a mean retention time of 0.5 - 1.0 s were observed in patients with acoustic neurinoma. The total beat rate varied strongly. There were on an average 13 beats/minute. Nystagmic eye movements and saccadic ocular movements always alternated.

A typical pattern of saccadic eye movements coud be found in cerebrovascular disorders. Very small saccadic ocular movements with an amplitude of less then 1,0 degrees and a short retention time (0.5 s) occurred in these cases. The total beat rate on average 15 beats/minute was higher than in the other groups.

No typical saccadic eye movements were seen in patients with multiple sclerosis. Both large amplitudes of more than 2 degrees and very small ones of 0.5 degrees were found. Individual values of the retention time and total beat rate also differed widely.

Only few isolated saccades could be found in patients with

peripheral vestibular disoders.

As it was expected, mainly nystagmic ocular movements occured. Examining and analyzing differnt positions of the body did not result in additional information.

CONCLUSION

The evaluation of saccadic ocular movements in addition to nystagmic eye movements plays a certain role in neurootologic diagnostics.

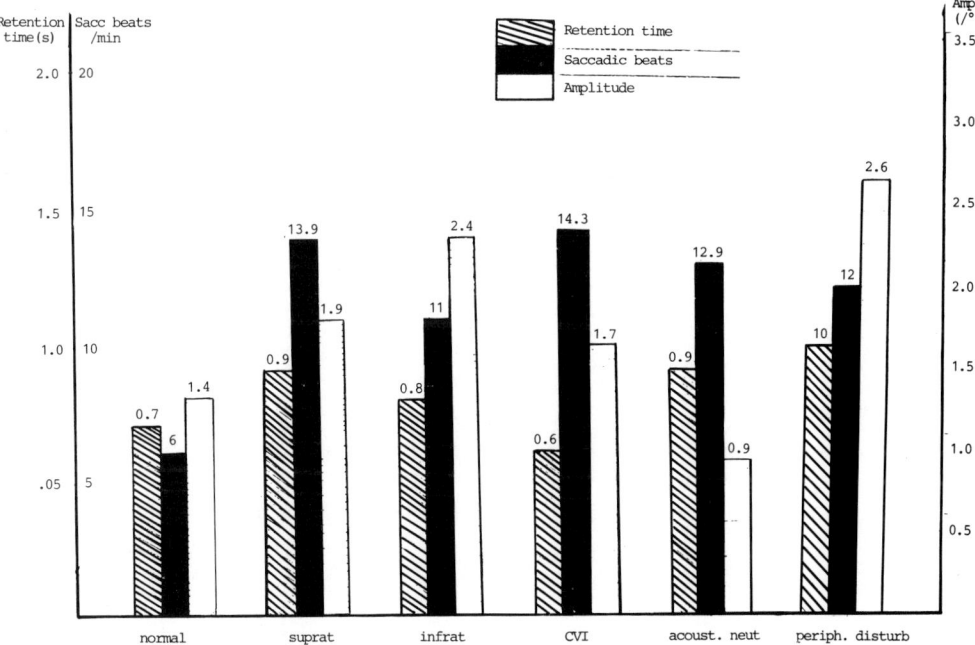

Fig. 1. Retention time, beat rate and amplitude of the square waves from verious neurootological disturbances

As illustrated in the figure, the parameters amplitude, total beat rate and retention time are suited to evaluate saccadic ocular movements during the registration of spontaneous eye movements for diagnosing central processes. The preliminary results presented in the paper require further studies.

THE PENG-APPARATUS WITH COMPUTER-AIDED EVALUATION MADE BY VEB KOMBINAT CARL-ZEISS JENA - FIRST CLINICAL EXPERIENCES

Prof. Dr.med. Dr.hc. H.R. GESTEWITZ
Militärmedizinische Akademie Bad Saarow, DDR

The reports of TOROK, GULLEMIN and BARNOTHY (1951) as well as of RICHTER and PFALTZ (1956), who were the first to use the photoelectrical principle of measurement for the continuous registration of ocular movements, were the basis of our works on the further development of photoelectronystagmography (PENG).

The purpose of our studies was to improve the PENG-method in close cooperation with industrial plants in that way that it can be generally applied in hospital and practice for the objective registration of ocular movements being of diagnostic importance.

The new PENG-unit made by VEB Kombinat Carl-Zeiss Jena (figure 1) consits of:
- measuring device for ocular movements in the form or spectacles (1)
- preamplifier (2)
- controller/power supply (3)
- 16-bit computer/IBM compatible (4)
- measuring cross for automatic calibration (5)
- multi-channel recorder/printer (6)

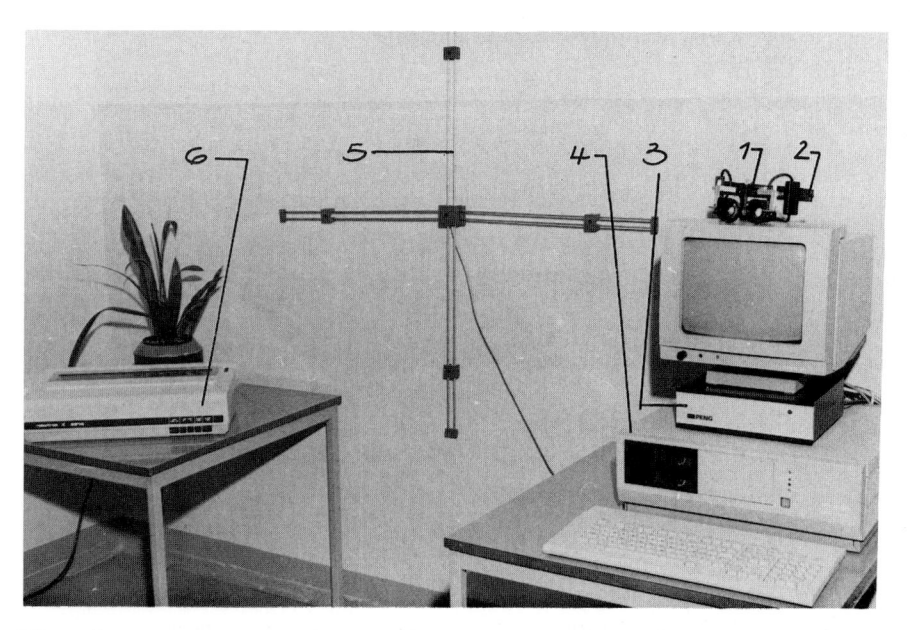

Fig. 1

First clinical test results obtained proved the following:
1. This apparatus being easy to handle in medical clinical practice allows the continuous, objective and simultaneous registration of all diagnostically important movements of both eyes as their computer-aided evaluation.
2. Photoelectrical converters allow to record the movements of both eyes in any position of the head and the body. The body of the patient can be in the state of rest (lying, sitting, standing) or in motion (walking, turning, other coordinated movements).
3. The PENG-unit allows the registration of small and smallest ocular movements up to amplitude of 0,1 degrees.
4. The technical arrangement enables eye movements to be recorded at an angle of vision of +/- 25 degrees related to the visual optic axis.
5. Movements of both eyes can be recorded continously and simultaneously while looking at visual target as well as in the case of complete elimination of any fixation.

Ocular movements continously recorded by means of the PENG-apparatus are evaluated by analyzing the individual data of the registration curves.

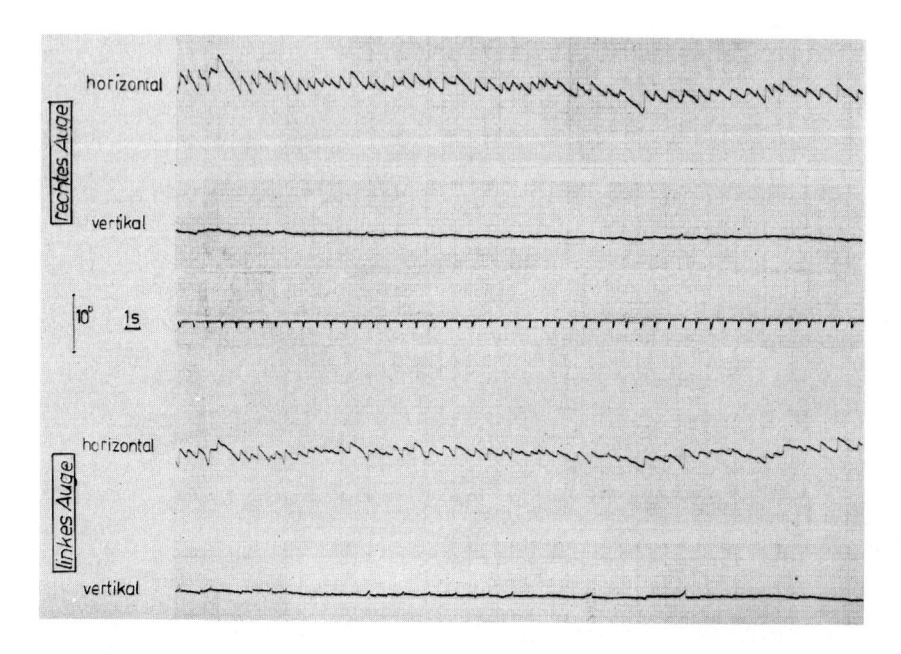

Fig.2. Horizontal spontaneous nystagmic ocular movements

The following parameters are evaluated:
- the form
- the direction
- the beat rate
- the amplitude
- the angular velocity of the slow component of the nystagmus and
- the duration of the nystagmic ocular movements.

On analyzing ocular movements it is important to evaluate the horizontal and vertical movements in their connection.
This allows to detect and evaluate ocular movements really occurred, including non-nystagmic ocular movements (figure 2).

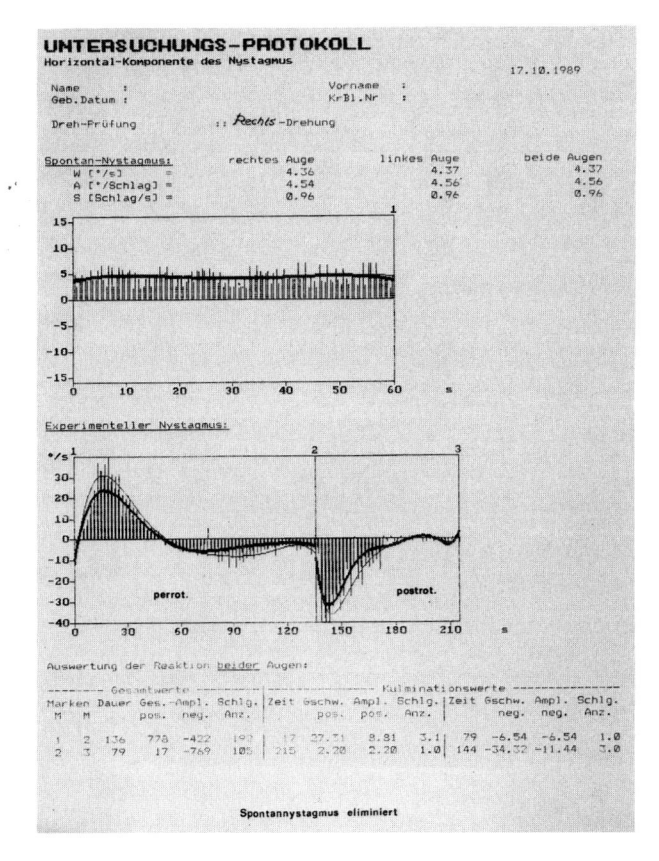

Fig.3. Computer-aided of a rotatory test by a patients with N.VIII-disorder (spontaneous nystagmic ocular movements to right)

Evaluating eye movement traces, using visual and/or manual methods, is very time-consuming.

Therefore, the PENG-apparatus from the VEB Kombinat Carl-Zeiss Jena is interconnected to a microelectronic evaluation unit.

Three evaluation program are available for the comprehensive as well as differentiated computer-aided analysis.
(1) Program for the evaluation of nystagmic ocular movements (figure 3)
(2) Program for the evaluation of smooth persuit eye movements
(3) Program for the assessment of waves and square waves.

Easy handling, high measuring sensitivity, no artifacts to a large extent and computer-aided evaluation are the advantages of the photoelectrical unit used for the continuous, objective and simultaneous registration of movements of both eyes.

VISUAL SUPPRESSION IN THE CALORIC AND ROTATORY TESTS

J DEBLEN, T LEDIN, L NOAKSSON, LM ÖDKVIST.

Dept of ENT, University Hospital, S-581 85 Linköping, Sweden.

ABSTRACT

The visual suppression (VS) ability was tested in patients with peripheral and central vestibular lesions and in patients with no permanent damage to the vestibular system. The VS quotient correlated to the maximum response in the caloric test, the bigger the response the more difficult to suppress it. The same results appeared even when the inter-aural differences were compared to VS differences. The VS in the caloric test compared reasonably well to the VS in rotatory tests. In some instances however, the rotatory VS test showed higher sensitivity, in that some patients with caloric VS gain of zero had an abnormal rotatory VS corresponding to their lesion. VS is an easy to use valuable tool to unveil some pathology in the posterior fossa. Rotatory VS tests are in some instances more sensitive to vestibular system lesions.

INTRODUCTION

In the electronystagmographic investigation it is very easy to include the visual suppression (VS) test. It is performed during the caloric response by lighting a small red lamp or light emitting diode in the dark room for ten seconds. The patient is instructed to foveate the lamp and thus suppress the vestibulo-ocular reflex (VOR). The quotient between the slow phase velocity (SPV) when fixating and during darkness is a measure of VS ability. Another way of more physiologically eliciting the VOR is by rotatory testing. In fact, caloric testing has been stated to be the equivalence of extremely slow rotatory testing with 0.003 Hz (Hamid et al 1987). The patient is instructed to fixate on a dot moving with the chair. The VS is then computed using the transfer function between the movement of the chair and the eyes. The VS has often been considered the same mechanism as smooth pursuit, which comprises the foveal fixation of a moving object (Leigh and Zee 1983). However, the systems are at least partwise different (Ödkvist et al 1988), albeit using many common neuronal pathways.

The present study, conducted in an everyday patient material, was intended to unveil the influence of the VOR responsiveness on the VS ability, and comparison between the VS during caloric irrigation and rotatory VS testing was made.

MATERIAL

One hundred and sixtyone patients referred for otoneurological investigation were included in the study. Patients were classified into three groups by diagnosis:

	N	Age (years) mean	SD	range
1. Peripheral vestibular disease	54	52.3	14.6	23-77
2. Central nervous system lesion	38	50.8	17.0	13-83
3. Transient vertigo - no permanent central or peripheral lesion diagnosed	69	47.5	14.5	11-74

All subjects underwent VS testing during the conventional caloric irrigation with electronystagmographic recording. In addition 48 of them (9 from group 1, 16 from group 2 and 23 from group 3) conducted VS testing in the rotatory chair.

CALORIC IRRIGATION

The VOR causes the eyes to move 180 degrees out of phase with head movement, thus keeping vision stable during head rotations. The sensing mechanism is the cupular detection of endolymph flux in the semicircular canals (Ewald 1892). One way of non-physiologically eliciting the VOR is by caloric irrigation. Bithermal (30 and 44 degrees C), binaural caloric irrigation was performed in darkness. Nystagmus was monitored by electro-oculography (EOG), both horizontal and vertical. The horizontal SPV was calculated (Henriksson 1956). Ag/AgCl electrodes were attached to the skin on the forehead (ground electrode), lateral to the eyes (horizontal movements) and above and below the left eye (vertical movements). Impedance was checked prior to measurement, with a maximum permissible level of 5 kohms. The apparatus was operated in DC mode (Thell and Ödkvist 1988). After each caloric irrigation of 30 seconds duration the maximum velocity of the evoked nystagmus response was calculated. This maximum response most often occurs within 60 seconds of irrigation cessation. When the nystagmus response had peaked, a very small red lamp was lit for ten seconds for the patient to fixate on. The velocity during this voluntary suppression was calculated. The VS gain is defined as the quotient between nystagmus SPV during and prior to lamp lightning.

ROTATORY TESTING

VS of the VOR may also be conducted, more physiologically, with rotatory testing (Larsby et al 1984). The subject sits in a hydraulic rotatory chair and is instructed to foveate a dot on a frame mounted on the chair 0.4 m in front of the eyes. The stimulus signals (duration 40 s) used are sinusoidal frequency sweeps 0-2.00 Hz with maximum angular velocities of 20 and 40 degrees per second, respectively, and a pseudorandom sum of sinusoids 0-2.00 Hz, with a maximum velocity of 40 deg/s. The eye position is measured with EOG, and the head velocity is measured with a rate sensor on a bite board. The measured EOG signal in response to rotatory stimulation is manually edited to remove artifacts and saccades, defined as voluntary or involuntary high speed movements of the eyes in order to fixate on a new target (Leigh and Zee 1983). The removed portions of the signal is replaced by a straight line with a slope that smoothly connects the two remaining parts of the signal.

The relation between the chair velocity and eye velocity, calculated as the differentiated inverted eye position, is evaluated using the transfer function between input (head velocity) and output (eye velocity in opposite direction). Symbolizing the input by x and the output by y, the terms gain, phase and coherence of a linear system are defined as follows (Bendat and Piersol 1971):

Let F(v) be the Fourier transform of signal v. By definition, the cross power spectrum G_{xy} and the auto power spectrum G_{xx} (and similarly G_{yy}) equal

$$G_{xy} = F(x) \, F^*(y) \quad \text{and} \quad G_{xx} = F(x) \, F^*(x)$$

where the asterisk denotes the complex conjugate.

The transfer function of the system, H, is defined as

$$H = \overline{G_{yx}} \, / \, \overline{G_{xx}}$$

giving a robust estimate in noisy environments. The bars on top of power spectra denote ensemble averages. In practice, averages in the frequency domain are often used. From this complex transfer function, the gain of the system, as a function of frequency, is calculated as the magnitude and the phase as the argument:

$$\text{Gain} = (HH^*)^{1/2} \quad \text{and} \quad \text{Phase} = \text{IMAG} \, (\log H)$$

where IMAG denotes taking the imaginary part, and log is the complex logarithm.

The coherence function estimates the relevancy of the computed transfer function and is defined

$$\text{Coherence} = \overline{G_{yx}} \, \overline{G_{xy}}^* \, / \, \overline{G_{xx}} \, \overline{G_{yy}}$$

where the need of averages is obvious. Otherwise, from the definition, the coherence would equal unity, at all frequencies.

DATA EVALUATION

The average nystagmus maximum SPV for both irrigation temperatures was calculated for each ear. The VS quotient average for each ear was calculated accordingly. In computing a maximum nystagmus SPV and VS ability of a subject, the values for both ears were averaged. However, if the quotient between the larger maximum velocity of either ear compared to the other was greater than an arbitrary limit of 2.5, the values of the most responsive ear was used instead of the average between ears. In case of very low nystagmus activity, a measured velocity value of zero, no VS quotient was calculated. In rotatory testing, two characteristics of each transfer function was calculated. Omitting the lowest frequency band, 0-0.25 Hz, and the highest, 1.75-2.00 Hz, the gain averages in both the lower three frequency bands, 0.25-1.00 Hz, and the three higher, 1.00-1.75 Hz, were computed.

The maximum velocity and VS ability were compared between groups. In each group, the dependence of VS ability on maximum nystagmus SPV was evaluated using linear regression. The difference in maximum SPV between ears was plotted versus the corresponding difference in VS ability to establish the influence of peripheral sensory organ responsiveness on the cerebellar suppression mechanisms. In the 48 subjects that conducted both rotatory and caloric tests, attempts to correlate the two VS abilities were made.

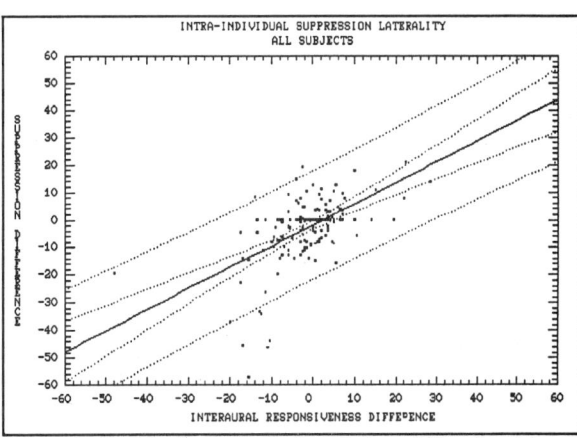

Intra-individual suppression laterality function.

Student's t-test was used to compare groups. The probability of correlation coefficients equalling zero was computed. The significance limit was 5%.

RESULTS

The maximum SPVs were 16.2 deg/s (SD 8.0) in group 1, 19.7 deg/s (SD 8.9) in group 2 and 18.3 deg/s (SD 9.9) in group 3. No significant differences were found between groups. The VS gain was 15.9 % (SD 17.8) in group 1, 18.7 % (SD 17.0) in group 2 and 8.4 % (SD 9.6) in group 3. Group 3 differed significantly from both group 1 (p<0.01) and 2 (p<0.001). Groups 1 and 2 did not differ.

Plotting the difference in maximum SPV between ears versus the corresponding difference in VS gain for all subjects revealed the intra-individual suppression laterality function (r=0.54, p<0.001, see figure). Splitting the analysis groupwise showed r=0.68 (p<0.001) in group 1, r=0.30 (NS) in group 2 and r=0.61 (p<0.001) in group 3. The relationship between maximum SPV and VS gain unveiled a mutual dependency in group 3 (r=0.52, p<0.001, see figure) and group 1 (r=0.38, p<0.01). However, in group 2 the relation was more obscure (r=0.19, NS).

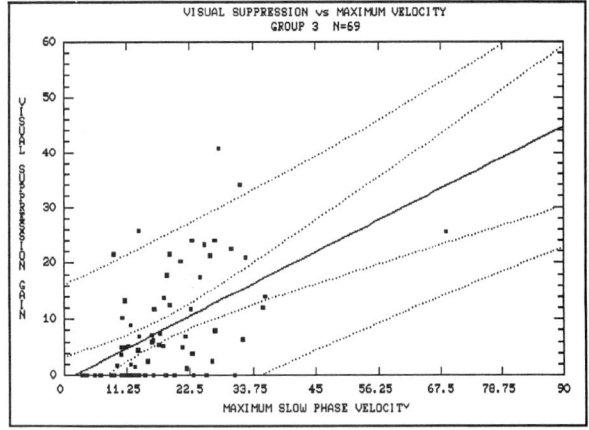

Maximum SPV vs VS gain in group 3.

The estimations of VS from the rotatory tests correlated well to caloric VS values. The presence of subjects with caloric VS of zero but having randomized rotatory VS gains as high as 35-40 % was noted. In sinusoidal testing with 20 deg/s maximum velocity the correlation coefficient was r=0.67 for low frequencies and r=0.66 for high frequencies, the corresponding values for 40 deg/s were r=0.73 and r=0.73. In randomized testing the correlations were slightly lower, r=0.55 and r=0.58, respectively. All these correlations are highly significant (p<0.001).

DISCUSSION

Visual fixation either suppresses or abolishes caloric nystagmus in normal subjects (Mahoney et al 1957, Collins et al 1962, Sokolovski 1966, Naito et al 1963, Demanez and Ledoux 1970). However, failure of VS is often found in cases reported as metabolic encephalopathies (Maccario et al 1972), cerebellar disease (Naito et al 1963, Hart 1967), brainstem disease (Naito et al 1963, Preber and Silfverskiöld 1960), posterior fossa lesions (Boniver and Demanez 1977, Alpert 1974, Hyden et al 1989) and psycho-organic syndrome due to chronic solvent exposure (Möller et al 1989). Experiments in animals and man have disclosed that acute intoxication with hydrocarbon solvents influences the VOR arc (Larsby et al 1976, Ödkvist et al 1980) and that solvents block the cerebellar inhibition of the VOR. In animals, the selective destruction of the cerebellar flocculus has been shown to permanently destroy the VS ability (Takemori and Cohen 1974).

The VOR is modulated by the cerebellum. There is often a conflict between VOR and fixation and pursuit mechanisms. The VOR is a broad frequency mechanism (Barr et al 1976, Barnes 1982, Larsby et al 1984), but the fixation and pursuit mechanisms operate mainly in the low frequency domains (Ödkvist et al 1988). The aim of both systems are to keep the field of vision stable in an ever moving world - the fixation and suppression mechanisms sometimes have to cancel the VOR. Studies of pathological VS and pursuit have indicated that the mechanisms are similar, but not equal (Ödkvist et al 1988).

In this study the VS of the better ear in caloric irrigation was calculated if the responiveness for the two ears differed by an arbitrary, not validated, factor 2.5 or more. The reason for this is obvious, as the results have shown that the VS gain is dependent on maximum nystagmus SPV, both in groups of subjects and when studying inter-aural differences. This may explain at least partwise the different normal VS gain limits in caloric testing aquired by others, e.g. 60-70 % (Alpert 1974) and 25-50 % (Demanez and Ledoux 1970). In Rhesus monkeys, a value of 50 % has been proposed (Takemori and Cohen 1972). The rotatory testing of VOR suppression is more physiological, but on the other hand does not evaluate each vestibular organ separately, which we have shown to be important. Though, inhibition originates in the same cerebellum, regardless of stimulus modality.

The finding of different VS levels from stimulating either ear is new. Obviously two factors are important in evaluating VS ability - one is the pathology of VS due to cerebellar dysfunction, the other is the correlation between the VOR response magnitude and the VS quotient. In order to correctly diagnose a defunct VS a coefficient has to be introduced, allowing a higher VS gain for more vivid caloric responses. This relation has to be explored in pure normal material of healthy subjects, presenting a sufficient spectrum of VOR response magnitudes.

REFERENCES

Alpert JN. Failure of fixation suppression: A pathologic effect of vision on caloric nystagmus. Neurology 1974: 24: 891-896.

Barnes GR. Visual factors affecting suppression of the vestibulo-ocular reflex. In: Functional basis of ocular motility disorders. Eds Lennerstrand G, Zee DS, Keller F. Oxford, Pergamon Press, 1982, p. 387.

Barr CC, Schulteis LW, Robinsson DA. Voluntary, non-visual control of the human vestibulo-ocular reflex. Acta Otolaryngol (Stockh) 1976: 81: 365-375.

Bendat JS, Piersol AG. Random data: Analysis and measurement procedures. Wiley-Interscience, New York, 1971.

Boniver R, Demanez JP. Interest of the study of the influence of ocular fixation during caloric tests in pontocerebellar tumors. ORL 1977: 39: 203-208.

Collins WE, Guedry FE, Posner JB. Control of caloric nystagmus by manipulating arousal and visual fixation distance. Ann Otol Rhinol Laryngol 1962: 71: 187-202.

Demanez JP, Ledoux A. Automatic fixation mechanisms and vestibular stimulation. Their study in central pathology with ocular fixation index during caloric tests. Adv Oto-Rhino-Laryng 1970: 17: 90-98.

Ewald JR. Physiologische Untersuchungen uber das Endorgan des Nervus Octavus. Wiesbaden, Bergmann, 1892.

Hamid MA, Hughes GB, Kinney SE. Criteria for diagnosing bilateral vestibular dysfunction. In: The vestibular system: Neurophysiologic and clinical research. Eds Graham MD, Kemink JL. New York, Raven Press, 1987, pp. 115-118.

Hart CW. Ocular fixation and the caloric test. Laryngoscope 1967: 77: 2103-2114.

Henriksson NG. Speed of slow component and duration in caloric nystagmus. Acta Otolaryngol (Stockh) 1956: Suppl 125: 1-29.

Hyden D, Larsby B, Ödkvist LM, Möller C. Visual suppression tests in acoustic neuroma patients. Acta Otolaryngol (Stockh) 1989: Suppl 468: 349-351.

Larsby B, Hyden D, Ödkvist LM. Gain and phase characteristics of compensatory eye movements in light and darkness. Acta Otolaryngol (Stockh) 1984: 97: 223-232.

Larsby B, Ödkvist LM, Hyden D, Liedgren SRC. Disturbances of the vestibular system by toxic agents. Acta Physiol Scand 1976: suppl 440: 157.

Leigh RJ, Zee DS. The neurology of eye movement. FA Davis Company, Philadelphia, USA,1983,pp 39-68.

Maccario M, Backman JR, Korein J. Paradoxical caloric response in altered states of conciousness. Neurology (Minneap) 1972: 22: 781-788.

Mahoney JL, Harlan WL, Bickford RG. Visual and other factors influencing caloric nystagmus in normal subjects. Arch Otolaryngol 1957: 66: 46-53.

Möller C, Ödkvist LM, Thell J, Larsby B, Hyden D, Bergholtz LM, Tham R. Otoneurological findings in psycho-organic syndrome caused by industrial solvent exposure. Acta Otolaryngol (Stockh) 1989: 107: 5-12.

Naito T, Tatsumi T, Matsunaga T, Matsunaga T. The effects of eye closure upon nystagmus. Acta Otolaryngol (Stockh) 1963: Suppl 179: 72-85.

Ödkvist LM, Thell J, Larsby B. A comparison between smooth pursuit and visual suppression. Adv Oto-Rhino-Laryngol 1988: 41: 109-115.

Ödkvist LM, Larsby B, Fredrickson JM, Liedgren SRC, Tham R. Vestibular and oculo-motor disturbances caused by industrial solvents. J Otolaryngol 1980: 9: 53-59.

Preber L, Silfverskiöld BP. Vascular paramedian pontine lesion associated with vestibulo-ocular disturbances. Acta Otolaryngol (Stockh) 1960: 51: 153-164.

Sokolovski A. The influence of mental activity and visual fixation upon caloric-induced nystagmus in normal subjects. Acta Otolaryngol (Stockh) 1966: 61: 209-220.

Takemori S, Cohen B. Visual-vestibular interaction: effects of vision in suppressing vestibular nystagmus. Society for Neuroscience: Program and Abstracts 1972:144.

Takemori S, Cohen B. Loss of visual suppression of vestibular nystagmus after flocculus lesions. Brain Res 1974: 72: 213-224.

Thell J, Ödkvist LM. Artifacts in electronystagmographic recordings. Acta Otolaryngol (Stockh) 1988: Suppl 455: 62-66.

Correspondence to: T Ledin, Dept of ENT, University Hospital, S-581 85 Linköping, Sweden.

OCULOMOTOR DISTURBANCES IN NORMAL CHILDREN LEARNING TO READ.

VICTOR GABERSEK

ENT department, Pr. B. Frachet, Avicenne Hospital, 125, rue de Stalingrad, 93000 BOBIGNY, France.

Electrooculographic (EOG) recording in children learning to read reveals the influence of numerous factors on oculomotor behaviour. Our results concern normal children from two different cultures, French and Arabic, who had one or more EOG examinations while learning to read at the beginning of the first year of primary school. Four tests were proposed: 1) Calibration of eye movements (Voluntary eye movements of 10°); 2) Pursuit eye movement with a pendulum; 3) Optokinetic test; 4) Ocular scanning/reading tests or reading-type tasks (the child must follow symbols without signification, arranged in 6 equal rows). Respecting the order of testing, 10 main points will be presented, showing the various aquisitions, losses and modifications of an oculomotor evolution in successive stages.

1) The Oculomotor Reaction Time (OMRT).

The OMRT is the time which elapses between the appearance of a visual stimulus and the beginning of an eye movement. In children we find a double genetic evolution: a) an increase of the gaze efficiency between 6 and 12 years (progressive decrease of the duration of OMRT). b) An establishment of privileged gaze direction (upwards) and , between 6 and 8 years, laterisation to the right . This lateralisation is independent of progress in learning to read but it seems to depend on the development of the spatial function. (fig.1).

2) The graphical variety of oblique eye movements on EOG tracings.

Thanks to convergence of electrical axes from corneo-retinal potentials (between cornea and the emergency of nervus opticus) the evolution of oblique eye movements may show, in EOG, 3 different graphical types for the same oblique eye movement according to the child.

a) The rotatory type (giving two isoelectric lines on horizontal monocular tracings) appear in 80% of pre-school children, in 63% of the elderly, and in 44% of patients 3 months after cranial injuries.

b) The rectilinear type (giving one isoelectric line on a horizontal monocular tracing) appears in occidental cultures first in right-up and left-down (oblique A) dominating towards 9 - 10 years, but in the Arabic culture right-down and left-up (oblique B) appears first. It is the oblique ocular movement seen in 100% of normal literate adults between 16 - 45 years. c) The intermediate type (with no isoelectric line) is necessary for going from the rotatory type (resulting from an oculocephalic association) to rectilinear type (a proof the an oculocephalic dissassociation which is absolutely necessary for rapid reading) and vice versa. We found it temporarily in 100% of children learning to read; durably in 73% of dyslexics (9 -14 years) in 90% of amblyopics and in 44% of patients up to 3 months following cranial injury. This evolution depends on the culture and on level of learning to read and on possible pathology.. The best tests to show this are calibration of eye movements and the optokinetic test.

3) The oculocorporal associated movements.

The oculocorporal associated movement results from visuomotor coordination between eye and head, eye and body or a body part. The most important are the oculopalpebral associated movement (5%) and the positional oculocephalic associated movements (10%). Both are pathological. They suggest the need for further medical investigation of connections to visual, vestibular, binocular etc factors. The first, oculopalpebral, hinders the appearance of saccades, the second, the cephalic position during the test, favors vision in upshoot in one eye and in downshoot in the other eye as with certain amblyopics. Both behaviours involve an ocular dyskinesis since the tracings show a modification of EOG amplitude and morphology. The frequency and rhythm can be normal. Other associated movements do not affect the test. For example, crossing the feet (oculopostural associated movement) is often a memory helper in the search for laterality. The ante- and retro-cephalic flexions (present also in elderly presbiopic persons) provoke ocular torsion and give greater gaze stability; moreover the eye movement can slip along the upper lid (anteflexion) or lower lid (retroflexion) like relying on a horizontal guide. The study of associated movements is part of all four tests.

4) The fovealization process.

The EOG tracing is very often perturbed during pursuit eye movement with the pendulum. Up to 80% if the child did not attend kindergarten; up to 90% in visual pathology where the explanation is simple: The oculomotor maturation can be stopped by a luminous retinal insufficiency or lack of retinal stimulation (corneal , crystaline lens or corpus vitreus opacity; anisometropia, strabismus) etc. The origin may be congenital, traumatic or spontaneously. But in the child whose evolution is normal, an aquired visuomotor activity can not regress, it can complete the evolution. In newborns the first organized, complex eye movement, the pursuit eye movement, would have a peripheral, perifoveal, subcortical origin (as in animals) where the movement of itself, in intense contrast, would elicit a reflex and ensure good test results. Around pre-school age a faulty pursuit eye movement suggest the process of fovealization which engenders sensibility to details and slight contrasts of the target. We have thus voluntary eye movements of ocular pursuit where the image of the target and not only its movement is actively realized in the brain.

5) The slow isolated clonus-type eye movement.

It presents a complex of 3 eye movements in rapid succession. The first of these eye movements is followed after latency (60 - 150 msec) by a biphasic eye movement ressembling a clonus. The first phase of the clonus-type eye movement always appears in the opposite direction to the tracking test target. The second phase, without latency, is always in the direction of the target, with velocity of the eye movement equalling that of the target. "Skipping" in the tracking test does not necessarily lead to a clonus-type eye movement, but a clonus-type eye movement is always preceded by a skipping movement with variable amplitude, faster than the pendulum and moving in the same direction. This clonus-type eye movement is present in amblyopics and in children as a transitory event (2O days) in the acute phase of neuroallergic illness.

6) Ocular grasping reflex.

This reflex may be elicited by monocular vision in the pursuit eye movement of the pendulum in 60% of amblyopics constantly and in 89% of children ,6 - 7 years old who had not attended kindergarten, occasionally. The adductional movement of the uncovered eye provokes a normal binocular response during the pursuit test but the abductional pursuit of the same eye gives stereotyped, saccadic, automatic, reflex , pursuit eye movements with short fixations (50 - 200 msec). In the optokinetic test the absence of the pursuit abductional eye movement (slow phase of optokinetic nystagmus) in the uncovered eye fails to give an optokinetic response directed toward the covered eye. However we note an increase of amplitude and frequency of the rapid phase of optokinetic nystagmus if it is directed toward the uncovered eye. In normal children this reflex disappears by the end of the first school year.

7) Inhibition of optokinetic response.

We observe 3 types of inhibition: 1) Immediate inhibition from the start of the test. (12% of children who did not attend kindergarten) which takes place right after the first slow phase of the expected optokinetic nystagmus. The gaze in the same direction as the moving stripes remains blocked on the border of the screen until the end of the test. It may be a reinforced fixation on the last passing stripe in an extreme lateral ocular position.. 2) Transitory inhibition. a) Transitory inhibition in the horizontal plane which was described above in ocular grasping reflex, suffices in normal children to permit a binocular vision to evoke the response. b) The rhythm of the response may be interrupted by a privileged gaze direction to any side of the stimulus. 3) Inhibition of optokinetic reactivity. The optokinetic reactivity is obtained with a sudden supraoptimal acceleration of the stimulation during 3 - 10 sec. In the absence of optokinetic nystagmus, the optokinetic reactivity is also absent.Normally in optokinetic reactivity the frequency of optokinetic nystagmus decreases and the amplitude increases. In monocular vision this modification is not visible if the optokinetic nystagmus beats in the direction of the covered eye; the nystagmus may keep the rhythm or decrease in frequency but the amplitude does not change. It may express a very diminished ocular grasping reflex.

8) Oculoglottic occurence.

During simultaneous recordings of phono- or glottograms and of eye movements during reading aloud the subject does not begin the phoneme at the same time as the ocular movement . This is logical since we know that this reading precedes by far the emission of perceived words through successive visual fixations on text. (The oculovocal span may go from minus 4 to plus 11 words).

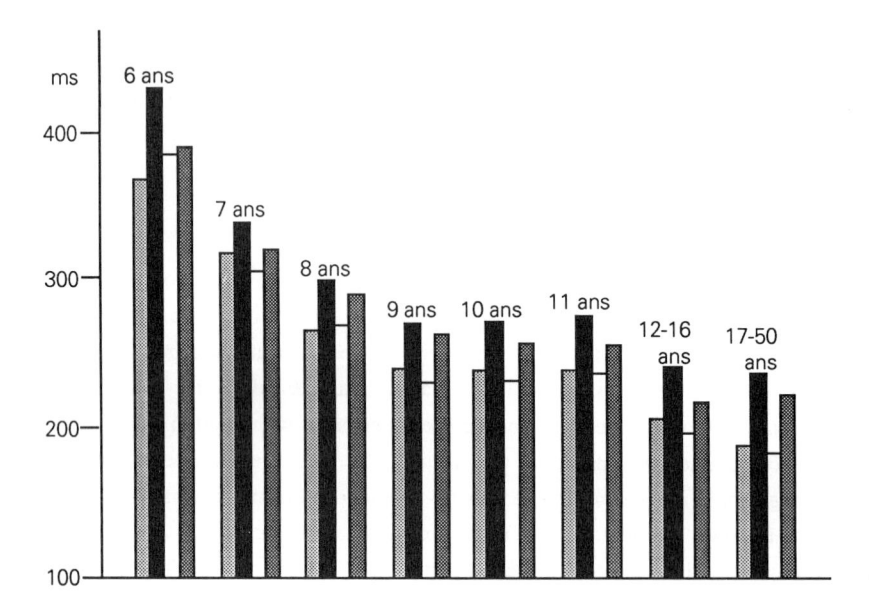

Fig 1. Averages of oculomotor reaction times (OMRT) : Establishment of genetic privileged gaze direction by occidental children. Each column represents from left to right averages of upwards, downwards, right- and leftwards OMRT.

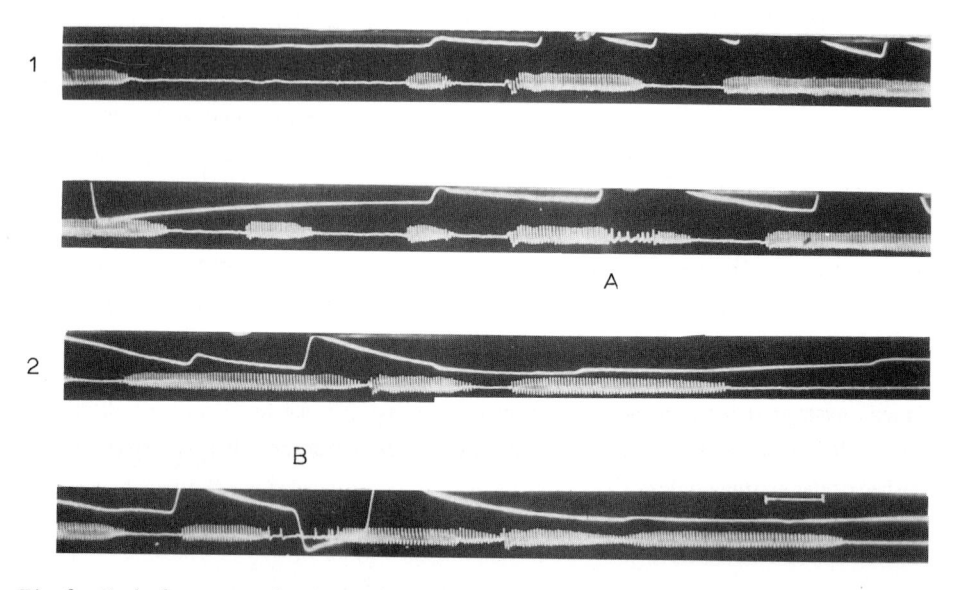

Fig 2. Each fragment slows simultaneous recording of eye movements and glottogram by reading aloud. 1. and 2 correspond to a first reading ; A and B to a second reading. The glottographical wave is interrrupted by an eye movement (A : situaiton 2) ; The oculoglottic occurence (B : situation 3). Time basis = 100 millisec).

Normally both activities bring into play not only two different functions respectively vision and speech , but refer to two different words. The appearance of eye movements is generally between 30 msec before and 20 msec after the phoneme. If the glottogram is clear we can say that speech is dominant but if the the glottogram wave is interrupted then the eye movements are dominant. 3 situations are possible: 1) The glottographical wave is spontaneously interrupted temporarily without ocular interference; 2) The glottographical wave is interrupted by an eye movement or blinking. In both cases after interruption the child finishes what he was saying without beginning the whole word again. 3) In an oculoglottic occurence the child will begin the whole word again. This is a very frequent sign in stutterers. (fig.2).

9) The incongruity of eye movements during reading.

Congruity expresses the binocular synergy of amplitude, frequency and direction of eye movements during reading or scanning eye movements like those of children who do not read. This is the ideal oculomotor behaviour of a normal literate adult. But the child in the 2 first school years or an illiterate adult will begin during his initiation to reading with a random alternating monocular predominance which signals the beginning of oculocephalic disassociation. This will be followed by alternating monocular predominance, which is determined by the direction of ocular exercice or by extreme laterality of typographical signs to fixate (The oculocephalic disassociation is practically terminated). The third and last stage furnishes two kinds of oculomotor processes: One leads to a constant incongruity with one eye directing; the other ,more frequent, could indicate a binocular behaviour. Both these situations will not hinder the development of rapid reading. The future dyslexic seems to follow a different course. The first two stages (alternating monocular predominance) cited above do not seem to appear in dyslexics.

10) Transitory ideomotor ocular apraxia.

If we inhibit the associated oculodigitogestual movement in the scanning test, 80% of the children who had not attended kindergarten, 2 1/2 months after the beginning of first school year, could not succeed in the test when they had to fixate signs arranged in a line. While each child believed he had fully followed instructions, in fact he did not fixate one sign after another, he skipped entire lines or , most frequently, skimmed over the signs without fixation and finished too soon, or he ran his gaze all over the text and he needed 4 times as long as a pupil at the end of the first school year. If we asked him to repeat the test, still believing he had done well, the child did it just as badly. We can say that the finger has become his ideomotor guide and substitutes for eye movements which are already associated with head movements and through them integrate in the accessory apparatus for vision. At end of the school year this apraxia disappears in normal children.

To sum up, we can say that the child's oculomotor behaviour in the first school year is not comparable with the normal adults. It has much in common with numerous pathological. syndromes concerning vision. The 10 points described above deal only with oculomotor aspects of reading mechanisms, and do not take into account cognitive and all sensory factors.

ELECTRICAL VESTIBULAR STIMULATION OF COCHLEAR IMPLANTED PATIENTS

BRUNO FRACHET, VICTOR GABERSEK, THIERRY VAN DEN ABBEELE, PIERRE TISON.

ENT Department, Pr. B. FRACHET, Avicenne Hospital, 125, rue de Stalingrad, 93000 Bobigny, France.

Two centuries ago (1790) VOLTA invented voltaic cells and 10 years later tested on himself the effect of a 50 volt galvanic current placed between his ears. In 1803 RITTER, with more than 100 volts, imitated VOLTA. They both experienced sound, painful and unpleasant sensations and vertigo.In 1820, PURKINJE used a 20 plate voltaic column (Cu- Zn, 20-25 volts) connected to two silver wires, which silver electrodes were attached to his fingers, themselves introduced into his ears. After sensation of a luminous phenomena, and metalic taste in the mouth, he felt a movement of dizziness in his head which seemed to move towards the direction of the Cu pole. He thus determined that direction of vertigo depended on the electrical pole. After 10 minutes, nausea, headache and drowsiness appeared, lasting for two hours after the end of the experiment. In 1855 DUCHENNE DE BOULOGNE used an active electrode with a salt solution in the outer ear and the indifferent electrode on the mastoid region. He found that sound sensations came when turning on or off current. Thus in galvanic stimulations, the cutaneous electrodes can be either bipolar and biauricular as showed by VOLTA, RITTER and PURKINJE, or else monopolar-monoauricular with Mastoid reference, as used by DUCHENNE DE BOULOGNE who already worked with alternating current. For 100 years, galvanic stimulation was the best recommended stimulation for study of nystagmus in neurotological investigations. Mastoid, stimulating electrodes have a 3 cm2 surface in order to limit pain. Galvanic current is applied with a 90 volt battery with constant flow. The intensity changes from 1 to 10 milliamperes (some authors up to 20 milliamperes) and current must be increased or decreased gradually and never interrupted suddenly. The patient is sitting, his head in BRUNING's first position, his eyes open thoughout the test in darkness or wearing FRENZEL glasses. The electronystagmographical (ENG) technique is not recommendet for galvanic nystagmus recording because an ocular rheogram is obtained and its amplitude is too great. In fact, rheogram jerks are synchronous with cardiac rhythm and mask nystagmic movements. This masking is due to the choroide playing the role of a physiological angioma (GABERSEK and JOBERT 1966)

The use of the photoelectronystagmographical method (PENG) of RICHTER and PFALTZ enabled us to find 2 different nystagmographical responses: 1) Nystagmic jerks with a frequency of 1 Hz and amplitude of 1°; the patient is in semi-darkness. 2) Real galvanic nystagmus of 5 to 8 Hz and amplitude of 5° in total darkness. Galvanic responses change with position of the mastoid negative electrode in the same subject, and from one subject to another indicating a certain

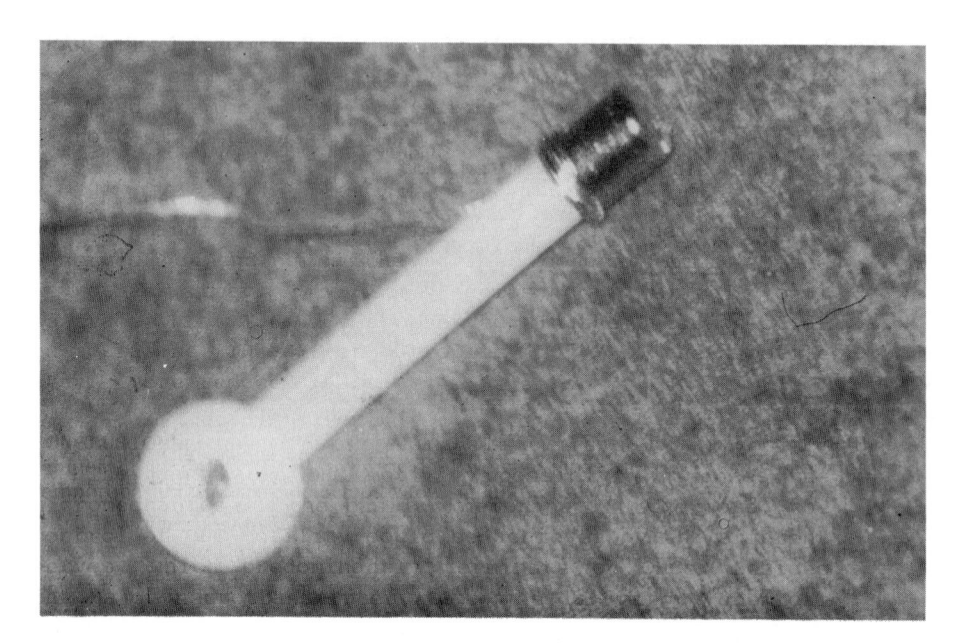

Fig 1) The cupule-shaped electrode and the incudo-vestibular prothesis.

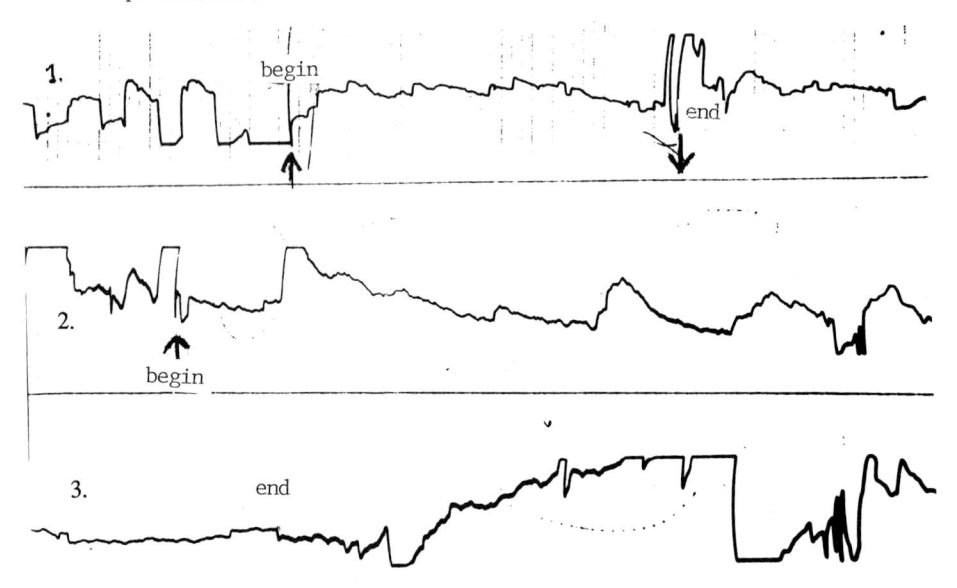

Fig 2) PENG recordings during galvanic stimulations in a patient with a right cochlear implants.
From top to bottom:1) 10° horizontal eye movement calibration and bipolar monauricular galvanic stimulation (implant is indifferent electrode : right galvanic nystagmus)
2) The implant is negative electrode : right galvanic nystagmus. 3) Left post-galvanic nystagmus.

selectivity of the stimulation. Double galvanic reactions were already pointed out by JENSEN (1896). One of those would be the real vestibular response, the other appearing only during a very intense stimulation giving clonical movements of extravestibular origin. However DOHLMAN'S works (1926) showed the persistence of normal galvanic responses after bilateral labyrinthectomy; the response disappears only after section of the vestibular nerve. HUIZINGA (1931) also removed SCARPA'S ganglion and obtained a weak response as he placed electrodes on the vestibular nerve. All these experiments on animals show that the response would be coming from peripheral neurons and that ocular galvanic response would have an extravestibular origin. This is also suggested by HENNEBERT (1950),DIX and HALLPIKE (1952), LEDOUX (1958), RISTOW (1960) etc. The best early PENG recordings in man are those of RICHTER and PFALTZ (1958). They showed a galvanic nystagmus with many inverted jerks, the amplitude does not excel 1° and the frequency 1 Hz. If this galvanic nystagmus is related to nystagmiform jerks of low amplitude obtained in semi-darkness, the question is: is this galvanic nystagmus of extravestibular origin? Real galvanic nystagmus should never have inverted jerks while uprighting the cupulae of the semi-circular canals could explain the "post-galvanic" nystagmus described by some authors.

100 years after DUCHENNE DE BOULOGNE, at the time of the first direct stimulation of the human auditory nerve (Eyries and al 1957), galvanic nystagmus presented less and less interest, whereas specific studies of stimulation of auditory nerve in total deafness began to evolve rapidly. This does not mean the end of galvanic stimulation of vestibule. Cochlear implants bring electrodes nearer to vestibular system and decrease electrical resistance. Cutaneous electrodes require resistances of 15 to 20 kohms, while an extracochlear electrode placed on the oval window decreases by 10 times this resistance. o,6 milliamperes are sufficient for good galvanic nystagmus.

Our electrode is an original device: a gold-shaped cupule electrode, on top of a teflon-piston, placed on the oval window. The surgical technique is identical to the usual stapedectomy for otosclerosis with its variants. The connection is transcutaneal wire-to-wire to an earring on the earlobe. This system offers an excellent stability of the electrode and the electrical resistance (fig.1).

In 5 patients with right cochlear implants we have obtained a nystagmus of low frequency (1 Hz) and of moderate amplitude (2-3°). At the end of each stimulation, we obtained a post-galvanic nystagmus lasting 9 sec. Changing poles does not evoke reverse nystagmus, but nystagmus of different morphology, frequency and amplitude (fig.2). It is interesting to observe that tinnitus, when present on the side of the implanted ear,changes side during stimulation. Rapid interruption of stimulus is followed by unpleasant musical sounds which echo for 10 to 20 seconds. Slower interruption, without steps, is followed by unmelodius sounds. In all cases, patients reporting tinnitus on the side of the implanted ear describe disappearance ot their tinnitus during stimulus on that side, with displacement of tinnitus on the other side. They also describe a slow deviation of their head opposite to galvanic nystagmus.

REFERENCES

1. Dix M.R.,Hallpike C.S.: The pathology,symptomatology and diagnosis of certain common disorders of the vestibular system . Ann.Otol.Rhin.Laryngol.1952,61:987-1016
2. Djurno A.,Eyries C.: Prothèse auditive par excitation electrique à distance du nerf sensoriel à l'aide d'un bobinage inclus à demeure. Press Med.1957,65:1417-1423
3. Dohlman G.F.: Some physical investigations on galvanic irritation on the labyrinth. Acta Otolaryngol. 1926,61:53-63
4. Duchenne de Boulogne: 1855,cited by Soussi
5. Frachet B.,Vormes E., Verschuur H.P.,Harboun-Cohen E.,Despreaux G.: Stimulation électrique de la fenêtre ovale: perspectives. Ann.Oto-laryngol. 1988,105:597-600.
6. Gabersek V., Jobert F.: L'enregistrement du nystagmus galvanique. Ann.Otolaryngol 1966,83:47-60
7. Hennebert P.E.: L' épreuve galvanique. Acta ORL Belgica 1950,4:409-417
8. Huizinga E.: De la réaction galvanique de l'appareil vestibulaire.Acta Otolaryngol.1931,15:451-468
9. Jensen P.: Uber den galvanischen Schwindel. Arch. ges. Physiol.1896,64:182-222
10. Ledoux A; Les canaux semicirculaires. Acta ORL Belgica,1958,12:1O9-346
11. Purkinje J.: Beiträge zur näheren Kenntnis des Schwindels aus heautognostischen Daten. , Med.Jahrb.d.K.K.österreich. Staates 1820,6:79-125
12. Richter H.,Pfaltz C.R.: Recherches électronystagmographiques sur la reaction vestibulaire galvanique. Conf. Neurol. 1958,18:370-378
13. Ristow: Tierexperimentelle Untersuchungen über den vestibularen Tonus. Arch. Ohr.Nas.Kehlkopfheilk.1960,176:792-793
14. Ritter H.: Über die Anwendung der voltaischen Säule. Neue J.d.pract.Arzneikunde 1803,17:30-1O8
15. Soussi Th.: Les implants cochléaires. Réhabilitation des surdités totales par implantation originale d'une électrode en cupule sur la fenêtre ovale .Med. Thesis, Paris 7, Fac. de Médecine Lariboisière Saint-Louis,1989:126p
16. Volta A.: On the electricity excited by more contact of conducting substances of different kinds. Trans.roy.Soc.Phil. 1800,90:403-431.

INFLUENCE OF THE HEAD-BODY POSITION ON OPTOKINETIC AFTERNYSTAGMUS

H.J.SCHOLTZ, A.W.SCHOLTZ, U.SIEVERT
Dept. of ORL, University of Rostock, Doberaner Str. 137, 2500 Rostock (DDR)

The optokinetic nystagmus (OKN) - evoked by movements of the visual surroundings - is mediated by two independent mechanisms. One depends on the retinal fovea and occipital cortex, the other one is mediated by the peripheral retina and nuclei, connected by the accessory optic tract. According to Magnusson et al. this subcortical OKN as well as the vestibulo-ocular reflex is believed to project to a velocity storage mechanism, which was compared to a leaking integrator. In this way visually and vestibular induced activity are retained by the velocity storage mechanism in order to maintain the ability of making compensatory eye movements and visual vestibular integration during low frequency movements and of contributing to the compensation of the VOR in the growing or lesioned individual.

In our recent investigations intended to prove the influence of different body positions on the OKN, we found a decrease in the slow phase velocity of the horizontal and vertical OKN, when the test was carried out in a posture different from the normal vertical head-body position.

According to the publications of Magnusson et al., the optokinetic afternystagmus (OKAN) reflects the subcortically mediated OKN. The cortical OKN is characterized by an abrupt onset and decay of the slow phase velocity (SPV), while the subcortical OKN shows a slow build-up and a following OKAN after cessation of the stimulus. With our previously described method of application of bright and dark stripes we expect a "combined" OKN, this means including the OKAN. The question is now, whether this OKAN can also be influenced by changing the head-body position in respect to the gravitational force.

MATERIAL AND METHOD

The examinations were carried out with 31 healthy persons (aged between 18 and 61 years) with a mean of 28,7 years, who had never suffered from ear or nervous diseases. They were fixed on a position table and had a semicircular screen at a distance of 70 cm before their eyes, on which an optokinetic striped pattern, consisting of 24 bright and 24 dark stripes, was projected by a stimulator over their heads.

In order to examine the horizontal OKN in right or left direction an optokinetic stimulation speed of $60°/s$ was applied for 10 seconds. Afterwards the light was switched off for 10 sec. These stimulation periods, consisting of 10 sec. stimulation and 10 sec. darkness, were repeated seven times, so that the test consisted of 8 trials in each direction. The darkness period after the last stimulation lasted 30 sec. During the periods of darkness the test subjects were requested to look straight ahead.

After the examination in the upright position, the horizontal head-body position of 90° was taken.

The OKN was recorded by means of photoelectronystagmography PENG 83 according to Gestewitz. The SPV of OKN and OKAN was calculated by a microcomputer. For the comparison between the upright and horizontal body position we took the maximum SPV of the OKN and the SPV of the OKAN during the second second after the light was switched off. The data from the first second were discarded, also for the calculation of the time constant of decay of OKAN, the other parameter we used. The time constant, which was determined from the slope of the line that relates the log of the SPV to the time, was determined from the course of the OKAN after the last stimulation and summarized for both directions.

Thus, the OKN and OKAN values obtained from 32 individual tests for each person were analyzed.

RESULTS

Two subjects showed no OKAN in the normal as well as in the horizontal body position. Table I summarizes the results obtained from 920 individual tests with 29 subjects.

TABLE I

Slow phase velocities of OKN and OKAN in different head-body positions (n= 920 trials)

n.s. = no significance

HEAD BODY POSIT:		SLOW PHASE VELOCITY	
		OKN(°/s)	OKAN (°/s)
0°	R	34,5	13,4
90°		33,1 n.s.	13,6 n.s.
0°	L	33,9	12,7
90°		32,2 n.s.	13,5 n.s.

The OKN in the normal position shows a slight preponderance to the right. The average maximum SPV amounts to 34,5°/s with the right nystagmus and 33,9°/s with the left nystagmus.

The same is true of the SPV of the OKAN, the average values of which were 13,4°/s for the right and 12,7°/s for the left direction. In the horizontal position the maximum SPV of the OKN decreased to 33,1°/s or 32,2°/s, respectively,

whereas the SPV of the OKAN remained unchanged (13,6 or 13,5°/s, respectively).
Due to the large inter-individual variants, the differences at the OKN are not
significant.

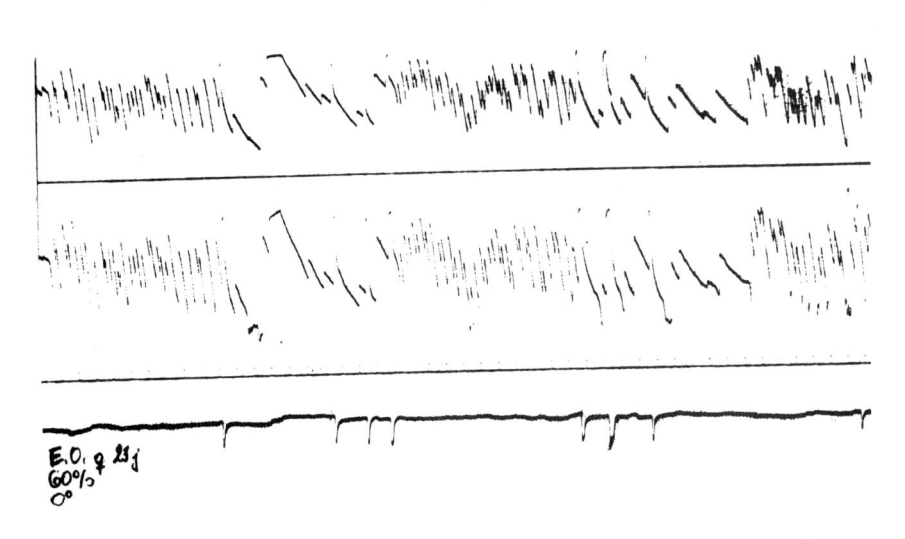

Fig. 1. PENG-registration of OKN in upright body-position (Stimulus 60°/s)

Fig. 1 and 2 show recorded examples with the respective computer evaluations at
the left or right nystagmus, respectively. The analogue curves of the OKN and
OKAN illustrate the minor differences in the upright and horizontal position.
The time constants amount to 10,4 ± 3,4 s in the starting and 11,2 ± 3,8 s
in the horizontal position, which means no significant difference here either.

DISCUSSION

Our results confirm previously reported observations, that the horizontal OKN,
in a body position different from the normal one, shows a lower SPV. The different
age structure of the present subjects groups with the resulting intrasubject
variability and a probable preponderance, does not, however, prove any significant differences.

The OKAN after a stimulation speed of 60°/s shows, in the normal position,
somewhat higher SPV values than reported for instance by Jele et al. and Tijssen
et al. In the horizontal head body position the SPV of the OKAN remains nearly
unchanged, whereas the time constant even rises insignificantly.

In an interpretation of the alteration of the OKN besides the influence of the
otolith organs an influence of the cervical proprioceptive activities cannot be
completely excluded. At the OKAN the conclusions are not clear. The influence
of the otolith organs seems to act on another pathway, so that we could find
rather an excitation of the eye movements. For the clarification of this problem,

an examination of patients with bilateral loss of the vestibular function is envisaged.

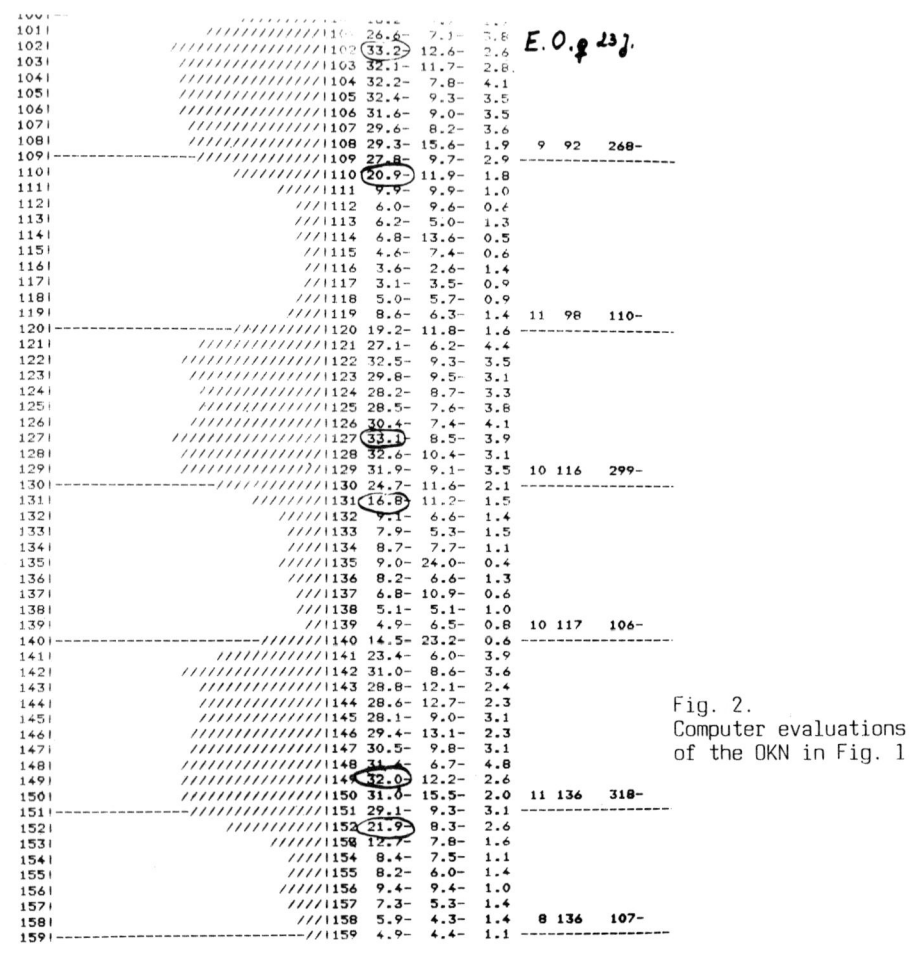

```
101|             ///////////////101  26.6-  7.1-  3.8    E.O.g 23J.
102|             ///////////////102  33.2- 12.6-  2.6
103|             ///////////////103  32.1- 11.7-  2.8
104|             ///////////////104  32.2-  7.8-  4.1
105|             ///////////////105  32.4-  9.3-  3.5
106|             ///////////////106  31.6-  9.0-  3.5
107|             ///////////////107  29.6-  8.2-  3.6
108|             ///////////////108  29.3- 15.6-  1.9    9  92  268-
109|-------------///////////////109  27.8-  9.7-  2.9 -------------
110|                ////////////110  20.9- 11.9-  1.8
111|                //////////111    9.9-  9.9-  1.0
112|                   /////112     6.0-  9.6-  0.6
113|                   /////113     6.2-  5.0-  1.3
114|                   /////114     6.8- 13.6-  0.5
115|                    ////115     4.6-  7.4-  0.6
116|                    ////116     3.6-  2.6-  1.4
117|                    ////117     3.1-  3.5-  0.9
118|                    ////118     5.0-  5.7-  0.9
119|                   /////119     8.6-  6.3-  1.4    11  98  110-
120|-----------------////////120    19.2- 11.8-  1.6 -------------
121|                ////////////121   27.1-  6.2-  4.4
122|                ////////////122   32.5-  9.3-  3.5
123|                ////////////123   29.8-  9.5-  3.1
124|                ////////////124   28.2-  8.7-  3.3
125|                ////////////125   28.5-  7.6-  3.8
126|                ////////////126   30.4-  7.4-  4.1
127|             ///////////////127   33.1-  8.5-  3.9
128|             ///////////////128   32.6- 10.4-  3.1
129|             ///////////////129   31.9-  9.1-  3.5   10 116  299-
130|-------------///////////////130   24.7- 11.6-  2.1 -------------
131|                ////////////131   16.8- 11.2-  1.5
132|                   /////132      9.1-  6.6-  1.4
133|                   /////133      7.9-  5.3-  1.5
134|                   /////134      8.7-  7.7-  1.1
135|                   /////135      9.0- 24.0-  0.4
136|                    ////136      8.2-  6.6-  1.3
137|                    ////137      6.8- 10.9-  0.6
138|                    ////138      5.1-  5.1-  1.0
139|                    ////139      4.9-  6.5-  0.8   10 117  106-
140|-------------///////////////140  14.5- 23.2-  0.6 -------------
141|                ////////////141   23.4-  6.0-  3.9
142|                ////////////142   31.0-  8.6-  3.6
143|                ////////////143   28.8- 12.1-  2.4
144|                ////////////144   28.6- 12.7-  2.3
145|                ////////////145   28.1-  9.0-  3.1
146|                ////////////146   29.4- 13.1-  2.3
147|                ////////////147   30.5-  9.8-  3.1
148|                ////////////148   31.4-  6.7-  4.8
149|                ////////////149   32.0- 12.2-  2.6
150|                ////////////150   31.0- 15.5-  2.0   11 136  318-
151|-------------///////////////151   29.1-  9.3-  3.1 -------------
152|                ////////////152   21.9-  8.3-  2.6
153|                   /////153      12.7-  7.8-  1.6
154|                    ////154      8.4-  7.5-  1.1
155|                    ////155      8.2-  6.0-  1.4
156|                    ////156      9.4-  9.4-  1.0
157|                    ////157      7.3-  5.3-  1.4
158|                    ////158      5.9-  4.3-  1.4    8 136  107-
159|-------------///////////////159   4.9-  4.4-  1.1 -------------
```

Fig. 2.
Computer evaluations of the OKN in Fig. 1

REFERENCES

1. Jell RM, Irland DJ, Lafortune S (1984) Human Optokinetic Afternystagmus Acta Otolaryng. (Stockh.) 98: 462-471

2. Leliever WC, Correia ML (1987) Further Observations on the Effects of Head Position on Vertical OKN and OKAN in Normal Subjects. Otolaryng. Head Neck Surg.1987: 275-281

3. Magnusson M, Schalen L, Pyykkö I, Enbom H, Henriksson NG (1988) Clinical Considerations Concerning Horizontal Optokinetik Nystagmus, Acta Otolaryng. (Stockh.) Suppl 455: 53-57

4. Scholtz HJ, Sievert U, Scholtz AW, Nakazawa H (1989) Einfluß der Kopfstellung auf den optokinetischen Nystagmus. IV.Symposium für Neuro-Otologie,Berlin (im Druck)

5. Tijssen MAJ, Straathof CSM, Hain TC, Zee DS(1989) Optokinetic Afternystagmus in Humans:Normal Values of Amplitude,Time Constant and Asymmetry.Ann.Otol. Rhinol.Laryng. 98: 741-746

© 1991 Elsevier Science Publishers B.V. All rights reserved.
Vertigo, nausea, tinnitus and hypoacusia due to head and neck trauma.
C.-F. Claussen and M.V. Kirtane, editors.

BRAIN ELECTRICAL ACTIVITY MAPPING A NEW FRONTIER IN NEUROOTOLOGY

ALES HAHN, CLAUS - FRENZ CLAUSSEN, DIETER SCHNEIDER, UWE FRAASS, BELA BÜKI

E. N. T. Clinics and Depts.of Otoneurology,
Universities of Prague, Würzburg and Budapest

SUMMARY:

In the department of Otoneurology at Würzburg University we introduced a new objective method for the evaluation of sensory function, BRAIN ELECTRICAL ACTIVITY MAPPING (BEAM) .
In detail are described responses to the rotatory as well as visual stimuli, a various pattern of Brain Mapps are presented.

KEY WORDS:

Brain Electrical Activity Mapping / Brain Surveyor / Visual and Rotational Stimuli

INTRODUCTION.

Vertigo, Nausea, Tinnitus and Hypacusia are very serious problems among the otoneurologic patients.
The sequentiel dynamic Electroencephalographic Mapping (Brain Electrical Activity Mapping) is a an objective method for the examination of spontaneous activity of the brain cortex as well as for the registration of the evoked activity .
Using this method we would be able to distinguish the major pathways which exist among different sensory structures in a greater detail and therefore recognize better their pathologic conditions.

MATERIAL AND METHODS :

At the department of Neurootology of the E. N. T.Clinic of Würzburg University of our research group uses an examination unit consisting of Encephaloscript ES 12 000 and a Brain Surveyor BS 2 400. Both equipements are produced by Picker - Schwarzer.
The Brain Surveyor operates with 32 Byte Processor allowing to record simultenous brain activity from the 16 channels.The equipment further provides also with very sensitive 14 ´´screen and 16 colours writer.
We are evaluating frequency as well as potential activities from the brain cortex which could be easily demonstrated in the shape of graphic maps.
For the paper presented we have used visual and rotatory stimuli.

For the examination of the **visual system** we initially examined *spontaneous activity* , which reveales a remarkable activity in the temporal region.
After a registration of the spontaneous activity *visualy evoked potentials* have been recorded. We are using a chessboard- pattern (Fig. 1) . In this type of stimulation a high positivity in the time period between 100 - 110 msec in the occipital region (electrodes O 1 and O 2) , lower positive activity in the parietal (P 4 and P 3) and temporal region.

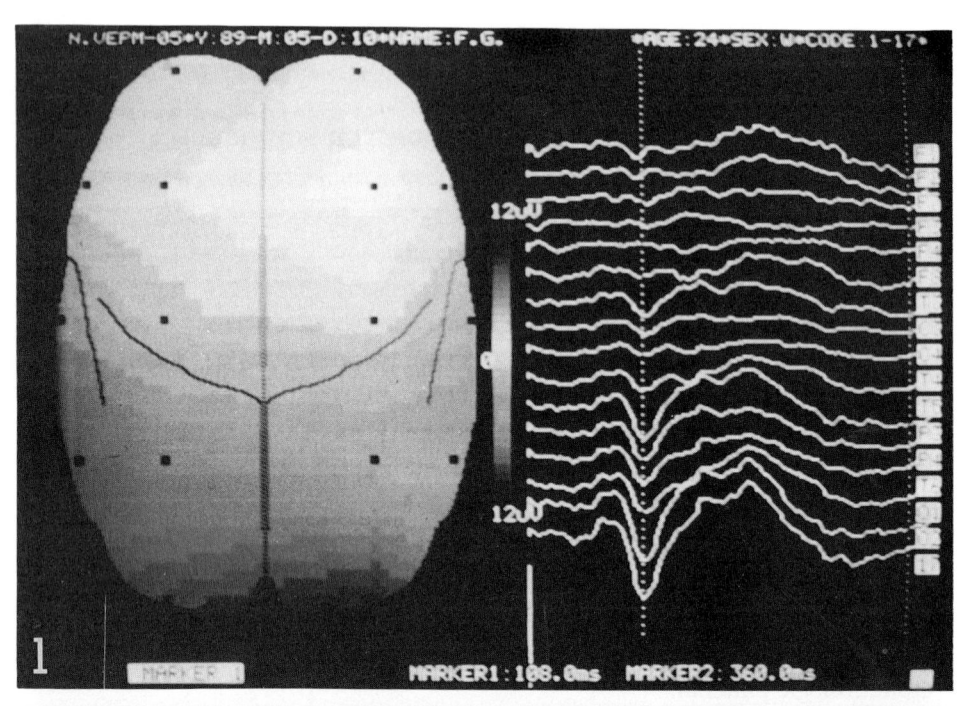

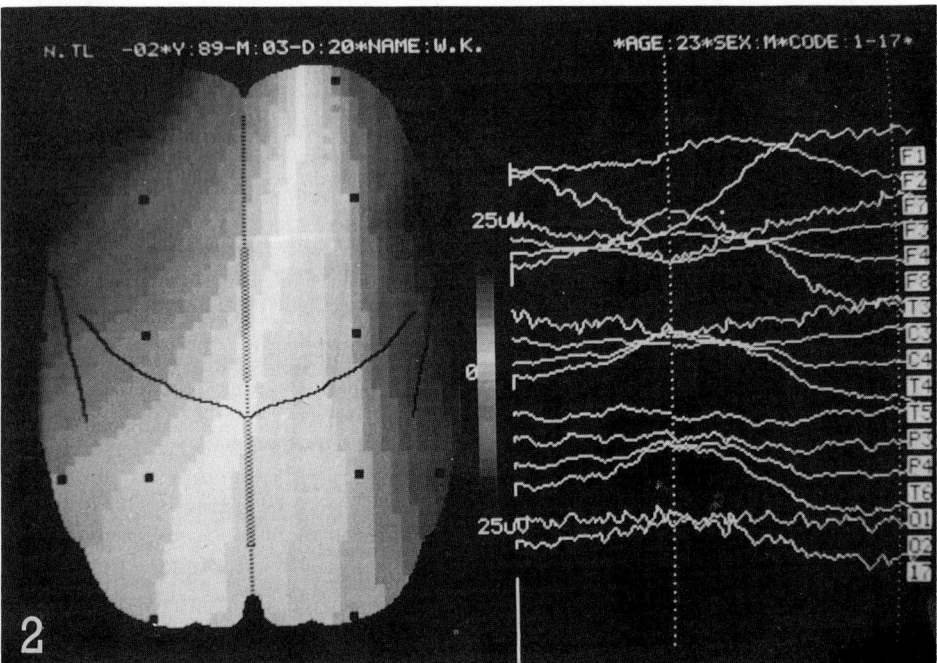

Fig.1.Visual evoked potentials (Chessboard- Pattern)

Fig 2. Visual Evoked Potentials (eye tracking test)

200 msec after stimulation a repolarisation in the occipital region is noticed as well as a small positivity in the frontal region.

Another stimulus is a digital tracking test. Assuming that the visual stimulus is directed from the right to the left in the time period at about 110 msec (Fig. 2) there is registrated a very high positivity in the fronto - temporal region (i.e. in the electrodes F 1,F 3 and T 3), while on the right side in the electrodes F 2, F 6 and T 4 a negativity is present. This situation is reversel if the optic stimuli are directed from the right to the left.

Thus in this situation the distribution of the potentials seems to be generated from the right to the left side and opposite. Applying the digital eye tracking stimulation in the vertical directionit is possible to registate a positive activity in the temporal region.

Generaring **rotatory stimuli** an electronically regulated rotatory chair with linear acceleration and velocity patterns is used. The perrotatory stimuli are recorded in the phase of the linear acceleration in which patient is linear accelerated with 3 ° / sec.-2 from 0 - 90 degree within 30 seconds. Then for 180 sec the chair is rotated constantly with angular velocity of 90 °/ sec. In this phase we register a perrotatory optokinetic nystagmus during the 30 seconds. Finaly an abrupt stop of the rotating chair with an angular deceleration of 270 ° / sec.-2 happens. The postrotatory nystagmus is observed during the period of 30 seconds.

Nystagmic eye movements are registrated mainly in the Delta Frequency Range i.e. in the frequency range from 0, 5 - 4, 0 Hz. We apply various filtres in order to separate the overlay of nystagmic activity from the rotatory evoked potentials. The most sensitive are the frequenties Theta (4 - 7 Hz) as well as Alpha(7 - 12 Hz) After right directed rotation a left nystagmus was observed; at the Brain Mapping picture we notice positive activity in the Theta and Alpha frequency ranges running along the skull towards to right side and also to the posterior part of the skull. This activity can be registered in the T 3, T 4 and T 6.

We were able to detect a substraction of the both hemispheres (Fig. 3.).

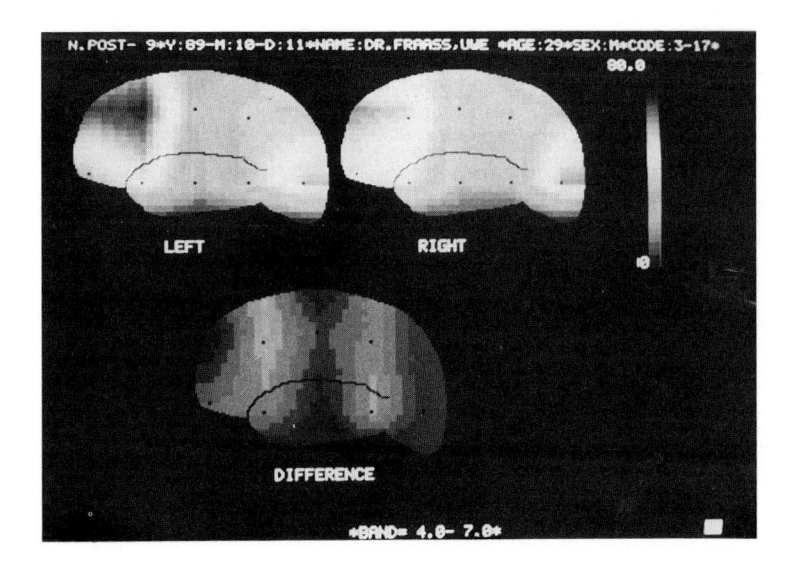

DISKUSSION :

Brain Electrical Activity Mapping provides new functional topics on neurootological topodiagnostics. Formely we only had two dimensions for projecting dysequilibriumum states in an objective manner, as Nystagmus and Body Sway.

Now we also can derive cortical activity patterns due to vestibular and/or ocular stimulations. Surprisingly topic imaging feature differences are unvealed between vertical optokinetic stimulation and chess-board visual evoked potentials on one the hand and horizontal optokinetic tracking stimuli as well as perrotatory horizontal nystagmus reactivities on the other hand.

Whereas the first two experiments lead to longitudinal superficial polarisation of the cortex, the latter two are depicting typical lateralisation on the polarisizing pattern.

Thus the differences from one temporal pool compared to the oposite are so obvious that they to be false analysed. Bertora a Bergmann (1987) have demonstrated by means of a method of corticaly evoked vestibular potentials of the rotatory chair that the main activity is to be found in the parieato - temporal cortex mainly in the range of the Theta band. These findings have also been proved in animal experiments of Hofferberth (1988).

Both of the authors however only applied small sections across the cortical surface due to the procedure of evoked potentials using only a pair of electrodes on each side of the skull.

Brain Electrical Activity Mapping enables to evaluate the cortical projection of sensory stimuli. According to our experiences this is a very promising method, which could in the near future bring many valuable informations about the pathologic conditions in otoneurology as well as in monitoring therapeutic al results.

REFERENCES:

Bergmannm J. M., Bertora, G .O.: Clinical Study of The cortical Electrical Activity During Supraliminal Vestibular Stimulations.
Acta AWHO, Vol. 6, 112 - 115, 1987.

Duffy, H. F.: Topographic Mapping of Brain Electrical Activity.
Butterworth, Boston, London, Durban, Singapure, Sydney, Toronto, Wellington, 1986.

Hofferberth, B., Zünkeler, T., Deitmer, M., Hirschberg, M.: Rotatory Evoked Potential in Normal and Labyrinthectomized Rabbits.
Adv.Oto - Rhino - Laryng., vol.41, pp.206 - 209 (Karger, Basel 1988).

Nieuwenhuys, R., Voogd, J., Huijzen, Ch. van .: The Human Central Nervous System,
Springer Verlag, Berlin, Heidelberg, New York, London, Paris, Tokio,
3rd Edition, 1988.

EXPERIENCES GATHERED SO FAR WITH THE INVESTIGATION OF THE DIRECTION CHANGING SOMATO-AUTOKINESIS

ERVÍN ČERNÝ
ENT Clinic, Prague /Czechoslovakia/

The term SOMATO-AUTOKINESIS /SAK/ describes the sensation of direction-alternating rotation of a subject's body, or direction-alternating deviations of the head and/or the trunk. This sensation may be accompanied by actual rotation or deviations. The ENT and psychological literature at our disposal offers no mention of this phenomenon.

To produce the SAK phenomenon the following conditions must be met: 1/ the elimination of somatosensoric cues, 2/ no mental activity, no reflections, no imaginations, 3/ concentration on the possible action of one's body in space /Fig. 1/.

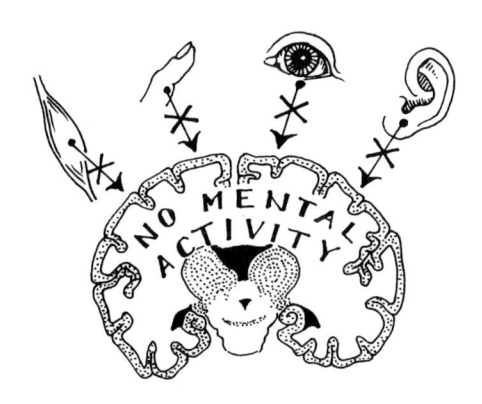

Fig. 1.

The experiment is carried out in a quiet room. The examined subject sits relaxed in a simple rotating chair, his eyes are closed and he reports his bodily feelings that arrive after a latency period of unspecified length. This may range from 30 seconds to 5 minutes or more. During SAK there are alternating sensations of rotation or deviation from one side to the other. These direction-alternating phases last from a few seconds to 2 minutes. In between the phases, there are intervals of several

seconds. The experiment lasts for 30 minutes. After the latency period, the examined subject may experience:
1/ either a direction alternating rotating sensation with or without rotating motion,
2/ or a direction alternating feeling of deviation of the head and/or trunk with or without deviating motion,
3/ more rarely, a soaring or sinking feeling,
4/ or alternation of rotating and deviating sensations.

To date we have examined 114 subjects /60 men, 54 women/ aged between 11 and 76. Most of them were between 18 and 25 years of age.

Of the total of 114 examined subjects, 83.4% experienced SAK. The SAK phenomenon was absent in 16.6% of subjects of whom 11.4% could not concentrate, 4.5% had a vestibular areflexia, and 0.7% suffered from multiple sclerosis.

In the position with outstretched arms there are 3 possibilities: a/ the subject deviates both his arms in the direction of SAK, b/ his arms move into the spread position, dropping and rising again, c/ the outstretched position remains unchanged.

In the Romberg position we observe alternating deviations forward-backward, to the opposite sides, less frequently also direction alternating rotation of the body around the surface of a cone whose apex is positioned between the soles of the subject's feet.

In walk, a deviation against the direction of SAK is observed /similarly as in the counter-rotating sensation following tests on a rotating chair/.

Side effects: some subjects report in SAK momentary sensations of loosing parts of their body, or of enlargement of the whole or parts of the body /bodily illusions/. In other cases they may have the impression of sitting much higher than they actually are, of being distant from the examiner, etc. /spatial illusions/.

We do not know the anatomical-physiological substance of the SAK phenomenon. We conclude that the elimination of a number of external and internal cues triggers off and brings to the surface of the brain certain sub-threshold sensoric activities which i.a. correspond with the function of the semicircular ducts and the utriculosacular system. Apart from subjective rotating and deviating sensations, these activities can produce, through cortico-reticulo-vestibulo-spinal projections, motoric effects in the groups of flexors - extensors or adductors - abductors. /Fig. 2/.

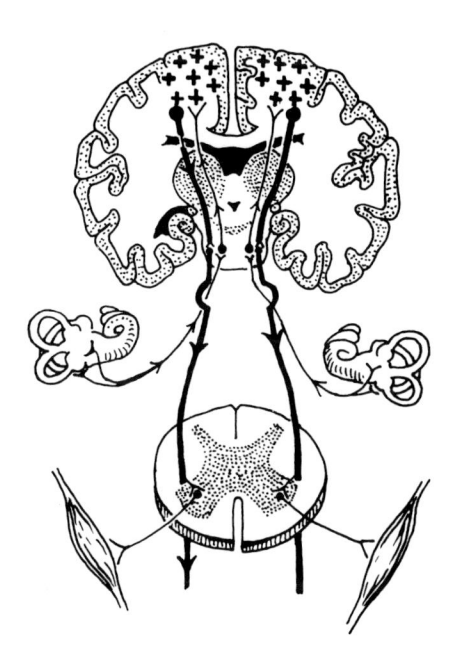

Fig. 2.
The alternating direction of these coordinated movements is probably controlled by centres in the substantia reticularis, similarly to what we expect to happen in the case of nystagmus alternans. Hopefully, further research will throw more light on this interesting problem.

REFERENCES

1. Černý E /1988/ Phenomenon of Spontaneous Postural Autokinesis in Alternate Direction. Čs Otolaryng 37:1-11

AUDITORY BLINK REFLEX IN CHILDREN WITH CEREBRAL PALSY

M. UZUNOVA, L. STAMATOVA
Research Institute of Pediatrics, Sofia, Bulgaria

INTRODUCTION

The contraction of orbicularis oculi muscle in response to different kinds of stimuli (visual, auditory, electrical and mechanical) forms the various typs of blink reflex. Electromyographical studies of the reflex is used in clinical practice to test the integrity of peripheral and central neural connections specifically related to the type of stimulation.

The most frequently used in neurophysiological studies is the electrically elicited blink reflex, but in small children the electrical stimulation may cause painful sensation, which limits its application. Auditory blink reflex has been demonstrated to be simple but sensetive method of indicating brainstem lesions (Tackmann et al., 1982) and has been proved to be useful for evaluation of brainstem function in perinatal neurological abnormalities (Yamada, 1984). Hemispheral lesions frequently cause changes in electrically elicited blink reflex closely resembling those observed in brainstem lesions (Kimura, 1974; Dehen et al., 1976; Dengler et al., 1982). It will be interesting to know auditory blink reflex changes in diffuse and bilateral hemispheric lesions in small children.

The purpose of this study was to describe changes in auditory blink reflex in infants and small children with cerebral palsy.

SUBJECTS AND METHODS

Ten children (6 boys and 4 girls) aged 3 months to 3 years, mean age one year and 4 months, were examined. All children were with quadiplegic form of cerebral palsy. Ten normal children matched for age and sex served as controls.

The blink reflex was evoked by auditory stimuli consisting of 1000 Hz tonr bursts with duration of 50 ms and an intensity 110 bB or less. The stimuli were delivered to both ears by means of earphones at random intervals, the least interval beeing 30 seconds. Electromyograms of the orbicularis oculi muscle were recorded by surface electrodes with small leading-off area. A ground electrode was located around the arm. Children lay supine with active electrode placed on the inferior eyelid and a reference electrode on the lateral surface ot the nose. The EMG signals were amplified, stored and after that read out and printed.

The latency of the reflex was defined as that of the first deflection of the EMG with an amplitude of 20mkV or more. The amplitude of the reflex response was its maximal peak-to-peak distance.

RESULTS

The mean latency of the blink reflex at 110 dB in normal children was 37,5 ms and varied between 28,3 and 43,0 ms. At this intensity the mean latency in children with cerebral palsy was 35,4 ms (range 27,0 - 46,4) and it did not differ significantly from the latency in normal children (p> 0,05).

The mean amplitude of the reflex responses at 110 dB in normal children was 168 mkV. At this intensity the mean amplitude of the responses in children with cerebral palsy was 320 mkV. A great variations in the amplitude was observed, which induced great standard deviations of the mean amplitude, but despite that in children with cerebral palsy the amplitude of the reflex response was significantly higher (p< 0,05) than in normal children. Reflex responses showed a decrease in latency and an increase in amplitude with an increase in stimulus intensity (Fig. 1).

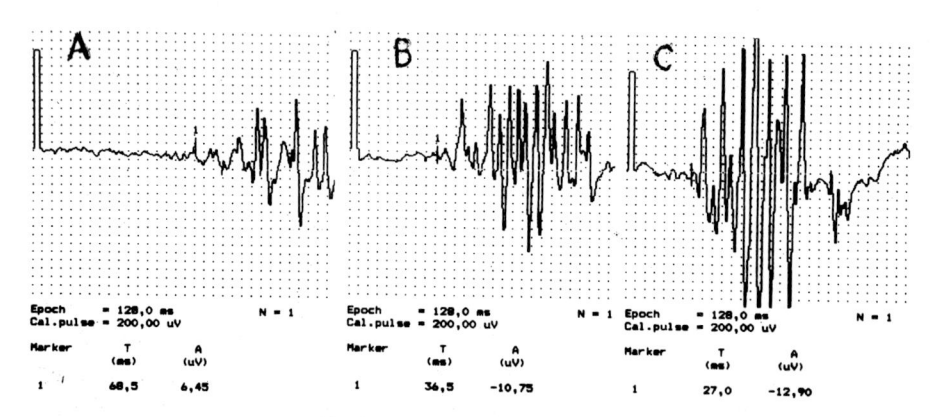

Fig. 1. The blink reflex responses decrease in latency and increase in amplitude with increse of stimulus intensity (from A to C). In A - latency is 68,5 ms; in B - 36,5 ms; in C - 27,0 ms

Even when stimulus intensity remained unchanged, the amplitude of the responses varied in wide range.The minimal response amplitude at maximal intensity in normal children was 77 μV and the maximal 420 μV. In the patient group the minimal amplitude was 175 V and the maximal - 643 μV.

The elicitability of the auditory blink reflex increased with increasing stimulus intensity. In all children with cerebral palsy an increased elicitability of the reflex was established compared with normal children. In 7 to 8 out of 10 consecutive maximal acoustic stimuli, applied in children with cerebral palsy, the blink reflex could be evoked, while in normal children only 3 to 4 stimuli out of 10 could be evoked, while in normal children only 3 to 4 stimuli out of 10 could elicit a reflex response.

An interesting finding was two components of the reflex response recorded in 3 children with cerebral palsy. Besides the response with the usual latency for auditory blink reflex, varying from 27 to 68 ms, there was an early one with latency 13 to 18 ms (Fig. 2). The form of this early response is biphasic or three-phasic and its amplitude varies between 25 and 430 μV.

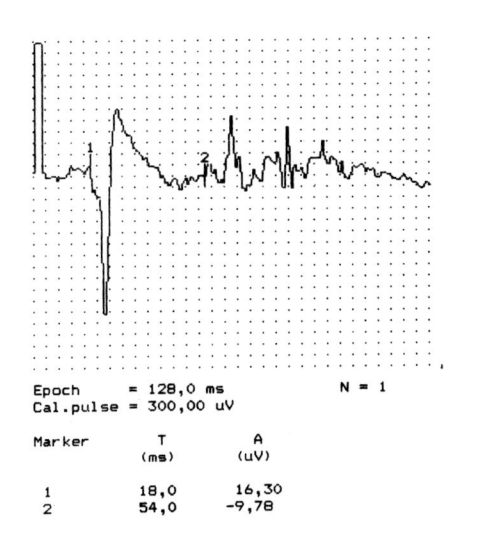

Fig. 2. Auditory blink reflex with two components - an early response with latency 18 ms, and late response with latency 54 ms.

DISCUSSION

The latencies determined in this study are similar to those reported by Yamada (1984) for auditory blink reflexes in newborn infants and adults.

The most prominent change found in children with cerebral palsy was the lack of habituation and an increased elicitability of the reflex. As the blink reflex elicited by acoustic stimulation is considered to be a consistent part of the startle reaction, the increased elicitability of the reflex in children with cerebral may be defined as an exaggerated startle reflex of startle disease (Suhren et al., 1966). The blink reflex arc for the acoustically evoked reflex is not exactly established but it is assumed that the reflex pathway is confined to the brain stem. The exaggerated blink reflex in cerebral palsy may be explained as an increased excitability of the neurones taking part in the reflex pathway, and especially that of nucleus reticularis pontis caudalis, as it is supposed to be a center of the audiogenic startle reflex (Leitner et al., 1980). In this respect our results corresponds to those reported by Shimamura (1973) for exaggerated startle reaction to click and electrical stimulation in children with cerebral palsy.

At present it is difficult to explain the origin of the early reflex response recorded in some of our patients. Such early response is typical for electrically and mechanically elicited blink reflexes and is conducted by oligosynaptic pontine pathway (Kimura, 1970). Further investigations will be necessary for clarifying their origin.

REFERENCES

1. Dehen H, Willer JC, Bathien N, Cambier J (1976) Electroenceph clin Neurophysiol 40:393-400
2. Dengler R, Kossev A, Gippner C, Struppler A (1982) Electroenceph clin Neurophysiol 53:513-524
3. Kimura J (1970) Arch Neurol (Chic) 22:156-161
4. Kimura J (1974) Neurol (Minneap) 24:168-174
5. Leitner DS, Powers AS, Hoffman HS (1980) Physiology and Behavior 25:291-297
6 Suhren O, Bruyn GW, Tuynman JA (1966) Journal Neurol Sci 3:577-605
7. Shimamura M (1973) In: Desmedt JE (ed) New Developments in Electromyography and Clinical Neurophysiology, Karger, Basel, vol. 3, pp 761-766
8 Tackmann W, Ettlin T (1982) Eur Neurol 21:264-269
9. Yamada A (1984) Brain & Development 1:45-53

HEAD SHAKING NYSTAGMUS AND RIGHT/LEFT VESTIBULAR ASYMMETRY

SACHIKO TAKAHASHI

from the Department of Otorhinolaryngology, Gunma University
3-39-15 Showamachi, 371 Maebashi, Gunma/Japan

SUMMARY

The relation between the three kinds of after nystagmus, namely postrotatory nystagmus (PRN), optokinetic afternystagmus (OKAN), and head shaking nystagmus(HSN) was investigated in 26 dizzy patients. The direction of HSN was in many cases consistent with the predominant direction of PRN or OKAN. The intensity of HSN showed positive correlation with the degree of directional preponderance in PRN but not in OKAN. Our data suggests that HSN is a simple but very sensitive test to detect the vestibular asymmetry.

INTRODUCTION

PRN, OKAN and HSN are known as after nystagmus in otoneurological field. They appear after the complete stop of the stimmulus as after discharge. Clinically it is very important that they reflect the vestibular asymmetry to some extent. According to our previous study HSN is directed to the intact side about 80 % of patients with unilateral vestibular lesion (1). It is also known in patients of unilateral vestibular hypofunction that PRN and OKAN are usually supressed toward the damaged side, while they are provoked almost normally toward the intact side (directional preponderance to the intact side). In this study we had compared the HSN, PRN and OKAN in dizzy patients to investigate the directional correlation of these nystagmus.

SUBJECTS AND METHOD

Subjects were 26 dizzy patients (17 to 75 y.o., 9 males). The patients of bilateral vestibular function loss were eliminated from the study. Eye movements were recorded by AC-electronystagmography (tc = 1.5 s) using silver-silver chloride electrodes. Vestibular tests were performed as follows. Except in OKAN the eye movements were recorded with closed eyes. 1) Spontaneous

a.

H S

b.

spont. nyst

left beating PRN
time constant

right beating PRN
time constant

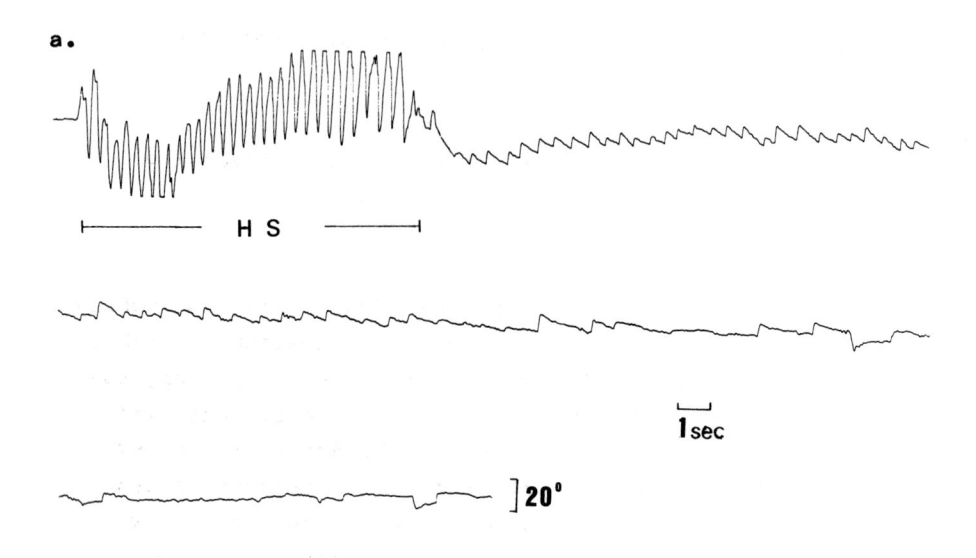

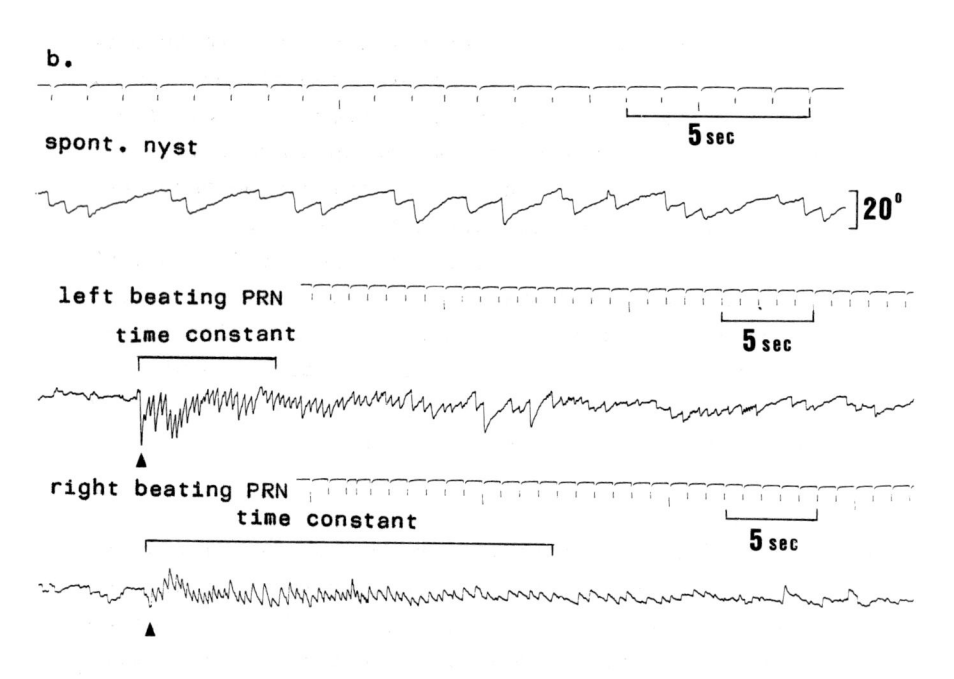

5 sec

5 sec

5 sec

1 sec

]20°

]20°

Fig. 1. YN 56 y.o. famale. HSN was elicited to right (a: temporal lead). Considering the influence of SPN to the left the PRN was clearly prolonged to the right (b: time constant of PRN was 7.5 sec to the left, 22 sec to the right).

nystagmus (SPN) was recorded with mental arithmetic for one minutes. 2) PRN was evoked by the sudden stop of chair after the constant-speed rotation of 90 deg/sec for one minute. 3) OKAN was evoked by sudden exstinguishing of the light when the accelarated rotation of full-field striped drum reached to 90 deg/sec. 4) HSN was evoked by shaking the head around the head axis with amplitude of 90 degrees 30 times in 15 sec. The directional preponderance was calculated using the duration in PRN and in OKAN (the subtraction of duration to the two directions was divided by their addition) as well as using maximal slow phase velocity in PRN. Slow phase velocity was not measured in OKAN, because the elicitation of nystagmus was irregular in some cases. To reduce the bias caused by SPN, the maximal slow phase velocity of HSN and PRN was linearly corrected by average slow phase velocity of SPN.

CASE REPORT

In a dizzy patient of uncertain origin (56 y. o. female) HSN was elicited to the right (Fig. 1-a). Bithermal caloric response was bilaterally symmetrical. Considering the SPN to the left, the time constant of PRN was clearly prolonged to the right with stronger intensity (Fig. 1-b). OKAN was also slightly prolonged to the right. This case was supposed to suffer from central imbalance and the HSN and PRN probably indicated the direction of effective velocity storage.

RESULTS

The Fig. 2 shows the relationship between the HSN, PRN and OKAN. In most of the cases the direction of HSN was identical with the predominant direction of PRN and OKAN. And the intensity of HSN, which is represented by maximal slow phase velocity, had positively correlated with the degree of directional preponderance in PRN (correlation coefficient: $r = 0.68$, calculated using duration as parameter, 0.46 using slow phase velocity). However, intensity of HSN and the degree of directional preponderance of OKAN did not show any significant correlation ($r = 0.30$).

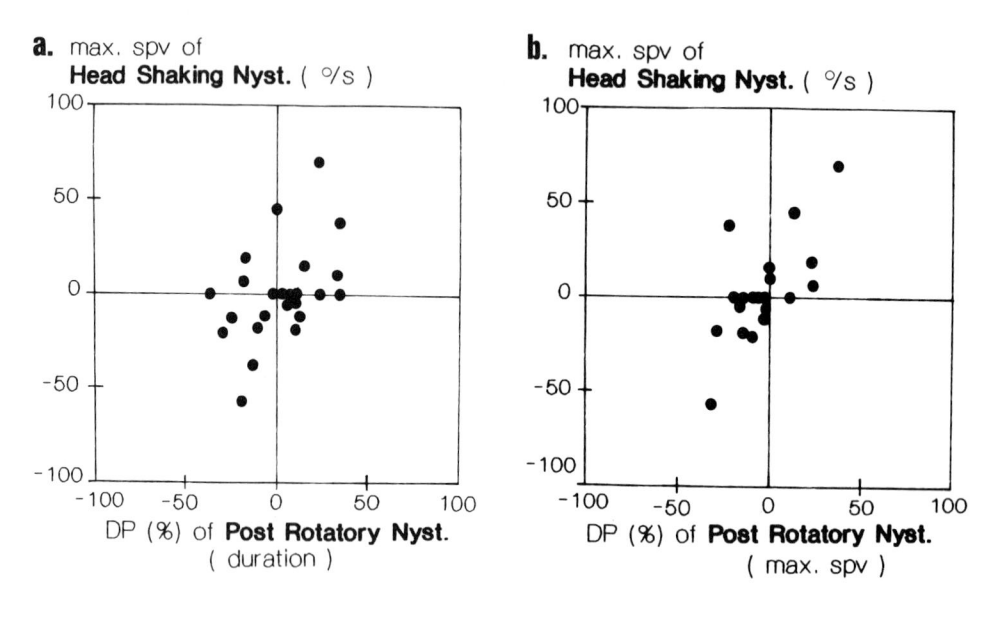

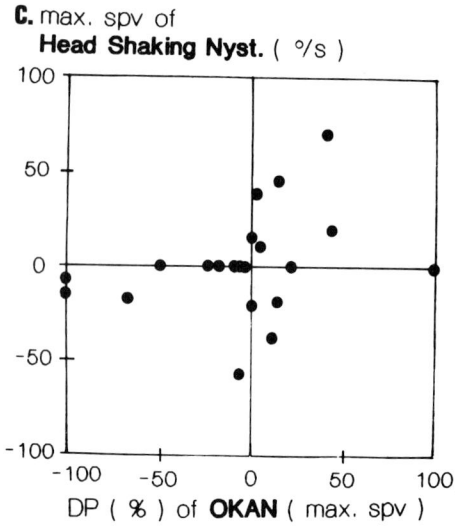

Fig. 2. Correlation between maximal slow phase velocity of HSN and directional preponderance of a; PRN (parameter; duration), b: PRN (parameter; maximal slow phase velocity) and c: OKAN. The right beating nystagmus and preponderance to the right are adjusted to be positive. A relative good correlation was observed in a and b (r = 0.68 and 0.46 respectively). Correlation was not significant in c (r = 0.30).

DISCUSSION

The positive correlation between HSN and PRN depends probably on the similarity of the generation mechanism.

The origin of HSN can be explained as follows. If the head is rapidly rotated to the right, the endolymphatic flow is directed ampullopetal in right lateral semicircular canal, which works as excitation, while ampullofugal flow of the opposite side works as inhibition. Ewald's second law states that the hight velocity vestibular excitatory inputs are more effective then inhibitory inputs, because the spontaneous vestibular firing rate of ca. 90 spikes/sec can be increased to as high as ca. 400 sec but only be decreased to zero. If the head is shaken rapidly to and fro in the patient with only one labyrinth, only the excitatory input from the remaining labyrinth is accumulated in the central vestibular system, which leads to the HSN beating toward the intact side.

The origin of PRN can be explained similarly. After the sudden stop of the chair from the rotation to the left, the cupula of the right lateral canal deviates ampullopetal and that of the left lateral canal, ampullofugal. Because ampulloperal flow is more effective in high velocity stimuli (Ewald's second law) the PRN is evoked to the right. In patients of unilateral labyrinthine lesion the PRN to the damaged side is strongly supressed because of the lack of the response from the damaged labyrinth. It leads to the directional preponderance of PRN to the intact side.

The unilateral labyrinthine hypofunction alone is not enough to explain the origin of HSN and PRN, since the time constant of these nystagmus last in many cases much longer than the cupula time constant, which is presumed to be about 6 seconds.

Another possible cause of HSN and directional preponderance of PRN is the asymmetric working velocity storage mechanism. The velocity storage mechanism perseverates the vestibular or ocular input and works to prolong the vestibular time constant. If the caloric response is bilaterally symmetrical and HSN and directional preponderance of PRN is provoked to one direction, they are considered to reflect the effective direction of velocity storage like in the patient in Fig. 1.

Between the HSN and OKAN the qualitative relation was only scarcely observed. Two reasons are thinkable. Firstly, since OKAN is evoked by pure optic stimulus, probably labyrinthine damage plays less important role to produce OKAN compared to HSN or PRN. Secondly, OKAN is, as widely recognized, very sensitive response. It is easily supressed by fatigue, sleepiness and tension of the subjects, which makes the quantitative analysis of OKAN very difficult. However in our population, if HSN was evoked, its direction was always consistent with the prolonged direction of OKAN. From this standpoint of view, OKAN and HSN reflect the same vestibular imbalance.

Caloric test is highly significant to determine the unilateral vestibular hypofunction. We have once compared HSN and caloric test results in 36 patients of unilateral labyrinthine lesion. In 30 cases (83 %) HSN beat toward the side of better caloric excitability. And the direction and intencity of HSN showed good correlation with the degree of canal paresis calculated with Jongkees formula ($r = 0.63$) (2).

PRACTICAL COMMENT ON HSN

Vertigo is generally based upon the vestibular asymmetry. The vestibular asymmetry is causes not only by unilateral labyrinthine lesions but also by central imbalance such as asymmetrical velocity storage mechanism. Head shaking test is sensitive in detecting vestibular asymmetry, but not specific in distinguishing peripheral hypofunction from central imbalance. The further caloric and rotatory tests are necessary to clarify the vestibular condition of patients.

REFERENCES
1. Takahashi, S. and Kamei, T.: The clinical significance of head shaking nystagmus; Vertigo, Nausea, Tinnitus and Hearing Loss in Cardiovascular Diseases. Elsevier Science Publishers B.V. 1986, p. 285-290.
2. Takahashi, S., Fetter, M., Koenig, E. and Dichgans, J.: The clinical significance of head shaking nystagmus is the dizzy patient. Acta Otolaryngol. (Stockh) 1990; 109:8-14

OCULOMOTOR STIMULATIONS IN A PATIENT WITH AN OCULAR EPILEPTIC EQUIVALENT.

VICTOR GABERSEK

ENT department, Pr. B. Frachet, Avicenne Hospital, 125, rue de Stalingrad, 93000 BOBIGNY, France.

Since Fere (1890) many authors have looked for links between epilepsy and vestibular disturbances and vestibular influence on the activation of epileptic crises, before the EEG era and since, using EEG procedure to find cortical representation of vestibular function. It was shown that focal epilepsy may induce oculomotor crises, that epileptic nystagmus refers to an oculomotor seizure manifestation and that an epileptic nystagmoid equivalent is associated with oscillopsy, visual hallucinations and vertigo. Other clinical investigations of eye movements associated with epileptic reflex discharges revealed particular eye deviation and behaviour in reading, in flash-induced nystagmus, intermitent photic stimulation, light touch, musicogenic epilepsy caused only by a discrete frequency band of church bells, blinking etc. Recently nystagmus retractorius has been associated with epileptiform activity. However the iconography in all these publications concerns mainly clinical and EEG observations with very few electronystagmographic (ENG) tracings.

We would like to introduce ENG potentiometric recordings in a 65 year old alert man presenting, since two years ago, ocular nystagmic crises every 15 minutes. The EEG in awake or sleeping state are normal. The MRI (Magnetic Resonance Imaging) shows patches in right cerebelar pedunculum and around both lateral ventriculi at the upper tentorial level. During crises the patient does not lose consciousness; he has visual, auditory and sensory motor troubles; he can move on flat ground but he can not find his way alone. Illuminated streets, a sunray through the shutters or through the forest lead to more frequent crises.

Concerning ENG tracings we can observe 3 types of nystagmus : A "basic" left-up nystagmus (outside of crises) which can be interrupted either by a right-up horizontal-rotatory nystagmus during calibration of 10° eye movements in all directions (Horizontal, vertical and oblique voluntary eye movements) (Fig 1), or by extreme excentric voluntary eye movements (Fig 2) and during optokinetic testing (Fig 3) or by a right-down oblique nystagmus during vestibular tests. Caloric test in left ear with cold water (Fig 4); Pendular moving tests (Figs 5 and 6). A crisis lasts about 20sec but the beginning of two crises can follow one after another at intervals of 5 and 15 seconds, extending duration wich however does not exceed 1 minute. Generally each crisis begins with right eye. The diagnosis was sclerosis multiplex and corticoid therapy made no improvement. Meprobamate was prescribed and a follow-up study will be made after one year.

64

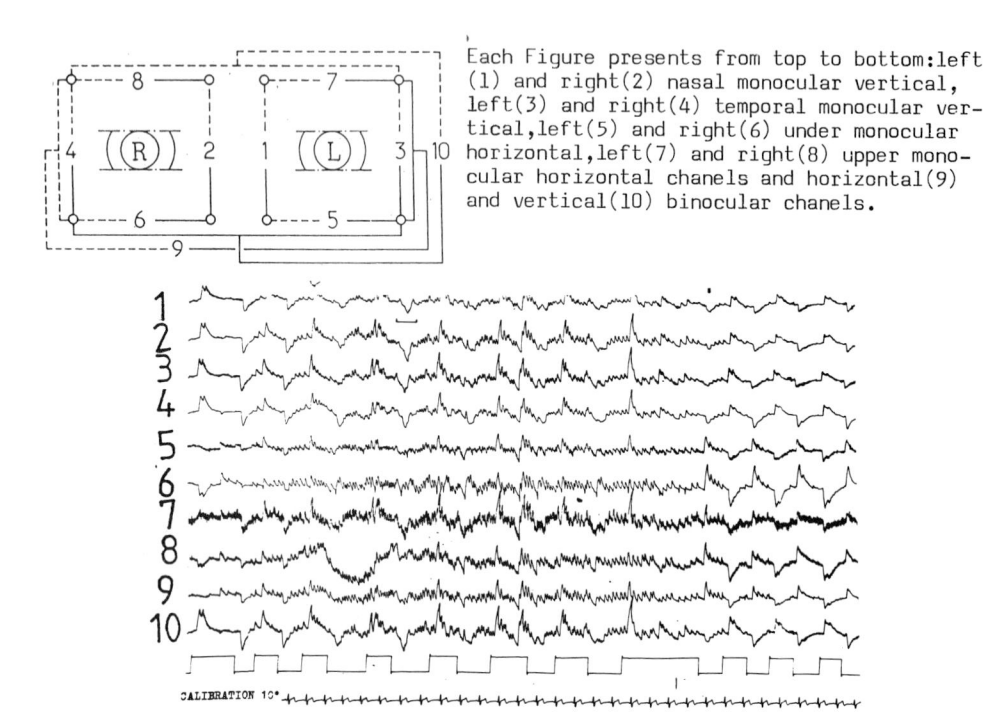

Each Figure presents from top to bottom:left (1) and right(2) nasal monocular vertical, left(3) and right(4) temporal monocular vertical, left(5) and right(6) under monocular horizontal, left(7) and right(8) upper monocular horizontal chanels and horizontal(9) and vertical(10) binocular chanels.

Fig 1: An Ocular Epileptic Equivalent Crisis (OEEC) of 20 sec appering by first right-up voluntary eye movement, introduces a right-up horizontal rotatory nystagmus with a hight frequency, which is superimposed on the calibration eye movements After 10 sec a skipping of calibration is shown. The voluntary eye movements reappear at the end of crisis. Cardiac rhythm is not perturbed.

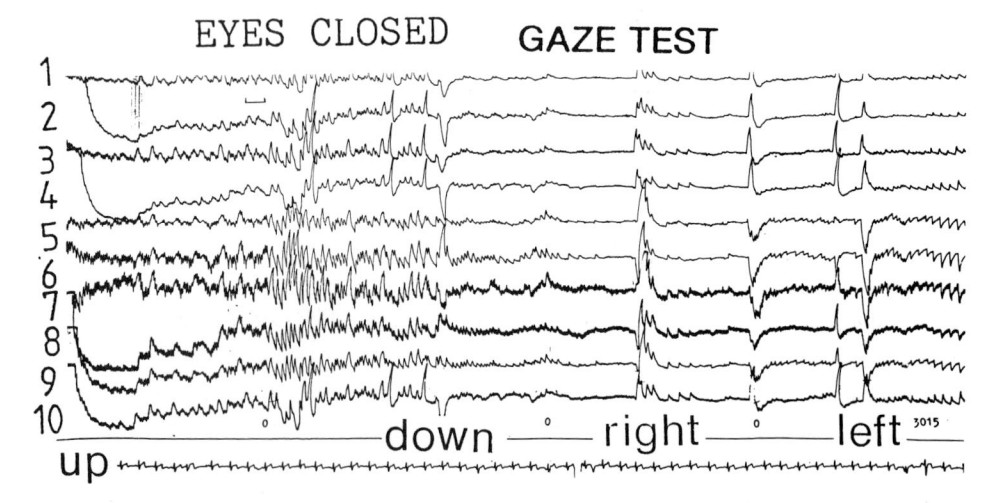

Fig 2: An OEEC of 20 sec appears after the upwards voluntary eye movement. The right-up horizontal rotatory nystagmus does not interrupted the test. After the crisis the "basic" left-up spontan nystagmus reappears. No modification on the cardiac rhythm.

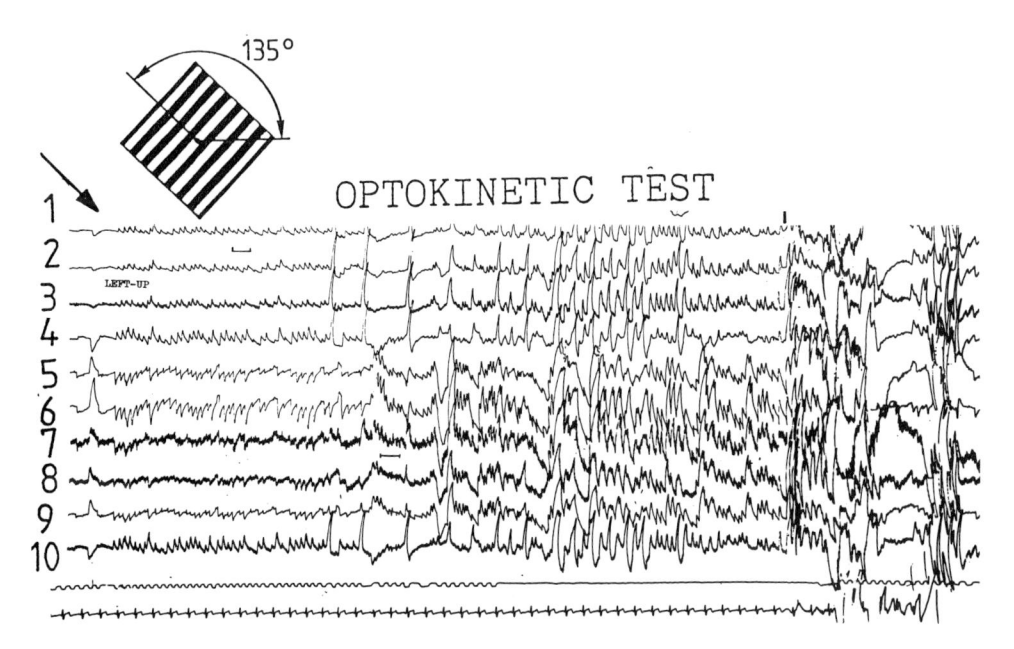

Fig 3: Left-up optokinetic response. OEEC of 30 sec with double sensory motor troubles. The right-upward horizontal rotatory nystagmus interruptes the left-up optokinetic response. We interrupt stimulation. Sensory motor trouble appears at the end of crisis. Then we put stimulation again and a new sensory motor trouble appears.

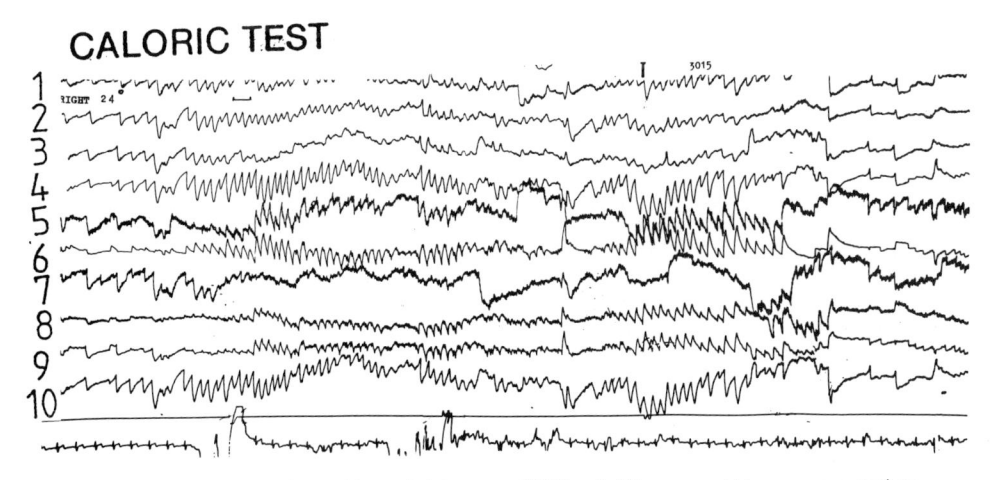

Fig 4: Caloric test 24° on the right ear, OEEC of 30 sec with sensory motor trouble. The left-downward caloric nystagmus is interrupted by a right-down obli que nystagmus(the trace 7 is isoelectric). The crisis begin on the right eye. Af ter the crisis the "basic" left-up spontan nystagmus appears. The cardiac rhy- thm is perturbed.

PENDULAR MOVING TEST

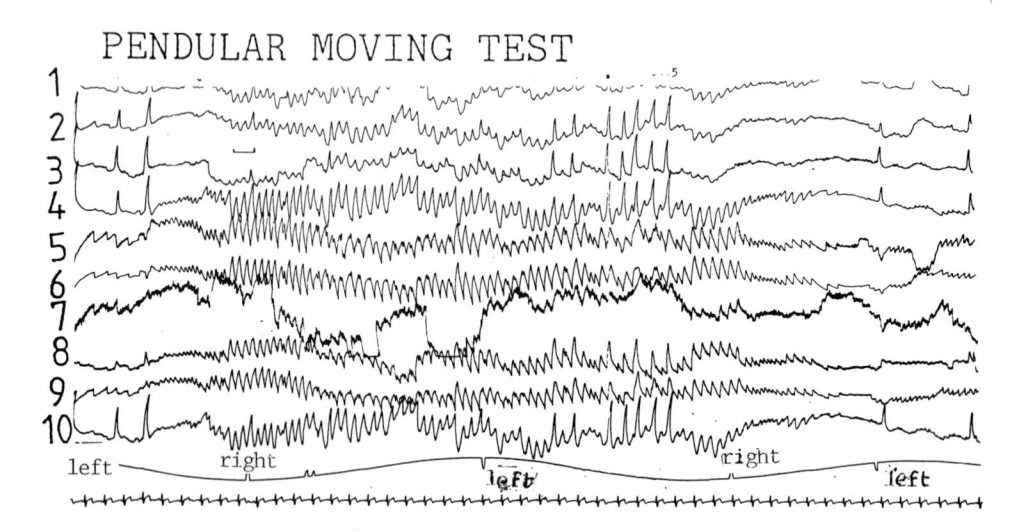

Fig 5: Pendular moving test. By rotatory movement to the left, the left vestibular nystagmus is replaced by a right-down oblique nystagmus (the trace 7 is isoelectric) with auditory and visual troubles. The duration of the OEEC is 30 sec.

PENDULAR MOVING TEST

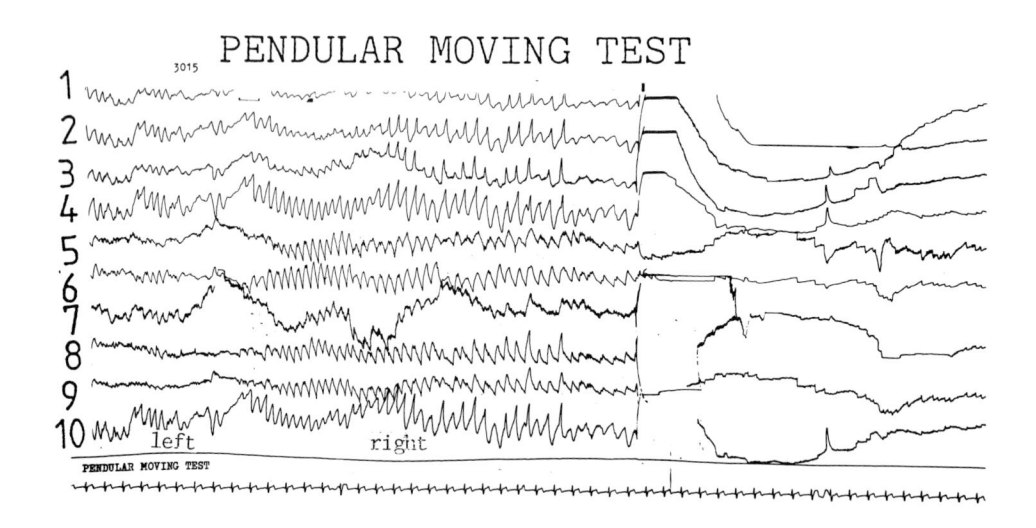

Fig 6: Pendular moving test at the end of the same response as in Fig 5. The OEEC of 20 sec appears and finishes with a sensory motor short head movement. After them the "basic" left-up spontan nystagmus reappears.

VERGENCE NYSTAGMUS PHYSIOPATHOLOGICAL CONSIDERATIONS ABOUT FIVE CASES

CAPUTO D*., CESARANI A°., ALPINI D., MINI M*

Institute Don C.Gnocchi Milan
Institute of Audiology University of Milan
ENG Laboratory Busto Arsizio Hospital

INTRODUCTION

Convergent or divergent nystagmus (ny) are unusual observations in neurotological practice but they are specifc signes of pretectal involvement. The aim of this paper is to report 4 cases with a convergent ny and a case with a divergent ny.

CASE HISTORIES

CASE 1 S.Maura, female, 46 yy. In 1970 left optic papillitis; in 1978 lower paresthesias; in 1984 left D5-D6 pain and hipoasesthesia; in 1984 dizziness.

Neurological conclusions: McAlpine probable Multiple Sclerosis or Poser laboratory supported defined MS.

Electronystagmographic findings: caloric ny was conjugated with hypereflexia and dysrithmias.

Optokinetic ny was low gained, conjugated, dysrithmic and hyposyncronous.

After horizonyal optokineteic stimulation convergent ny was recorded.

Ny was disconjugated with a prevalence of left eye movements.

Ny lasted 40" and it was present at the end of every OK stimulation.

CASE 2

R.Maria Paola, female 34 yy; in 1976 upper limbs paraesthesias; in 1977 transiet diplopia; in 1978 right optic neuritis; form 1979 slowly progressive gait impairment convergence was absent.

Neurological conclusions: defined Multiple Sclerosis.

ENG findings : bilateral disconjugated gaze nystagmus; disconjugated dysrithmic caloric ny with a second phase.

Convergence ny appeared either after OK stimulation or during caloric second phase.

In booth conditions it was more rithmic and regular in left eye.

CASE 3

A.Ferdinando, male 44 yy; in 1972 right optic neuritis; in 1975 left optic neuritis; in 1980 persistent oscillopsia and lateral gaze diplopia; from 1980 gait impairment and urologic disorders.

Neurological conclusions: defined Multiple Sclerosis.

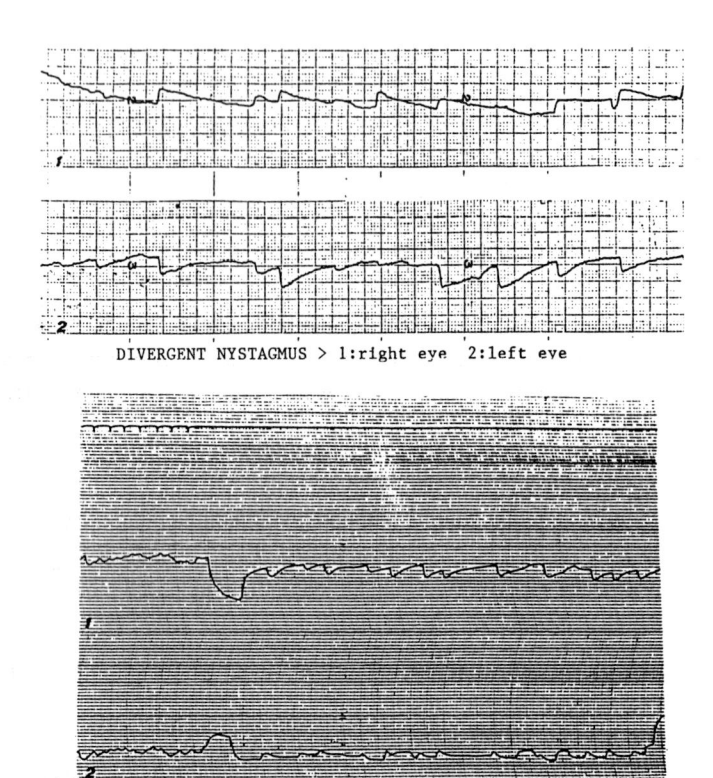

DIVERGENT NYSTAGMUS > 1:right eye 2:left eye

CONVERGENT OPTOKINETIC AFTERNYSTAGMUS (OKAN)

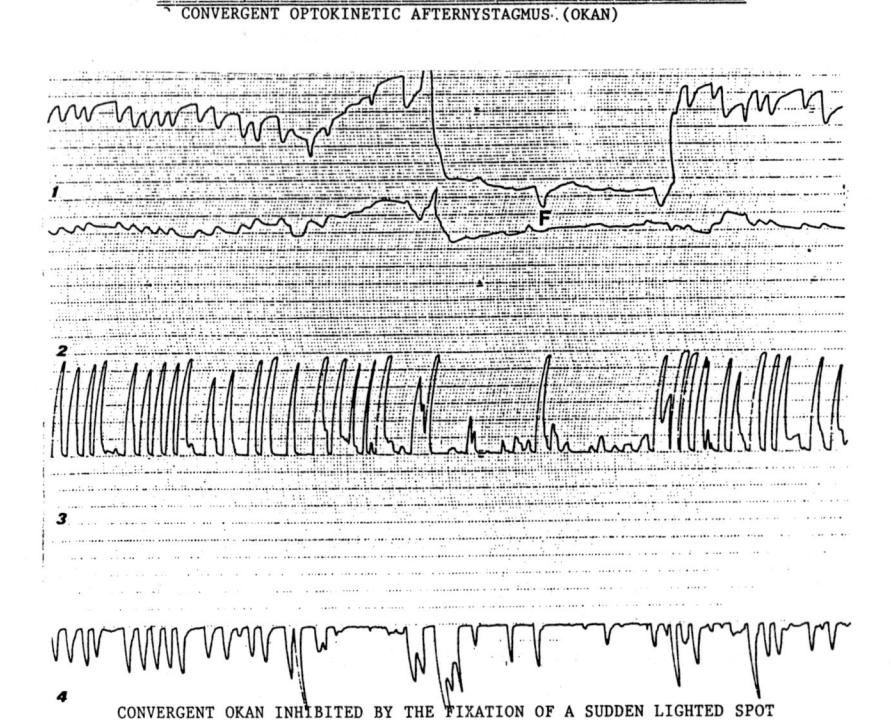

CONVERGENT OKAN INHIBITED BY THE FIXATION OF A SUDDEN LIGHTED SPOT

ENG findings: bilateral disconjugated gaze ny, hiperreflexic, disconjgated dystrithmic caloric ny; convergent OK after ny (OKAN), prevalent in right eye, easily inhibited by fixation of a light spot.

CASE 4

Z.Giovanni, male, 52 yy. from 1968 slowly progressive paraparesis; from 1980 urological disorders; in 1985 right lateral diplopia for a week cnvergence was absent.

ENG findings: spontaneous ny was absent; OKN was conjungated while groups of 10-15 convergence ny beats appeared during vertical stimulation either upward or downward.

At the end of OK stimulation convergence ny lasted 10.

In every case no retractorious ny was observed.

CASE 5

A.Giuseppe, male, 32 yy; In 1985 right optic neuritis; in 1986 ataxia and dysartria; 1987 gait disorders; in 1988 lateral gaze diplopia.

Neurological conclusions: defined Multiple Sclerosis.

ENG findings: spontaneous horizontal bialteral gaze disconjugated ny; during recording in the dark groups of divergent beats were observed, in frontal gaze.

PHISIOPATHOLOGICAL CONSIDERATIONS

Vergence eye movements are slow, taking as long asa second for completation.

The reaction time for fusional vergence mevements is about 160 msec and for accomodation vergence movements about 200msec.

Vergence movements carry the eyes in opposite directions to enable binocular fixation of a single object.

Some analysis suggest that the fusional vergence sub-system is under a continuos from of control as in the pursuit system.

Convergence ny usually correlated to restractorious ny and they are considered signes of pretectal involvement.

First description was at the turn of the century. In the following decades many examples were described although it is sufficientely rare for pubblications.

The convergence ny is not usually spontaneous but it is induced by manoeuvres such as attempted convergence, upward gaze or attempted production of vertical OKN. In man it is usually observed in pt with tumours of the pineal gland and colliculi. It has been described also in vascular disease including arterio-venos malformation.

It has been also in documented in encephalitis and in Multiple Sclerosis even it is not an usual finding.

In the physiopathological plane eye movement recordings and ENG studies have shown that the convergent movements are not normal vergence movements.

Infact in many pt. responses to conventional vergence stimuli are impaired or absent. From EMG data it had been concluded that the ocular movements of convergence ny result from synchronous innervation of opponenent pair of rectus muscles. The well know Ochs paper (1979) showed that the opposed adductions have velocities of glissades. Ochs proposed that opposed adductions saccades arise out of the dynamic overshoot mechanism divergence ny is extremely rare and occur in pt. with hindbrain lesions often with downward anomalies. It has been observed in a pt. witha tumor of cerebellar vermis(Cogan 1959) in a pt. with silvian cysticercosis, in some pt. with MS.

In the physiopathological plane the same pathways of convergence ny are involved, but the cases reported in literature are very few and there is no systematical studies this kind of ny.

Regarding the cases reported in this paper is interesting to releave that in all cases convergence ny was recorded as an optokinetic after ny and in one case a caloric second phase.

It may be hipotized an involvement of vestibular nuclei and/or projections in the generation of these convergence (and divergent) ny.

Unfortunely all the pt. were affected with a disseminated MS and precise correlations between site of lesion and ny are not possible.

REFERENCE

1. Cogan D.G.Convergence Nystagmus Arch. Ophtal. 62 (2) 161-165, 1959
2. Dufour A., Brusa M;, Formenti A.: il Nigstagmo divergente Considerazioni e studio ENG del caso osservato. Ann. Laring. Otol. Rinol. Faringol. 76 (4) 411-419, 1978.
3. Furtado D./ Nystagmus disjonctif convergent Rev. Neurol. 94, 335-350, 1956
4. Ochs A.L., Stark L., HoytW.F., D'Amico D.: Opposed adducting saccades in convergence-retraction Nystagmus. Brain 107, 497-508, 1979.
5. Reineck R.D., Vergence Disorders. In Lennerstrand G., Zee D.S., Keller E.L. (eds) Functional basis of ocularmotor disorders, p. 101-108, Pergamon Press Oxford, 1982.
6. Schor C.M., Vergence eye movements: basic aspects. In Lennerstrand-Zeekeller op. cit. p. 83-92
7. Smith J.L., Zieper I., Gay A.J., Cogan D.G. Nystagmus retractorius. Arch. Ophtal. 62, 864-867, 1959.

A NEW CONCEPT OF MENIERE'S SYNDROME

DR. L.H. HIRANANDANI
Madam Cama Road, Bombay-400 039.

Meniere's Syndrome is accepted classically as a result of hydrops of the membranous labyrinth. It is characterized by symptoms of giddiness, tinnitus and deafness. Audiological investigations reveal perceptive hearing loss and positive recruitment phenomenon. Vestibular function tests show hyper-response in the acute stage. The response diminishes in the quiescent phase of the disease.

Various aspects of this syndrome have been discussed by several clinicians and research workers since it was first described by Prosper Meniere in 1861. The description of his symptomatology has been accepted, but adequate evidence is not available to suggest the real aetiological factor or the immediate and late pathological changes occuring in the labyrinth. This is because it is not a fatal disease. Most of the data is the result of clinical experience and investigations.

From my experience of 50 years in the field of Ear, Nose, Throat, I have come across many cases of meniere's and I have come to certain conclusions :

(1) Hydrops is not the only aetiological factor. Even that has not been proved. But there are definitely other causes. These are : (a) Vascular pathology, (b) Allergy, (c) Hormone disturbances similar to what occures in migraine, (d) Syphilis - is not so common now, and (e) Viral neuronitis or labyrinthitis.

Why actually hydrops suddenly occurs - no one knows. Allergy has been considered as the factor. In my experience I have only come across one strong supporting evidence. The patient had severe urticaria and that was followed by Meniere's Symptoms. The patient immediately responded to corteco-steroid therapy. In other cases of hydrops, where I have prescribed the drug, all cases have not responded to the treatment. I, therefore, conclude that allergy is not the only cause of hydrops.

I came to the conclusion of vascular pathology 35 years ago and I like to mention here my conclusions. The internal auditory artery is the end-artery and there is no other anastomotic vessel. The blood supply of the labyrinth can be compared to blood supply of the myocardium and brain. We are aware of pathological changes which can affect the heart and brain. Due to high blood pressure, high cholesterol and diabetes, there can be spasm of the coronary artery resulting in anginal pains. There can be thrombosis of the artery producing infarct. If these changes can occur in the coronary vessels, similar changes can also occur in the internal auditory artery and/or its branches.

In 1968 - Dr. Axelsson, a physiologist from Sweden described the blood supply of labyrinth and on the basis of his description, I could support my findings. If due to the factors mentioned in case of coronary are present, auditory artery can go into spasm which produces reversible symptoms. But if thrombosis occurs, there can be permanent damage of the labyrinth. The artery divides into cochleo-vestibular and vestibular branches. The cochleo-vestibular branch divides and supplies cochlea and vestibule. So the main artery may not be affected, but any of its branches may be involved resulting in only cochlear or only vestibular Meniere's. Every clinician is aware that we can get such cases and that is why I call them cochleo-vestibular Meniere's, cochlea Meniere's and Vestibular Meniere's.

The hydrops can also involve the whole canal or only the cochlea. Hydrops cannot involve only the vestibule because the fluid is produced in the cochlea. All this can be explained on hydro-dynamics of the labyranthine fluid.

I had one case only which suggests that migrainous pathology is one of the causes of Meniere's. A patient used to suffer from migrainous headaches for years and always used to have aura of the impending attack. But last time instead of getting the headache, he developed Meniere's.

There was one case which I clinically diagnosed as haemorrhage in the labyrinth. Patient developed malaria and was administered quinine. He developed haemoglobinuria followed by vestibular symptoms. Within next three months he developed dead vestibules which did not respond even to ice-cold water. It is 40 years and he still has to walk with a stick, because his both canals have been destroyed.

I have come across several cases of syphilis, which produce total destruction of the cochlear part of the labyrinth resulting in total deafness. Viral disease similar to Bello Palsy has also been the factor.

All the investigations though have enlightened us but we can never come to the conclusion whether the lesion is retro-cochlear or cochlear. Even C.T. Scan cannot conclusively prove the pathology, but M.R.I. has helped tremendously to know whether the lesion is retro-cochlear. There is one symptom and I call it clinical recruitment. If that symptom is present, we can definitely say that it is a cochlear lesion. If a patient says that a loud sound upsets him, then SISI test will prove it and we can practically 100 per cent say that the lesion is cochlear.

When patients ask me about the prognosis, I always say G.O.K.(God Only Knows). Because I reiterate that we really do not know what pathological changes are actually taking place during the attack. May be very soon P.E.T. (Positron Emission Tomography) will demonstrate the real pathology.

Because we do not know the actual cause, various treatments have been like hitting in the dark. Leave aside the retro-cochlear lesion-tumour, but for cochlear pathology, treatment has been anti-vertigenous drugs and vasodilators. Though vasodilators will be beneficial in cases of vasular pathology but when hydrops is the cause which is the result of vasodilation of stria-vascularis, the vasodilator drugs can only worsen the symptoms.

We have as yet no appropriate drug for migraine. Sudden serotonin (Autacoid-Local Hormone) deficiency is the cause so far known but administration of Serotonin in cases of migraine has neither proved beneficial nor without risk. My treatment for cochlear lesion has been as follows :

1) Anti-vertiginous drugs.

2) Vasodilators and CO_2 inhalations only in cases of vascular pathology. In addition, the preventive measures as we adopt in cases of coronary disease like control of blood pressure, reduction of cholesterol and control of diabetes. In cases of persisting uncontrollable symptoms and if the hearing loss in one ear is more than 70 per cent, I do labyrinthectomy. If the hearing is good, then I do duct decompression and later vestibular neurectomy. CO_2 is the known physiological vasodilator for vessels of brain. It is used as carbogen (95 per cent Oxygen and 5 per cent CO_2).

In cases of cervical spondylosis, I believe neck traction to provide mobility to cervical vertebrae is not the answer. Instead the aim should be to strengthen the muscles attached to cervical vertebrae. This is achieved by asking the patient to make all possible neck movements against resistance. The therapy has been beneficial in my cases.

INFLUENCE OF ASYMMETRIC PERIPHERAL VESTIBULAR ACTIVITY ON OPTOKINETIC AFTER-NYSTAGMUS IN MAN

KRISTER BRANTBERG and MÅNS MAGNUSSON
Department of Otorhinolaryngology, University Hospital of Lund, Lund, Sweden.

INTRODUCTION

Optokinetic nystagmus (OKN) is generated by the retinal slip of the image. In man, OKN is evoked by two mechanisms: the cortically mediated (or fast) mechanism, which is probably identical to the pursuit-system (1), and the subcortical (or slow) mechanism (2). The subcortical component of OKN is reflected in the optokinetic after-nystagmus (OKAN).

The initial slow phase eye velocity of OKAN has been demonstrated to be closely related to the gain in the vestibulo-ocular reflex (VOR) (3,4). The VOR gain (i.e. eye velocity / head velocity) are dependent on the functional status of the vestibular endorgans and nerves. Consequently one would expect changes of activity in the peripheral vestibular apparatus also to cause changes in OKAN, hence, asymmetric vestibular function can be suspected to cause asymmetries in OKAN.

Galvanic stimulation of the vestibular nerves induce an asymmetric vestibular input and may cause nystagmus. However, if the stimulus is low enough, there is no nystagmus or sensation of vestibular stimulation.

In the present study horizontal OKAN was evaluated with and without galvanically induced changes in peripheral vestibular activity. The aim was to ascertain whether minute changes in peripheral vestibular activity, which do not produce spontaneous nystagmus, cause asymmetries in the initial velocity of OKAN.

SUBJECTS

The study comprised twenty naive subjects (14 males, 6 females, mean age 34.5 years, range 25-45). None of the subjects had any history of cochlear, vestibular or central nervous disorders. Alcoholic beverages and drugs of any kind were not allowed for 24 h before the test.

METHODS

Horizontal optokinetic stimulation was given by whole-field optokinetic drum (90 deg/s for 60s). The subjects was instructed to stare at the moving stripes. Eye movements were recorded by a DC electro-oculografic technique and transcribed simultaneously by an ink-jet recorder (Mingograph 81, Siemens-Elema, Stockholm). The recording was ended 60 seconds after termination of the optokinetic stimulation by turning off the light.

A bi-polar, bi-aural galvanic stimulation of low amperage (1mA) to the vestibular nerves was administered by 3.5 x 4.5 cm large carbon-rubber electrodes (CEFAR AB, Lund, Sweden) placed on the mastoids. The cathode was in all subjects placed behind the right ear and the anode behind the left, thus generating increased activity in the right vestibular nerve compared to the left(5). Continuous galvanic stimulation was given during the optokinetic stimulation as well as during the recording of OKAN.

Initial velocity of OKAN was evaluated as the slow phase eye velocity two seconds after the end of the optokinetic stimulus. Asymmetry was calculated as the directional preponderance (DP) for OKAN generated by drum-rotation towards left ($OKAN_L$) and right ($OKAN_R$). DP = ($OKAN_L$ - $OKAN_R$) / ($OKAN_L$ + $OKAN_R$).

Student's t-test for paired data was used to evaluate the differences in DP for right-beating OKAN with and without galvanically induced increased activity in the vestibular nerve.

A difference of $p<0.05$ was considered significant.

RESULTS

At galvanic stimulation alone, no continuous feeling of vertigo or rotation was reported, and no galvanically induced nystagmus was recorded in darkness.

At optokinetic stimulation alone the mean initial velocity of OKAN in response to drumrotation towards left was 8.1 deg/s, SD 7.2 and in response to drumrotation towards right 7.6 deg/s, SD 6.2 (Fig. 1). The mean DP for right-beating OKAN within the individual subject was was -0.03, SD 0.40.

At simultaneous galvanic and optokinetic stimulation the response to drum rotation towards left and right was 9.3 deg/s, SD 7.2 and 6.0 deg/s, SD 5.1 respectively (Fig. 1). The mean DP was 0.25, SD 0.41. Thus, there was a significant increase in DP for right-beating OKAN at galvanic stimulation, that is, a stronger response after OKN with the fast phase beating towards the cathode, compared with optokinetic stimulation alone ($p<0.05$).

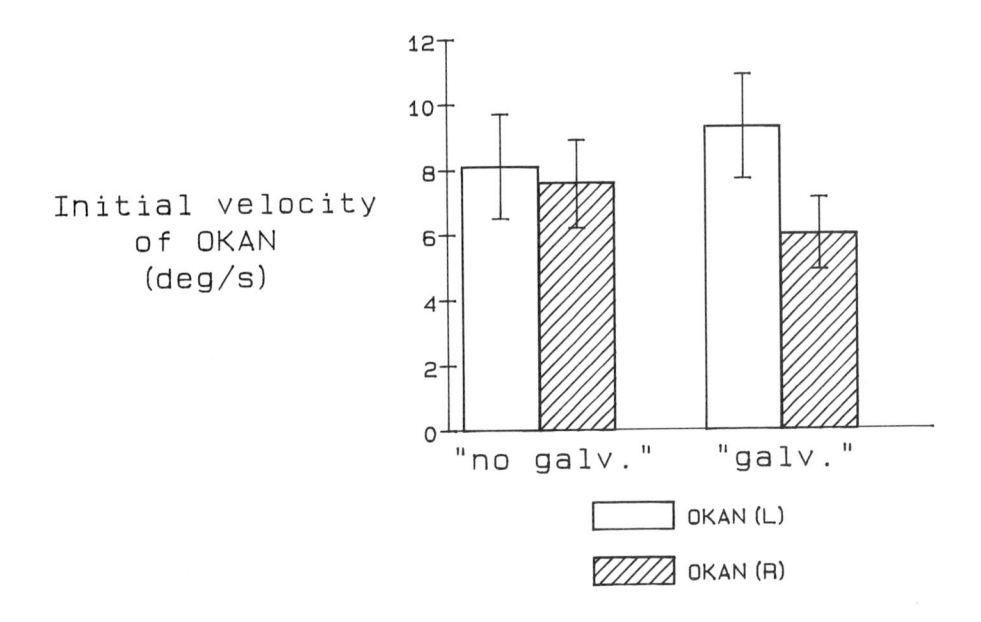

Fig. 1. Asymmetric OKAN at galvanic stimulation ("galv.) compared to optokinetic stimulation alone ("no galv."). Means and SEM for initial slow phase eye velocity of OKAN following drum rotation towards left (OKAN(L)) and right (OKAN(R)) are given.

DISCUSSION

In the present study it was found that galvanically induced activity changes in the peripheral vestibular apparatus, which did not cause spontaneous nystagmus in darkness, caused changes in initial slow phase velocity of OKAN.

At galvanically induced increased activity in the right vestibular nerve there was a significant increase in directional preponderance for right-beating OKAN, compared to optokinetic stimulation alone. These findings are commmensurate with the demonstrated close relation between the VOR gain and the initial slow phase velocity of OKAN, and suggests that the tonic vestibular input is not only important for the function of the vestibular system, but also for the optokinetic system.

When investigating a vestibular side difference we still relay on the caloric test. However, the magnitude of the caloric response may only loosely be related to peripheral lesion severity, because caloric irrigation tests exclusively the low frequency response of mainly the lateral canal and it's afferents (6). Since asymmetry of OKAN seems to reflect small asymmetries in peripheral vestibular function, testing OKAN may offer another possibility to study and evaluate vestibular side difference in peripheral vestibular disorders in man (7).

REFERENCES

1. Leigh RJ, Zee DS. (1983) The neurology of eye movement. Philadelphia, FA Davis Co, pp 69-88

2. Honrubia V, Downey WL, Mitchell DP, Ward BA, Ward PH. (1968) Experimental studies on optokinetic nystagmus. II. Normal humans. Acta Otolaryngol (Stockh) 65:441-448

3. Lisberger SG, Miles FA, Optican LM, Eighmy BB. (1981) Optokinetic response in monkey: Underlying mechanisms and their sensitivity to long-term adaptive changes in vestibulo-ocular reflex. J Neurophysiol 45: 869-889

4. Zasorin NL, Baloh RW, Yee RD, Honrubia V. (1983) Influence of vestibulo-ocular reflex gain in human optokinetic responses. Exp Brain Res 51:271-274

5. Courjon JH, Precht W, Sirkin DW. (1987) Vestibular nerve and nuclei unit responses and eye movement responses to repetitive galvanic stimulation of the labyrinth in the rat. Exp Brain Res 66:41-48

6. Hamid MA, Hughes GB, Kinney SE. (1987) Criteria for diagnosing bilateral vestibular dysfunction. In: Graham, Kemink, eds. The vestibular system: Neurophysiologic and clinical research. New York, Raven Press, pp 115-118

7. Brantberg K, Magnusson M. (1990) Galvanically induced asymmetric optokinetic after-nystagmus. Accepted in Acta Otolaryngol (Stockh)

GABA$_A$ RECEPTORS INDUCE HYPERPOLARIZATION IN OUTER HAIR CELLS OF THE GUINEA PIG COCHLEA

ALFRED H. GITTER, PETER K. PLINKERT AND HANS P. ZENNER

Department of Otolaringology, Silcherstr. 5, Eberhard-Karls-Universität, D-7400 Tübingen, FRG

INTRODUCTION

Several lines of evidence indicate that gamma-aminobutyric acid (GABA), the main inhibitory neurotransmitter of the central nervous system (CNS), is also released from the olivo-cochlear efferent neurons reaching the outer hair cells (OHCs) (KLINKE, 1986; ALTSCHULER and FEX, 1986; EYBALIN et al., 1988).

By means of two monoclonal antibodies, we were able to visualize GABA$_A$/benzodiazepine receptors at the basal pole of OHCs and the tonotopical arrangement of the receptors along the basilar membrane (PLINKERT et al., 1989). In the present paper, we report electrophysiological evidence for GABA$_A$ receptors in OHCs of the guinea pig cochlea. GABA$_A$ receptors consist of chloride channels which are activated, i.e. their opening probability increases, when the extracellular GABA concentration is raised; this causes membrane hyperpolarization. Therefore, we investigated the cell potential of isolated OHCs *in vitro* in the presence of various concentrations of bath-applied GABA and other substances that modulate GABA receptor current.

MATERIAL AND METHODS
Outer hair cell dissociation

Healthy colored guinea pigs with body weights of approximately 250 g and a positive Preyer's reflex were decapitated. Thetemporal bones were quickly removed and cooled to 4° C. Then, the lateral wall of the cochlea was opened and the membraneous labyrinth was explanted. In a cell-culture dish, each cochlear turn was dissected with a sharp-pointed needle. The procedure yielded several dozens of morphologically intact OHCs. To avoid any alteration of membrane proteins, enzymes were not used in this study. If the cells were not completely separated, the dissociation was accomplished by gently sucking the tissue into a 5 μl-pipette (Eppendorf) and then flushing it into fresh tissue culture medium. Single viable OHCs were kept in a 52 mm-diameter, round cell-culture plastic dish containing 5 to 6 ml Hanks' MEM tissue culture medium (pH 7.4, buffered with 4.2 mmol/l NaHCO$_3$ and adjusted to 300 mOsm/kg) and observed under an inverted microscope (Leitz). The experiments were made at room temperature (23° C).

Patch-clamp technique
Patch-clamp experiments in the whole-cell configuration were performed as described by MARTY and NEHER, 1983. Recording pipettes were pulled from soft-glass capillaries (Hilgenberg, Malsberg, FRG) with 1.5 mm outer diameter. Silver silver-chloride electrodes connected pipette and bath with the patch-clamp amplifier (List electronic, Darmstadt, FRG). Pipettes were filled with saline solution containing (concentrations in mM): K-gluconate 160, EGTA 1, HEPES 3; $CaCl_2$ 0.6484; pCa=7, pH=7.2, adjusted with 4.9 mM KOH. When filled with this solution, pipettes typically had resistances of 5 MΩ (range: 3 to 10 MΩ). Before the pipette was attached to the cell, the pipette's voltage was adjusted to nullify the current flowing to the bath. The voltage inside the pipette was taken to be -5.8 mV with respect to the true bath potential, because of the diffusion potential at the pipette's tip which was measured independently in control experiments.

RESULTS

Isolated OHCs were perfused *in vitro* during whole-cell recording with i) cell culture medium, ii) culture medium containing test substances and iii) culture medium containing an elevated potassium concentration (9 mmol/l sodium were substituted with, potassium resulting in a final K^+ concentration of 15 mmol/l). The latter was used as a control. Due to the use of low-resistance electrodes, the intracellular compartment was dialyzed. An exponential function $V(t) = V_e - (V_e - V_a) \exp(-t/\tau)$ was fitted to the time course of the measured potential during the dialysis period. OHCs with final potentials V_e more negative than -56 mV were further used. Cells with more positive potentials usually showed morphological defects. The dialysis time constant τ of intact cells was 28.9 ± 10.4 s (mean ± SD, n=41) and the final potential V_e was -70.5 ± 5.2 mV (mean ± SD, n=46). The negative cell potential was close to the K^+ Nernst equilibrium potential, because the cell membrane of OHCs contains predominantly K^+ conductanes (GITTER et al., 1986). The response to changes of the external bath solution was tested using a perfusate with an increased K^+ concentration. This control was performed in all experiments after perfusion with the test solution. The elevated K^+ concentration induced depolarization of 18.9 ± 1.7 mV (mean ± SD, n=44) in accordance with a predominantly K^+-permeable cell membrane. GABA was applied extracellularly in concentrations of 10^{-8} M, 10^{-6} M, 10^{-5} M, 10^{-4} M and 10^{-3} M. This induced cell membrane hyperpolarizations of -0.75 ± 0.35 mV (n=2), -2.0 mV (n=1), -2.0 ± 0.4 mV (n=4), -2.9 ± 0.9 mV (n=4), respectively (mean ± SD). Depolarizations were not observed. Clorazepate (TRANXILIUM, Midy Arzneimittel, Munich), which increases the probability of GABA-receptor channels being open, enhanced the hyperpolarization. GABA (10^{-6}M) with clorazepate (2.5 10^{-5} M) caused a hyperpolarization of 8.3 ± 1.3 mV (n=8). Picrotoxin, which blocks GABA-receptor channels, decreased the transmitter-induced voltage change. GABA (10^{-6}M) with clorazepate (2.5 10^{-5} M) and picrotoxin (10^{-4} M) resulted in a hyperpolarization of only -2.0 ± 1.0 mV (n=3).

DISCUSSION

Extensive studies of $GABA_A$-receptors in the CNS revealed that the receptor complex is composed of a GABA binding site, a chloride ionophore and, in most cases, a regulatory unit, the benzodiazepine receptor (Schoch et al., 1985; Möhler et al., 1989). In the CNS, $GABA_A$ receptors regulate chloride currents across the cell membrane. Stimulation results in a conformation change of the receptor molecule and, opening of a chloride channel. Inward current carried by Cl^- leads to membrane hyperpolarization. An interesting synergism exists between the action of benzodiazepine, barbiturate and GABA. Benzodiazepines enhance allosterically GABA effects by increasing the opening probability of the chloride-channel (MÖHLER et al, 1989). Recently, we demonstrated the presence of integral proteins creating GABA-ergic receptors on the surface of OHCs. Using two monoclonal antibodies directed against the α- and β-subunit of the $GABA_A$/benzodiazepine receptor, we visualized these two epitopes at the basal membrane of isolated OHCs. The observed immunoreactivity of the post-synaptic membranes indicated the presence of a post-syaptic $GABA_A$-receptor complex. A functional characterization of the GABA/benzodiazepine receptor was achieved in our patch-clamp experiments. Receptor activation by the chemical messenger GABA was followed by a dose-dependent hyperpolarization of the cell membrane. These GABA responses were enhanced by the benzodiazepine clorazepate and inhibited by the GABA-receptor channel blocker picrotoxin. Inhibitory GABA receptors on OHCs, which are arranged tonotopically along the basiliar membrane, may be part of a control circuit that modulates the biomechanics of the cochlea (Gitter et al., 1988).This view is in accordance with electrophysiological experiments of KLINKE and OERTEL (1977), in which the GABA antagonist picrotoxin induced a partial blockade of effects resulting from the electrical stimulation of the olivocochlear nerves at the floor of the fourth ventricle.

Technical assistance of C. König is gratefully acknowledged.

REFERENCES
1) Altschuler, R.A. and Fex, J. (1986) Efferent neurotransmitters. In: Neurobiology of Hearing: The Cochlea. Eds.: R.A. Altschuler, D.W. Hoffman and R.P. Bobbin. Raven Press, New York
2) Eybalin, M., Parnaud, C., Geffard, M. and Pujol, R. (1988) Immunelectron microscopy identifies several types of GABA-containing efferent synapses in the guinea-pig organ of Corti. Neurosci. 24, 29-38
3) Gitter, A.h., Frömter, E. and Zenner, H.P. (1986) Membrane potential and Ion channels in Isolated Outer Hair Cells of Guinea-pig Cochlea. ORL J. Otorhinolaryngol. Relat. Spec. 48, 68-75
4) Gitter, A.H., Plinkert, P.K. and Zenner, H.P. (1988) Origin of adaptation and amplificaiton processes in the mammalian cochlea. In: Vertigo, nausea, tinnitus and hypoacusis in metabolic disorders, pp. 197-200
5) Hamill, O.P., Bormann, J. and Sakmann, B. (1983) Activation of multiple conductance state chloride channels in spinal neurons by glycine and GABA. Nature 305, 805-808
6) Klinke, R. (1986) Neurotransmission in the inner ear. Hearing Res. 22, 235-243
7) Klinke, R. and Oertel, W. (1977) Evidence that GABA is not the afferent transmitter in the cochlea. Exp. Brain Res. 23, 311-314
8) Marty, A. and Neher, E. (1983) Tight-seal-whole-cell recording. In: Single channel recordings. Edited by B. Sakmann and E. Neher, Plenum Press, New York
9) Möhler, H., Malherbe, P., Sequir, J.M. Bannwarth, W., Schoch, P. and Richards, J.G. (1989) Location, Structure, and Sites of Synthesis of the $GABA_A$ Receptor in the central nervous system. In: Allosteric Modulation of Amino Acid Receptors: Therapeutic Implications. Edited by E.A. Barnard and E. Costa, Raven Press, Ltd. New York
10) Plinkert, P.K., Möhler, H. and Zenner H.P. (1989) A subpopulation of outer hair cells possessing GABA receptors with tonotopic organization. Arch. Otorhinolaryngol. 246, 417-422
11) Schoch, P., Richards, J.G., Häring, P., Takacs, B., Stähli, C.,Staehelin, T., Haefely, W. and Möhler, H. (1985) Co-localization of $GABA_A$ receptors and benzodiazepine receptors in the brain shown by monoclonal antibodies. Nature 314, 168-171

α-BUNGAROTOXIN BINDING TO NICOTINIC ACETYLCHOLINE RECEPTORS IN THE MAMMALIAN COCHLEA

PETER K. PLINKERT, ALFRED H. GITTER AND HANS-PETER ZENNER

Department of Otolaryngology, Silcherstr. 5, Eberhard-Karls-Universität, D-7400 Tübingen 1, FRG

INTRODUCTION

Active mechanical processes are postulated to explain the amplification and sharp tuning of the sound-induced vibration of the basilar membrane. The morphological basis is seen in outer hair cells (OHC) with their remarkable capability for motile responses to various stimuli (1,2,3,4). The predominant olivo-cochlear efferents reaching the OHC regulate these energy-requiring processes. The signal transfer from the efferent nerve terminals to OHC is achieved by a chemical messenger, which is released into the synaptic cleft. Thus the neurotransmitter and its postsynaptic receptor on OHC plays a key role in our understanding of the transduction process. To investigate whether acetylcholine (ACh) is the efferent neurotransmitter at OHC we performed immunocytological, biochemical and physiological experiments with the isolated sensory cells. The dissection of the mammalian OHC was performed according to the method described by ZENNER et al., 1985 (6). The isolation was carried out in the absence of proteolytic enzymes to avoid alterations of membrane proteins.
The presence of choline acetyltransferase and ACh-esterase, necessary for the synthesis and breakdown of ACh led to the suggestion that ACh might be the efferent transmitter (7).
Furthermore, FEX and ADAMS (1978) demonstrated that effects caused by the electrical stimulation of the crossed olivo-cochlear bundle could be blocked with intracochlear application of α-bungarotoxin (α-bgtx) (8). The exact identification and characterization of this synapse was however still missing.

IMMUNOCYTOLOGY OF ACETYLCHOLINE RECEPTORS ON OHC

Using two monoclonal antibodies (mAb) we searched for ACh-receptors (AChRs) on isolated OHC. The immunoglobulins were directed against external and internal epitopes of the α-subunit of nicotinic AChRs. In our study, staining of the primary antibody was performed with the peroxidase reaction. Using these two antibodies, receptor epitopes were visualized at the basal end of OHC (9). The specific binding of the mAb directed against cytoplasmic epitopes was only followed after pretreatment with Triton-X-100 in order to
permeabilize the outer cell membrane for the antibodies. Both immunoglobulins showed a characteristic brown staining at the basal pole of the isolated sensory cell. Using digital image enhancement a cup-like arrangement of AChRs was often observed at the lower pole of OHC. The presence of extra- and intracellular receptor epitopes demonstrates, that OHC possess transmembraneous AChR-molecules. The localization at the basis of OHC corresponds to electronmicroscopic pictures, which demonstrated the typical morphological appearance of the efferent nerve endings in this region.

TONOTOPICAL ACHR DISTRIBUTION

The turn-selective isolation of the auditory sensory cells exhibited a decreasing baso-apical receptor distribution. The mAb 35, known to react with extracellular domains exhibited a positive staining in the basal turn in 55 % OHCs. In the second turn, immunoreactivity decreased to 48 %, in the third to 38 % and the apical turn, only 25 % of the sensory cells showed the characteristic brownish staining. Similar results were obtained with the mAb 155 which was directed against the cytoplasmic receptor epitopes (10).

α-BUNGAROTOXIN BINDING ON OHC

To further elucidate the nature of the AChR-epitopes found immunocytologically, we performed biochemical studies with radiolabelled α-bgtx. The isolated OHC were incubated at room temperature with ^{125}J-bgtx in final concentrations of 1 to 100 nM. Then, the cells were centrifuged in an air-driven ultracentrifuge, and the supernatant was discarded. The sediment was washed twice with buffer to eliminate free toxin. Finally, the samples were counted in a scintillation counter. Nonspecific binding was checked by preincubating OHCs with "cold" α-toxin (10 μM) prior to the addition of the radiolabelled compound. The data for the specific α-bgtx binding were calculated from the total minus the unspecific α-toxin binding. A typical receptor binding curve showed that the saturation level is reached at 80 nM. It can be calculated, that about 0.02 fM bungarotoxin bind to each OHC, representing equal amounts of nicotinic AChRs. Thereby, we estimate a number of roughly 10^7 binding sites per OHC.

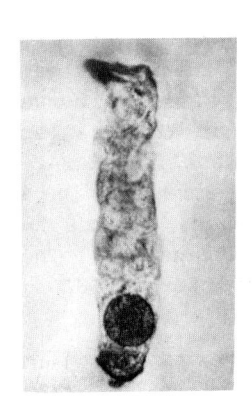

Fig. 1 Visualization of intracellular AChR-epitopes on OHC with mAb 155. Similar results were obtained with mAb 35 directed against extracellullar epitopes (not shown).

Fig. 2: AChR-immunoreactivity using the antibodies mAb 155 and 35 in the different turns of the cochlea.

TRANSMITTER INDUCED OHC MOTILITY

To demonstrate the physiological function of the observed nicotinic receptors we applied the neurotransmitter ACh ($10^{-4} - 10^{-5}$ M) or its analoque Carbachol ($10^{-4} - 10^{-7}$ M) to the basal pole of isolated OHCs by means of a micropump. With a resolution of 0.4 μm a shortening of the viable isolated sensory cell could be observed, depending on the applied concentration of the neurotransmitter. In some cells, a maximal cell contraction of 1.6 μm was observed. In the presence of d-tubocurarine (10^{-4} M) and atropine (10^{-4} M), these motile events were reduced (10).

CONCLUSION

The remarkable OHC motility possibly influences the micromechanics of the basilar membrane. Furthermore, the control of OHC-motility could be achieved by the efferent nerves, which predominantly terminate on OHCs. Besides the major neurotransmitter ACh, the inhibitory chemical messenger GABA may be released from the efferent nerve terminals to influence the biomechanics of the basilar membrane. Recently, we were able to visualize $GABA_A$-receptors on OHC. These receptors were arranged in a tonotopical distribution, which was, however, inverse to the AChR arrangement along the basilar membrane (11). The identification of the efferent neurotransmitter at OHC is a step forward in our understanding of hearing.

REFERENCES
1. Neely, S.T. and Kim, D.O. (1983) Hear. Res. 9: 123-130
2. Zenner et al. (1985) Hear.Res. 18: 127-133
3. Zenner, H.P. (1986) Hear. Res. 22: 83-90
4. Ashmore, J.F. (1987) J. Physiol. 338: 323-347
5. Zenner, H.P. (1988) Acta Otolaryngol. (Stockh) 105: 39-44
6. Zenner et al. (1985) Laryng. Rhinol. Otol. 64: 642-648
7. Klinke, R. (1986) Hear. Res. 22: 235-243
8. Fex, J. and Adams, J.C. (1978) Brain Res. 159: 440-444
9. Plinkert, P.K. (1989) Laryng. Rhinol. Otol. 68: 450-455
10. Plinkert et al. (1990) Hear. Res. 44: 25-34
11. Plinkert et al. (1989) Arch.Otolaryngol. 246, 417-422

GENERAL ASPECTS
OF HEAD AND NECK TRAUMA

POSTTRAUMATIC DYSEQUILIBRIUM

CLAUS FRENZ CLAUSSEN, ERIKA CLAUSSEN

Neurootological Reserch Center, Kurhaustr. 12, 8730 Bad Kissingen, Germany

INTRODUCTION

Injury to the head is one of the common causes of vertigo and dizziness. The severity of the posttraumatic symptoms depends on the extend of the damage to the brain including the presence or absence of otobasal fractures, trauma to the orbit and/or trauma to the neck including the cervical spine. More than 20 years back we were confronted in occupational medicine that only 2 percent of the officially accepted occupational hazards are falling accidents. However, 20 % of all the fatal occupational hazards recorded in the Federal Republic of Germany were falling accidents. The severity of the traumas in the falling accidents has forced the West German labour control authorities (Berufsgenossenschaften) to working out a special preventive decree (Unfallverhütungsvorschrift, Grundsatz 41 "Arbeiten mit Absturzgefahr") for selecting special risks in a preventive measure. Thus, cranio-corpo-graphy has been introduced as an objective and quantitative equilibrium test with an instant test recording of the vestibular spinal performance.

The diagnosis of a head injury is not difficult, as it is always memorized by the patient, who will report about it in the neurootological history. Usually the neurootologist does not see the victim during an unexplained or an overt posttraumatic coma. He gets already the reports about the lacerations or contusions or brusis. With request he is supplied with the x-rays from a general or special surgical department, which have revealed possible fractures. Frequently also the echoencephalograms, the CT-scans and the NMR scans are available in severe cases.

Cranial nerve palsies with a damage to the cranial nerves occurs in a bout 5 % of head injuries. The olfactory, facial and acoustic nerves are most commonly effected. In the field of neurootology we frequently find that a complete or partial recovery is a rule except for lesions of the olfactory nerve, as well as for ruptures oder dissections of the 8th nerve. Also focal cerebral lesions with hemiplegia, aphasia or other focal localized damage to the brain or especially the brainstem may occur in suffering of severe head injuries. Especially the focal lesions to the brainstem lateron complain for a long time for vertigo and dizziness.

The posttraumatic syndromes include headaches, dizziness, irritability, restlessness, inability to concentrate, increased sweating, depression and other personality changes. They occur in more than one third of the victims of head injuries. These symptoms, however, do not seem to be related to the severity of injury of the brain being attributed to minor derangement of cerebral function or to psychological reactions. Especially dizziness and vertigo may undergo a self sustaining cycle of development. When only seeing the patients one to ten years after the trauma, it may become very difficult to sorting out the various aspects in the etiology of his so-called posttraumatic dysequilibrium complaints.

MATERIAL AND METHODS

Based on our clinical records, which are available in our neurootology division at the university head center of Würzburg, we are classifying our patients into 5 groups, i.e., verified otobasal fracture, verified cerebral contusion, clinically treated cerebral concussion, clinically treated minor head trauma and head trauma without a following medical treatment. The last group is rather complicated to handle as it may contain minor head traumas as well as severe head traumas in cases who dissimulated.

We have evaluated 9.190 neurootological case reports from our neurootological data bank NODEC IV. There we found that 2.515 cases, i.e. 27.37 %, reported about an earlier head-neck-trauma. More detailed classifications of the trauma were possible in 2.297 cases, i.e. 24.99 %. The trauma classification is represented in table 1.

RESULTS

Medical trauma classification in 2.297 neurootological patients suffering from posttraumatic vertigo after a head and neck trauma.

TABLE I

CLASSIFICATION OF TRAUMA

Classification of the trauma	n	%
Otobasal fracture	108	4.70 %
Cerebral contusion	123	5.35 %
Cerebral concussion	819	35.66%
Minor head trauma, medically treated	1247	54.29%
Head trauma without subsequent medical treatment	1138	49.54%

In younger, still professionally working patients, the insurance relevant causes of the accident have been classified according to occupational hazard, sports accident, home accident and traffic accident. The results are represented in table 2.

TABLE 2

CLASSIFICATION OF TRAUMAS IN NEUROOTOLOGICAL PATIENTS WITH RESPECT TO VARIOUS INSURANCE COMPETENCES.

Trauma group	Cases
Traffic accidents	556
Occupational hazards	279
Home accidents	219
Sports accidents	84

Vertigo and dizziness, which mainly lead the posttraumatic patients to see a neurootologist, can be very late residual symptoms. Even an otobasal fracture or a verified cerebral contusion may appear at the neurootologists only after years (see table 3).

TABLE 3

TIME DELAY BETWEEN HEAD AND NECK TRAUMA AND THE FIRST NEUROOTOLOGICAL INVESTIGATION BECAUSE OF THE RESIDUAL POSTTRAUMATIC VERTIGO.

Trauma classification	Trauma before weeks	Trauma before months	Trauma before years
Otobasal fracture	29	41	38
Cerebral contusion	15	29	79
Cerebral concussion	48	120	651
Minor head trauma, medically treated	36	149	1.062

Every case of the whole data bank underwent a thorough history taking by our neurootological history scheme NODEC. The total sample of 2.515 patients with residual posttraumatic symptoms after head injuries where requested for their basic vertigo signs (see table 4) and also with respect to their vertigo provoking mechanisms (see table 5). The incidence of the typical signs is always compared with the incidence in the total sample of 9.190 cases in NODEC IV. During the recent years especially the data bank NODEC IV has proofed to be a standard of neurootological symptoms and equilibriometric findings.

TABLE 4

VERTIGO SYMPTOMS IN 9.190 NEUROOTOLOGICAL PATIENTS OF NODEC IV AND 2.515 POSTTRAUMATIC NEUROOTOLOGICAL CASES.

Symptom	NODEC IV 9.190 = 100 %	Head-Neck-Trauma 2.515 = 100 %
Rocking	39.54 %	43.84 %
Lifting sensation	5.22 %	6.50 %
Rotatory vertigo	35.90 %	39.94 %
Falling tendency	20.20 %	24.14 %
Blackout	20.23 %	26.30 %
Instability	36.40 %	41.10 %

TABLE 5

VERTIGO TRIGGER MECHANISMS IN 9.190 NEUROOTOLOGICAL PATIENTS OF NODEC IV AND 2.515 PATIENTS AFTER HEAD AND NECK TRAUMA.

Symptom	NODEC IV 9.190 = 100 %	Head-Neck-Trauma 2.515 = 100 %
Kinetosis	10.11 %	11.79 %
Turning the head	24.80 %	29.23 %
Bending	23.09 %	29.71 %
Getting up	37.31 %	44.11 %
Gazing towards one side	6.82 %	8.66 %

All our patients underwent a functional neurootological and equilibriometric examination. Thus we tried to assess the location and nature of the functional degeneration underlying the posttraumatic residual vertigo symptoms. The objective and quantitative equilibrium investigation included an analysis of the cranio-corpo-gram, thus obtaining a record of the gait and standing patterns by means of a radar image like photogram of the light tracings from the head and the shoulders during stepping and standing.

An analysis of the optomotor equilibrium mechanisms has been reflected by electronystagmography, using monaural bithermal caloric stimulation and the evaluation through the butterfly calorigram of Claussen or the binaural vestibular ocular reflex testing with supraliminal perrotatory and supramaximal postrotatory stimulation using the rotatory intensity damping test of Claussen. Furthermore prognostically important signs like vestibular recruitment or decruitment have been evaluated through the vestibular stimulus response intensity comparison (VSRIC). Thus a mosaic of various functional findings enabled us to objectively document in more than 90 % of all the posttraumatic vertigo cases a functional deviation which verified the subjective complaints. The efficacy of the various test procedures applied is represented in table 6. The high incidence rate of objective functional findings releaves the majority of the posttraumatic cases, especially after years from the stigma of malignering.

TABLE 6

POSITIVE NEUROOTOLOGICAL FINDINGS BASED ON 4 OBJECTIVE AND QUANTITATIVE EQUILIBRIOMETRIC TESTS IN 9.190 NEUROOTOLOGICAL PATIENTS (NODEC IV) AND 2.515 PATIENTS WITH RESIDUAL POSTTRAUMATIC VERTIGO SYMPTOMS.

Neurootological test	% pathological findings in NODEC IV	% pathological findings in patients with head and neck trauma
butterfly calorigram	63.44 %	64.63 %
rotatory intensity damping test	62.62 %	52.16 %
vestibular stimulus response intensity comparison	69.22 %	65.74 %
cranio-corpo-gram (step-test)	58.90 %	57.56 %

Table 6 only gives the result for the total sample. They do not differ significantly between the whole sample of NODEC IV and the group of head-neck-trauma patients. However, much higher incidence rates of functional disorders are found in subsamples. In the cases with otobasal fractures, forinstance, positive finding in the butterfly calorigram is seen even years after the fracture in 72,73 %. Years after a cerebral contusion this incidence rate lies at 75,71 %. In cases with a cerebral concussion this finding amounts years after the trauma still to 66.67 %.

A pathological rotatory intensity damping test is seen in 70.37 % of the otobasal fracture patients, even years after the trauma. This figure only amounts to 66.67 % weeks after the trauma. In patients with cerebral concussions, this finding amounts to 51.02 % after years, whereas after weeks it still lies at 63.64 %. Pathological findings in the vestibular stimulus response intensity comparison still amounts years after otobasal fractures to 72.41 %, whereas it lies after weeks at 71.43 %. Thus it remains rather unchanged over the time. In cases with cerebral contusion, this finding amounts weeks after the trauma to 88.99 %, then it slightly decase to 76.56 % years after the trauma. The cranio-corpo-gram of the stepping test shows weeks after the otobasal fracture in 73.33 % pathology, which decase to 53.57 % after years. In cases with cerebral contusion, the positive stepping test cranio-corpo-grams amount weeks after the trauma to 87.50 %, then this figure decase to 64.81 % years after the trauma.

Our results show that the classical opinion that the posttraumatic symptoms especially due to cerebral concussion and milder head injuries should rather quickly disappear and that now long lasting signs can be attributed to minor derangements of cerebral functions cannot be supported any longer. Our findings, based on a systematic neurootological network investigation, exhibit a very differentiated picture in the individual cases. Due to the aging process and other diseases affecting our patients, even minor posttraumatic lesions can turn into more progressive degenerative states in the neurosensorial system. Similar data are available for our patients suffering from head trauma due to whiplash accidents.

REFERENCES:

1. Barany, R (1906) Untersuchungen über den vom Vestibularapparat des Ohres reflektorisch ausgelösten rhythmischen Nystagmus und seine Begleiterscheinung. Mschr. Ohrenheilk. 40, 193-297

2. Barany R, Wittmaack K (1911) Funktionelle Prüfung des Vestibularapparates. Fischer-Verlag, Jena

3. Claussen C.-F (1970) Über eine Gleichgewichtsfunktionsprüfung mit Hilfe der Cranio-Corpo- Graphie (CCG) und Polarkoordinaten im Raume. Arch.klin.exp.Ohr.-,Nas.-Kehlk.Heilk., 196, 256-261

4. Claussen C.-F (1981) Schwindel - Symptomatik, Diagnostik, Therapie. Edition medicin & pharmacie, Dr.Werner Rudat & Co., Hamburg

5. Claussen C.-F (1985) Presbyvertigo, Presbyataxie, Presbytinnitus. Springer-Verlag, Berlin, Heidelberg, New York, Tokio, 1985.

6. Claussen C-F, Claussen E (1986) Forschungsbericht Cranio-Corpo-Graphie (CCG) - Ein einfacher objektiver und quantitativer Gleichgewichtstest für die Praxis. Schriftenreihe des Hauptverbandes der gewerblichen Berufsgenossenschaften eV, D 5205 St. Augustin

7. Romberg H (1848) Lehrbuch der Nervenkrankheiten.
   Springer-Verlag, Berlin, S. 184-191

8. Unterberger S (1938) Neue objektive registrierbare Vestibulariskörperdrehreaktionen, erhalten durch Treten auf der Stelle. Der Tretversuch.Arch.Ohr.-,Nas.-,Kehlk.Heilk. 145, 273-282, 1938.

9. Claussen C-F, Tato JM (1973) Equilibriometria Practica.
   Hasenclever, Buenos Aires

10. Claussen C-F, v. Schlachta I (1972) Butterfly Chart for Caloric Nystagmus.
    Arch.Otolaryng., 96, 371-375

11. Claussen C-F, De SaJV (1978) Clinical Study of Human Equilibrium by Electronystagmography and Allied Tests.Popular Prakashan, Bombay

12. Claussen C-F (1985) Presbyvertigo, Presbyataxie, Presbytinnitus.
    Springer-Verlag, Berlin, Heidelberg, New York

13. Claussen C-F, Aust G, Schäfer WD, v.Schlachta I (1986) Atlas der Elektronystagmographie. Edition medicin & pharmacie, Hamburg, 1986.

14. Fitzgerald G, Hallpike, CS (1942) Studies in Human Vestibular Function: Observation on the Directional Preponderance of Caloric Nystagmus Resulting from Cerebral Lesions.

15. Hallpike, CS (1956) The Caloric Tests.

16. Henriksson NG.(1956) Speed of Slow Component and Duration of Caloric Nystagmus. Acta Otolaryng. (Stockh.), Suppl. 125,

17. Henriksson NG , Jahneke JB, Claussen C.-F (1969)
    Vestibular Disease and Electronystagmography.
    Press Company, Studentlitteratur, Lund/Schweden

NEURORADIOLOGICAL ASPECTS OF POSTTRAUMATIC BRAIN LESIONS

HELGA GRÄFIN VON EINSIEDEL

Neuroradiologie*, Institut für Röntgendiagnostik, Klinikum rechts der Isar der Technischen Universität München, *Möhlstraße 28, D-8000 München 80

Computed tomography (CT) is the first and most important diagnostic procedure in a head injured patient, who is persistently unconscious from the beginning or who develops unconsciousness later on. CT immediately and reliably demonstrates a wide variety of intracranial pathology as listed in Table I.

TABLE I
CLASSIFICATION OF HEAD INJURIES

I. Intracranial extracerebral hemorrhage
  epidural hematoma
  subdural hematoma
    - acute
    - subacute
    - chronic
    - hygroma
  subarachnoid hemorrhage
II. Blunt brain injury
  focal
    - cerebral concussion
    - cerebral contusion
    - intracerebral hemorrhage
    - laceration
	diffuse
	  - brain swelling
	  - brain edema
	secondary
	  - ischemia
	  - herniation
	  - venous thrombosis
	  - carotid-cavernous
	    sinus fistula
	III. Open head injury
	  depressed injury
	  penetrating/perforating
	    injury
	  CSF fistula
	IV. Late sequela of head injury

INTRACRANIAL EXTRACEREBRAL HEMORRHAGE

The characteristic CT appearance of an acute epidural hematoma (EDH) is a biconvex hyperdense mass lesion in the course of the middle meningeal artery. A skull fracture is present in 90% of cases. Since most EDH result from arterial bleeding, they are rapidly growing, leading to a marked midline shift and ventricle compression. Displacement and compression of the aqueduct cause widening of the contralateral ventricle which may be confined to the temporal horn. With further progression the medial temporal lobe herniates into the tentorial nodge with consecutive midbrain compression (Fig.1). Most EDH occur in the temporoparietal region. EDH in the posterior fossa often expand to the supratentorial compartment (Fig.2).

Subdural hematomas (SDH) typically have a crescent shape. They usually cover a major portion of the brain surface, because blood can freely spread in the subdural space. They either result from ruptured bridging veins or from arterial bleeding caused by a hemorrhagic contusion. Besides the most common location over the convexity, SDH are seen in the interhemispheric slit or covering the tentorium.

Chronic SDH can occur weeks or months after a minor head injury. About 20% of chronic SDH are isodense on CT. They can have an enormous space occupying effect and yet, the patients symptoms may be minor, because the mass has slowly developed.

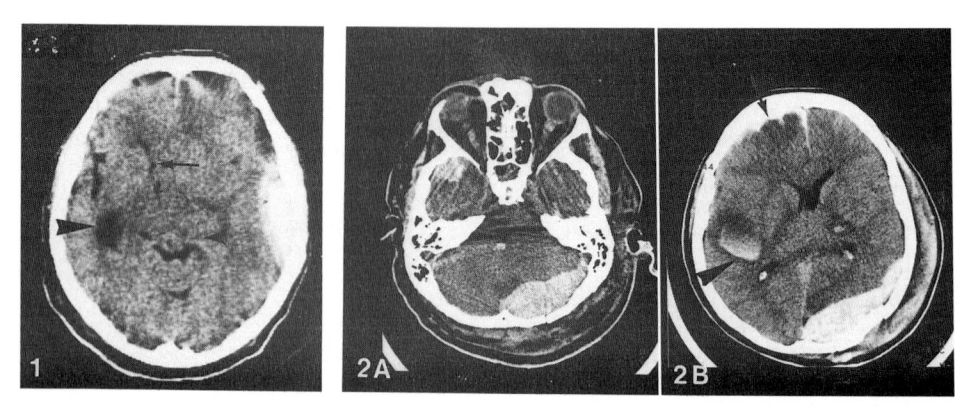

Fig. 1. Secondary brain stem compression following acute epidural hematoma. Axial CT scan shows biconvex EDH, marked midline shift (—▶), compression of ambient cistern and midbrain (▶), displacement of temporal lobe and widening of contralateral temporal horn (▶).

Fig. 2. Acute epidural hematoma in the posterior fossa (A) with supratentorial extension (B) in coup-contrecoup injury. Axial CT scans three days after trauma. Skull fracture and extracranial tissue swelling indicate the site of blow (A,B). The contrecoup lesion consists in hemorrhagic cortical contusion, subarachnoid and subdural hemorrhage (B —▶) and in intracerebral hematoma (B ▶).

Subarachnoid hemorrhages are usually combined with contusions (Fig.2B). They can be located in the basal cisterns or in the sulci of the convexity.

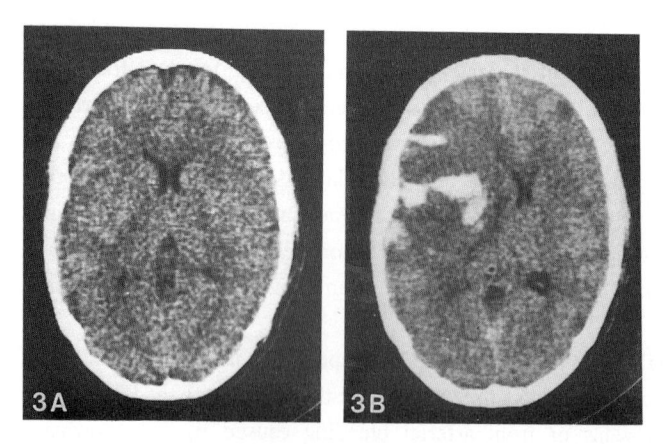

Fig. 3. Delayed traumatic hemorrhage. Axial CT scans. Six hours after trauma CT is entirely normal (A). Twenty hours later a large space-occupying hemorrhagic contusion has developed (B).

BLUNT BRAIN INJURIES

Cerebral concussions do not lead to morphological damage.

The predilection sites of a cerebral contusion are the basal frontal lobes and the temporal poles. Contusions may be defined to the cortex or involve subcortical structures. Besides edema they usually show some hemorrhagic infiltration. Contusions can be located at the immediate site of the impact (coup lesion) or at the opposite site (contrecoup lesion) or both (Fig.2).

Intracerebral hemorrhages occur in the white matter of the hemispheres, in the basal ganglia or in the brain stem. Hemorrhagic contusions and intracerebral hemorrhages may appear with a delay of one or two days with a prior normal CT (Fig.3).

Between the first and third week post trauma a disruption of the blood brain barrier occurs at the periphery of a contused area. At this time there will be enhancement of contrast material. In brain injury a contrast CT is usually not performed. However, it may give important information as small cortical contusions can be missed by plane CT and are only demonstrated by a contrast enhancement. In acute and subacute brain injuries, magnetic resonance (MR) imaging is not the procedure of choice. Yet, the distribution of contusional bleedings and especially brainstem involvement are better displayed than with CT, at least in the subacute stage where bleedings show a bright signal on T1-weighted images due to the blood break-down product methemoglobin (Fig.4).

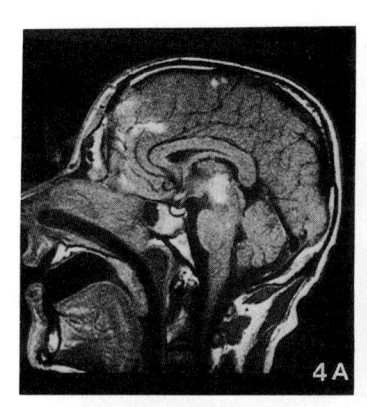

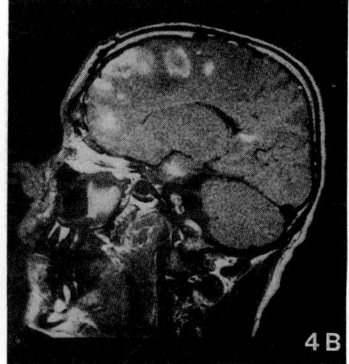

Fig. 4. Multiple hemorrhagic contusions seven days after severe head injury. Midsagittal (A) and parasagittal (B) T1-weighted spin-echo images show numerous bright lesions at the predilection sites of brain contusions, i.e. in inferior and polar portions of frontal and temporal lobes, in the midbrain and pons.

Following brain injury diffuse changes may occur. Brain swelling is expected to be due to hyperemia secondary to vasoparalysis. The ventricular system is slit like, the external fluid spaces are not visible and the widening of the intracerebral vessels can be demonstrated after contrast injection. The brain swelling disappears after a day or so and control CT's will show the spinal fluid spaces to have returned to normal.

In the acute stage generalized brain edema can not be differentiated from brain swelling. However, in contrast to brain swelling, edema damages the white matter which finally results in ventricular dilatation.

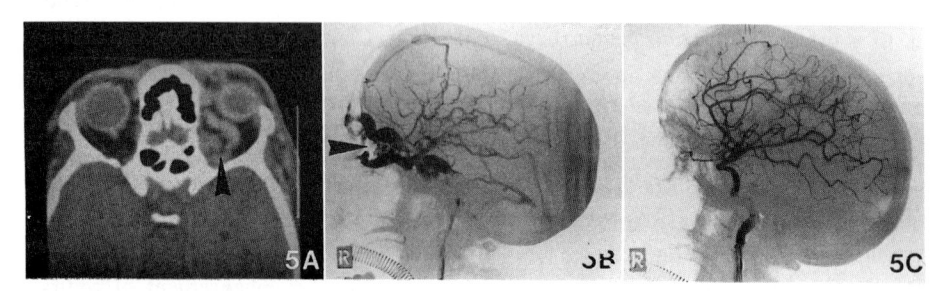

Fig. 5. Posttraumatic carotid-cavernous sinus fistula. Axial CT scan (A) and lateral subtraction carotid angiogram (B) show tortuous intraorbital veins (▶) and dilated calvarial veins. No intracranial carotid circulation. After interventional treatment with three detachable ballons placed in the cavernous sinus, the fistula is closed with preservation of the carotid artery (C).

Among the secondary traumatic lesions, ischemia is the most common. It may i.e. follow transtentorial herniation. The posterior cerebral artery which runs around the cerebral peduncle may then be compressed by the parahypocampal gyrus leading to an infarction in the corresponding vascular territory.

The characteristic findings of posttraumatic hypoxia i.e. in combination with a trauma of the lungs are infarctions in the boundary zones between the territories of the anterior, middle and posterior cerebral arteries.

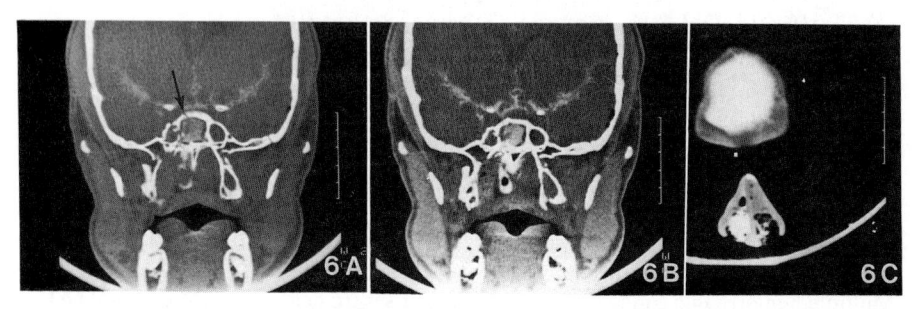

Fig. 6. CSF fistula following frontobasal trauma. CT cisternography. Coronal CT scans show right-sided fracture in the sphenoid body (A →), contrast material in the spenoid sinus (B) and in the right-sided pledget inserted in the nose (C).

Carotid-cavernous sinus fistulas develop by tearing of the carotid artery in the cavernous sinus portion. After days or months characteristic symptoms occur consisting in a pulsating exophthalmus, chemosis and ptosis. CT is diagnostic in demonstrating dilated intraorbital veins (Fig.5). These fistulas are treated by transarterial positioning of detachable ballons in the cavernous sinus.

OPEN HEAD INJURIES

Among open head injuries depressed trauma and cerebrospinal fluid (CSF) fistulas do occur while penetrating and perforating injuries are a rare event in peace, at least in european countries. Depressed fractures with dural laceration always show an underlying brain contusion.

CSF fistulas are diagnosed by CT-cisternography. By this method even very small fractures of the frontal base are detected as well as the point of leakage (Fig.6).

LATE SEQUELA OF HEAD INJURY

In most cases a brain contusion or a larger intracerebral hemorrhage will lead to a circumscribed substance loss and is detectable lifelong. However, residues have not necessarily to be seen. Small globular hemorrhages are known to be resorbed without detectable brain damage and this is also encountered in some larger hematomas (Fig.7).

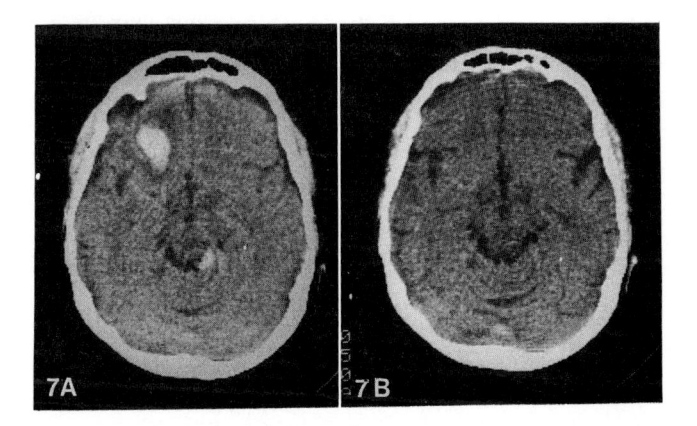

Fig. 7. Complete resorption of traumatic hemorrhages. Axial CT scans. Right frontal and left dorsolateral midbrain hemorrhage four days after head injury (A). Three months later hematomas are completely resorbed without leaving a parenchymal defect (B).

The residuum of an intracerebral hemorrhage will be a hemosiderin accumulation which, in contrast to CT, can be visualized with MR. On T2-weighted spin-echo images hemosiderin shows up by a low signal intensity. Old temporobasal contusions may be hard to detect on CT images because of bone artifacts in the middle fossa. In these cases again MR is helpful, especially if performed in the coronal orientation (Fig.8).

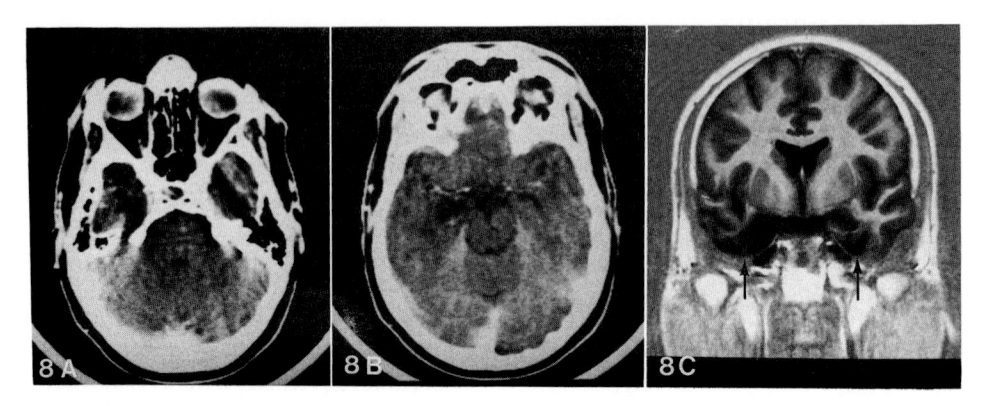

Fig. 8. Old temporal lobe contusions. Axial CT scans show residual damage in the right temporal lobe only (A,B). With coronal T1-weighted inversion-recovery MR bilateral temporobasal lesions are detected by low signal intensity (C →).

CT is the procedure of choice in acute and subacute brain injuries while MR is the preferable diagnostic tool in the investigation of late sequela, especially in those patients in whom no CT was performed in the early posttraumatic period and who present with a normal CT later on.

SEQUELAE OF INJURIES OF THE TEMPORAL REGION

RAIMUND P. FIRSCHING, ABBAS KARIMI-NEJAD
Klinik für Neurochirurgie, J. Stelzmannstr. 9, 5000 Köln 41, Federal Republic of Germany

To discuss sequelae of injuries of the temporal region a classification of head injuries and specific neurophysiologic findings will subsequently be presented:

CLASSIFICATION

The purpose of a classification of head injury is to specify the kind and severity of a lesion sustained. There have been numerous attempts at a classification in the past history[10]. Considering either treatment or prognosis, for practical reasons, classification of head injuries may be divided into two basic categories: 1.Morphological lesions. 2.Impaired cerebral function.

Morphological lesions

The location of a lesion following head injury has been used to specify the kind of head injury. In addition to lesions of the skull, of the dura mater, of the brain parenchyma and the vessels there may be an extracerebral haematoma or multiple injuries. Combinations of these are the rule. Some intracranial haematomas develop several hours, days or weeks after the injury. Within one hour epidural haematomas have hardly reached a siginificant size, while subdural haematomas are usually fatal, when they become space occupying within one hour[6].

Impaired cerebral function

Obviously the clinical course is not always determined by the morphological lesions, as some patients die inspite of the absence of gross pathomorphological lesions and others survive even grotesque skull fractures without major sequelae. Numerous coma grades and scales have been suggested for an early assessment, the most prominent being the Glasgow Coma Scale[12]. The 4-level 'Coma Scale' as suggested by Frowein[5] has stood the test of time. Other coma scales have been recommended elsewhere[1,11]. While the early evaluation of neurologic deficits after head injury serves to determine prognosis as related to survival, the evaluation of the overall social capability months and years after the injury may be used for a retrospective classification of brain tumors from the clinical course. The Glasgow Outcome Scale[8] has proved to be most useful and reli-able for this purpose and has therefore been adopted worldwide.

SPECIFIC NEUROPHYSIOLOGICAL FINDINGS

Registration of evoked potentials has become popular, as they provide objective data from a comatose patient, who cannot tell, what he hears, feels or sees. They have proved useful in 3 ways: First: assessment of prognosis. Second: the diagnosis of lesions of the auditory, somatosensory or visual pathway. Third: Diagnosis of brain death.

Prognostic value of evoked potentials:

Of the somatosensory (SEP), visual (VEP) and auditory evoked potentials (AEP) the SEPs proved to have the closest correlation with outcome distinguishing survival or nonsurvival. In a series of 76 patients with head injury: The bilateral loss of somato-sensory evoked potentials was associated with a 95% mortality. Normal somatosensory evoked potentials were associated with a 76% survival. The initial loss of evoked potentials of any modality, somatosensory, visual or auditory, was associated with a fatal outcome with only a few exceptions[3].

Diagnostic value of BAEP in temporal lesions:

All of 76 comatose patients with bilateral loss of BAEP died with 2 exceptions: One was a 74 year-old male, who had had a peripheral hearing loss before he sustained a head injury. The other was a 34 year-old male with a congenital complete hearing loss on the right. He suffered a petrous bone fracture on the left and reproducible BAEPs could not be obtained from either side. Sadly, he turned out to be deaf bilaterally when he regained consciousness.

In 11 patients the BAEP was completely absent unilaterally with an ipsilateral petrous bone fracture. Thus we concluded that in petrous bone fractures loss of hearing function is mostly not caused by a lesion of the auditory nerve but of the ear.

Brain death

The 40 Hz AER is a middle latency auditory evoked potential, first described in 1981 by Galambos and coworkers[7]. Clicks delivered to one ear repetitively at a rate of 40 Hz evoked a sinusoidal response with the appropriate montage of electrodes and filter settings. Varying the stimulating frequency to 20, 30, 50, 60, 70 etc. Hz it became apparent that the amplitude of the response was maximal at 40Hz.

The reason for this is still unclear, and the location of the generator of the 40 Hz AER is not known. In our series of 76 patients we compared the 40 Hz AER to the BAEP. In most cases loss or preservation of the BAEP coincided with the 40 Hz AER. In a few exceptional cases, however, it did not[2].

As wave V of the BAEP is normally generated no later than 6.4ms after the stimulus and the normal 40 Hz AER latency of the first peak (P1) may be as late as 9.3ms, we concluded that the generator of P1 is probably further up the auditory pathway than the generator of wave V. The inferior colliculus has been suggested as the generator of wave V. As purely temporal lesions have no effect on the 40 Hz AER, midbrain/thalamic structures have been suggested as a likely site of the generator[4]. This would explain the examples of contradictory findings of the 40 Hz AER and the BAEP we have found: In upper pontine lesions the BAEP was partly preserved but the bloc of the auditory pathway was complete and the 40 Hz AER was not preserved. The bloc of the auditory pathway may be incomplete in some lesions during the process of developing brain death. The volley passing through may not be enough to produce a BAEP but enough to produce the 40 Hz AER, which may be more sensitive possibly because of a resonance phenomenon. Therefore the recording of the 40 Hz AER in addition to the BAEP during the development of brain death may be advisable.

To summarize the neurosurgical management of injuries of the temporal region, no more than one hour should pass until CT and eventually the evacuation of a haematoma can be carried out[6,7]. Depending on the further clinical course of events, delayed haematomas, chronic subdural haematomas and depressed skull fractures and otorrhea must not be overlooked. Evoked potentials have proved to be valuable for the diagnosis of a lesion of the auditory pathway, for the assessment of prognosis and for the declaration of brain death.

REFERENCES

1. Benzer A, Mitterschiffthaler G, Prugger M, Rumpl E (1987) Innsbruck-Koma-Skala versus Glasgow-Coma Scale. Notfallmed 13:41-50

2. Firsching R (1989) The brain-stem and 40 Hz middle latency auditory evoked potentials in brain death. Acta Neurochir 101:52-55

3. Firsching R, Frowein RA (1990) Evoked potentials in head injury. In: Advances in Neurotraumatology. Ed.: Vigouroux. in press

4. Firsching R, Luther J, Eidelberg E, Brown WE, Story JL (1987) 40 Hz - middle latency auditory evoked response in comatose patients. Electroenceph clin Neurophysiol 67:213-216

5. Frowein RA. (1976) Classification of coma. Acta Neurochir 34:5-10

6. Frowein RA, Firsching R (1990) Classification of head injuries. In: Injuries of the brain and skull, Handbook of clinical neurology. Eds.: Vinken, P. and Bruyn, G., North-Holland publ. comp., Amsterdam, Oxford, American Elsevier publ. comp. co. inc., New York, Vol 23, in press

7. Galambos R, Makeig S, Talmachoff P (1981) A 40 Hz auditory potential recorded from the human scalp. Proc Natl Acad Sci 78 (4):2643-2647

8. Jennett B, Bond M (1975) Assessment of outcome after severe brain damage. Lancet I:480-484

9. Karimi A, Sanker P (1990) Traumatische intrakranielle Hämatome. In: Platt, Vosschulte, Fahlbusch (eds.), Handbuch der Gerontologie, Vol. 4, Fischer, Stuttgart

10. Muller G (1976) Classification of head injuries. In: Injuries of the brain and skull. Handbook of clinical neurology. Eds.: Vinken, P. and Bruyn, G., North-Holland publ. comp., Amsterdam, Oxford, American Elsevier publ. comp. co. inc., New York, Vol 23, pp 1-23

11. Starmark JE, Stålhammar D, Holmgren E, Rosander B (1988) A comparison of the Glasgow Coma Scale and the Reaction Level Scale (RLS85). J Neurosurg 69:699-706

12. Teasdale G, Jennett B (1974) Assessment of Coma and impaired consciousness. Lancet II, 81-84

HEAD TRAUMA WITH ASSOCIATED VERTIGO

Wallace Rubin, M.D.

Clinical Professor Otorhinolaryngology and Biocommunication
Louisiana State University School of Medicine
New Orleans, Louisiana

Patients who have sustained a head injury with a temporal bone fracture ususally have some neurologic symptoms at the time of the accident. These neurological symptoms may mask the auditory and vestibular symptoms. On awakening from unconscious- ness if such has been present, patients with transverse temporal bone fractures will be aware that there is no hearing on the involved side. Shortly after the accident, there will be complaints of dizziness and findings of spontaneous nystagmus. Most patients are seen a number of days following the injury. There is, by this time, no question about the complete unilateral hearing loss on the side of the injury, and sufficient time has elapsed for improvement and of the vestibular complaints. Evaluation of this kind of patient will reveal a complete sensorineural hearing loss on the side of the injury. Spontaneous nystagmus and a complete loss of vestibular response on the side of the injury can also be confirmed on testing.

Since the eight cranial nerve has been severed, then no corrective treatment is possible. Most patients compensate for their dizziness within three to six months and need no further help in this regard. During the time of compensation, sympto- matic therapy for the dizziness may be indicated. Explanation as to the cause of the problem and the reasons for the inability to correct the situation are important for the patient.

In the patient with a longitudinal temporal bone fracture, there is a history of head trauma with or without basal skull fracture and other neurologic symptoms. There may or may not be specific complaints referable to the eighth cranial nerve. If they are present, the severity of the complaints depends on the time that the patient is seen in relation to the accident. The longitudinal temporal bone fracture can cause bleeding into the middle ear cavity. Blood can therefore be found in either the ear canal or in the middle ear. There can also be a perforation of the tympanic membrane. The patient may or may not have a hearing loss and, in many instances, complains of dizziness which is more marked on head movement. The patient may not complain of dizziness until allowed to move around in bed or allowed to be out of bed following the control of the more serious systemic and neurologic problems.

Sophisticated radiography reveals the longitudinal fracture through the temporal bone. There may be hearing loss, although the hearing may be within normal limits. If there is a hearing loss, the patient may have a mild sensorineural involvement, which may be primarily high tone or a conductive hearing loss of various degrees. Vestibular evaluation may reveal a positional nystagmus. The direction of the positional nystagmus will have no localizing value in terms of the ear involved. There may be a reduced vestibular response on the side of the fracture, depending on whether the fracture line has extended through a semicircular canal. In most individuals these symptoms persist for months and even years. The control of the vertiginous problem is primarily symptomatic. This, incidentally, is the kind of patient in whom there can be recurrent episodes of meningitis as a result of cerebrospinal fluid leakage through a fracture in the tegmen.

Many individuals who suffer head injuries with no basal skull fracture complain of dizziness that is persistent, annoying, and difficult to control. These patients frequently have not had the benefit of a complete evaluation to confirm the source of their complaints. The site of damage to the vestibular system may be in the ear opposite the side of the injury. More than likely the anatomic difficulty is neurovascular or vascular in origin. The abnormalities may involve both the auditory and vestibular mechanisms. In most instances, though, the findings are related predominantly to the vestibular mechanism.

Auditory evaluation is usually normal, and the vestibular evaluation reveals either a spontaneous or positional nystagmus. There may also be a reduced vestibular response on the side of the trauma. In many instances, in addition to the spontaneous or positional nystagmus, the ABB or SBB caloric response may reveal an asymmetry or preponderance. This might indicate that the brainstem or central control areas are involved. It is most important that an adequate explanation of the problem be presented to the patient and that vestibular habituation exercises be utilized to help the brain recycling for compensation of the vestibular symptoms. Vertigo following head injury of this kind is usually of long duration and may not respond well to any mode of therapy.

ENG recordings are an absolute requirement for confirmation of vestibular diagnosis in whiplash injuries, head trauma with longitudinal fracture of the temporal bone, and head trauma without fracture.

FRACTURES OF THE SKULL BASE

FUNCTIONAL COMPLICATIONS AFTER THE OTOBASAL FRACTURE

LUTZ KESSLER

Department of Otorhinolaryngology, Medical Academy "Carl Gustav Carus" Dresden, Fetscherstrasse 74, DDR-8019 Dresden (GDR)

INTRODUCTION

The number of the patients with skull base fracture has increased remarkably in the recent years. The greatest reason for it is considered to be the increase of the traffic accidents. Our clinical experience proved the increasing tendency not only in otobasal fractures but also in rhinobasal fractures. Most of the victims were young male adults. Especially the motorbike drivers were frequently encountered.

One must always keep in mind that one fifth of the patients of skull base trauma are suffering from polytrauma. The injuries in chest and abdomen are accompanied most frequently.

The intracranial bleeding can lead the patients to the fatal course and consequently it is mostly feared. It could occur even long time after the preceding injury. The computerized tomography helps us to detect the intracranial bleeding in its early stage and can enable us to treat the patients in the proper time.

The skull base fracture most always be considered as the combined injuries of cranium, brain and sensory organs.

The long lasting functional complications of otobasal fracture are typically: 1. hearing impairment, 2. dysequilibrium and 3. facial paresis.

As it is well known, the otobasal fracture is distinguished between the longitudinal and transvers fracture. The prominent symptoms of the pyramidal longitudinal fractures are manifested through the injuries of the middle ear such as external ear bleeding or conductive hearing loss. On the other hand the main symptoms of pyramidal transvers fractures are characterized by the injury of inner ear such as vestibular function loss. The facial nerve is affected much more frequently in transvers fractures than longitudinal fracture. Sometimes otobasal fracture occurs in combination with rhinobasal fracture. Bilateral otobasal fracture is also possible.

RESULTS OF EXAMINATION IN EARLY STAGE

Eighty five patients of otobasal fractures were treated in ward in the Department of Otorhinolaryngology of the Medical Academy "Carl Gustav Carus" in Dresden from 1973 to 1988. The dominating number of the vistims (38 cases, 45 %) were found to be in second and third decade of liefe. The rate of the male patients amounted to 82 % (Fig. 1).

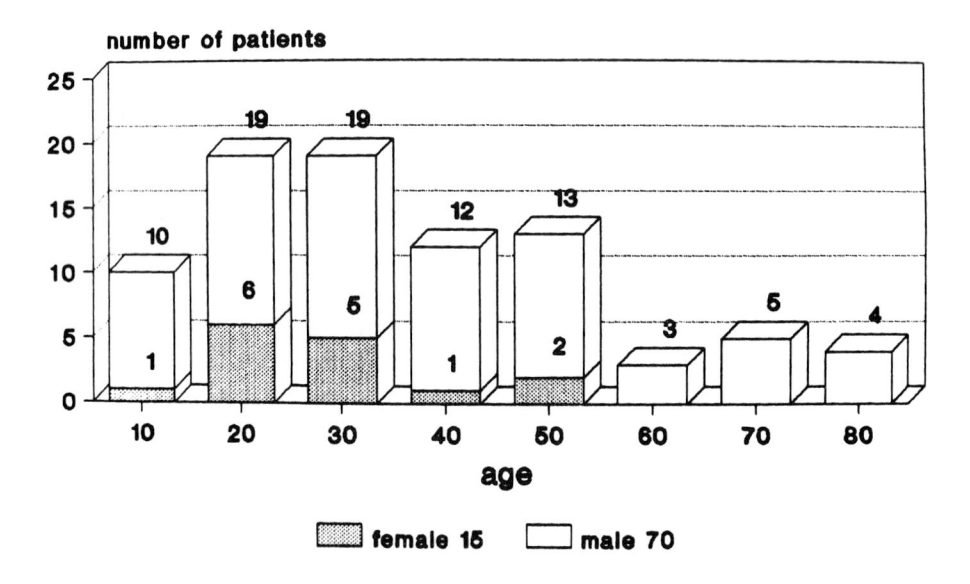

Fig. 1. Distribution of sex and age in 85 patients with otobasal fracture.

The most frequent cause of the otobasal fractures were traffic accidents in 55 % (47 cases). The rate of the patients who drunk alcohol prior to the accident was considerably high (Fig. 2).

Among the 85 patients, 74 patients (87 %) suffered from the longitudinal fracture and the remaining 11 (13 %) the transvers fracture. The injuries were unilateral in all patients. In 12 patients the otobasal fracture was combined with the rhinobasal fracture (Fig. 3).

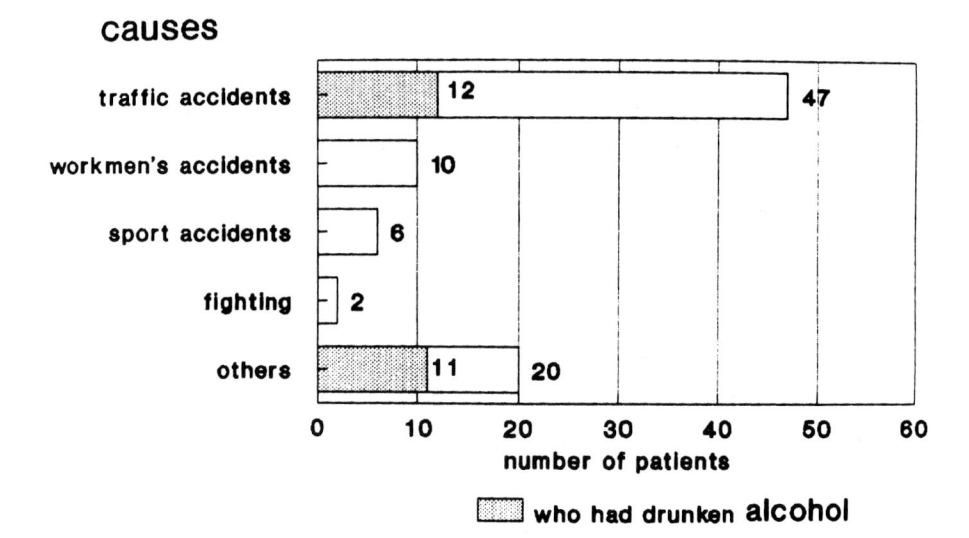

Fig. 2. The cause of the otobasal fracture in 85 cases

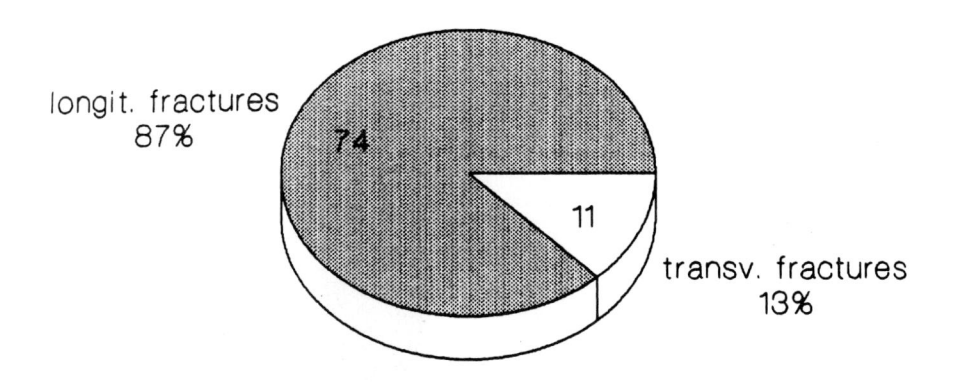

Fig. 3. The form of otobasal fractures in 85 Cases

In consequence bleeding or discharge of cerebrospinal fluid from the external ear canal was observed in 68 patients (80 %). Hearing impairment was found in 64 cases (75 %). Cerebral nerve palsy - mostly of the facial nerve - occured directly after the accident in 60 cases (71 %). However only 10 patients (12 %) complained of dizziness (or vertigo) or showed nystagmus after the injury. 33 patients (39 %) with otobasal fracture lost counsciousness after the accident.

RESULTS OF EXAMINATION IN LATE STAGE

Sixty patients of otobasal fracture, who were hospitalized in our clinic, came to the controlling examination lately. The onset of the accident was at least 6 month prior to the examination with the average of 2.5 years. The patients underwent: 1. the physical examination, 2. otoscopy, 3. audiometry, 4. facial nerve function test and 5. vestibular function test.

24 of the patients (40 %) were free of complaints. Among the 36 patients, who had complaints or showed symptoms, conductive hearing loss was found in 29 patients, facial paresis in 8. The unilateral vestibular function loss combined with deafness was found in 7 patients (Fig. 4).

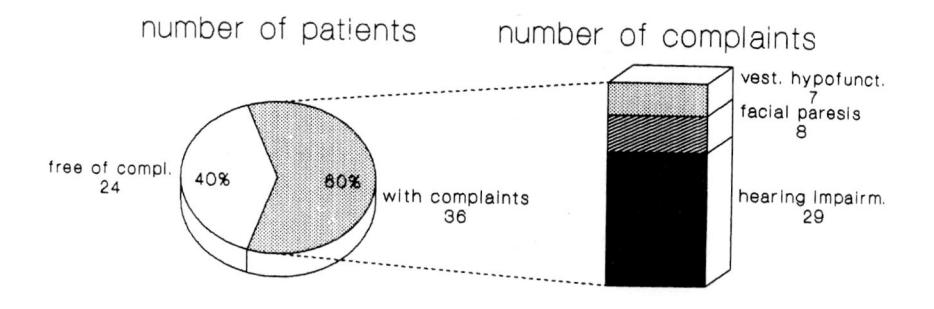

Fig. 4. Complaints of 60 patients after the otobasal fracture.

The good recovery tendency of peripheral facial paresis after the fracture was noteworthy. Among the 39 patients, who showed facial paresis shortly after the accident and were called to the controlling examination, facial paresis was recognized in only 8 patients, 7 of whom were the patients of transvers fracture.

Surprisingly at the time of the controlling examination spontanous nystagmus was no more to be seen in all of the 7 patients of transvers fracture with total vestibular function loss. It is considered to be due to the central vestibular compensation, because the caloric response of the damaged side remained unevoked even in the repeated examination.

SUMMARY

Otobasal fracture belongs to one of the rare diseases in the field of otorhinolaryngology. The most frequent cause is a traffic accident. The dominating vistims are the young male adults. Pyramidal longitudinal fracture is encountered much frequently than transvers fracture. According to our late examination results the dizziness the patients with pyramidal fracture decreased remarkably within a few month due to the central compasation mechanism. The peripheral facial paresis caused by the pyramidal longitudinal fracture showed also preferable tendency of spontaneous recovery.

BEHAVIOUR OF THE SPEECH ANALYSIS AFTER FRONTO-BASAL SKULL FRACTURES

H.G. DIEROFF, G. SCHUHMANN, JENA, DDR

The basis of the present study is a paper of the year 1975 in which we tried to prove central hearing damage in cases of fronto-basal skull fractures. At that time we used some tests of subjective audiometry of central hearing damage such as pure-tone hearing level, direction audiometry, dichotic speech discrimination test according to Feldmann; furthermore we tried to differentiate between central and peripheric damage in cases of a positive dichotic speech discrimination test with the help of impedance measurement. Measurements taken in 23 adults showed only a slight damage in the high-frequency range of the conventional audiogram but there was diminished direction hearing as a result of a possible central lesion.

Our experience enabled us to concentrate the test programme. In the meantime we have developed a distorted speech test based on the Freiburg speech test, whereby only the words were distorted. This test makes the proof of central hearing possible in a very efficient way.

The distorted speech audiometry is an excellent instrument to diagnose central hearing damage and a sign of degeneration in hearing nerve. The results of speech discrimination of non-distorted and distorted words with an intensity of 50, 70 and 90 dB on the attenuator of the speech audiometer are expressed as a quotient in persons with normal hearing, conductive or combined hearing loss with only slight sensorineural damage; here we found a distortion quotient from 1,1 to 1,49. In cases of sensorineural hearing losses the distorsion quotient is mostly fluctuating about 2 - 3. But it can attain very high values of 20 and more or infinite. The high values are caused either by a degeneration of the hearing nerve as in cases of acoustic neurinoma or by central hearing loss. Thus in cases of elderly patients we can see a clear increase of the distorsion value after the 60th year of life. Our present investigations are based on results in 22 persons. We found a good agreement of the results in the pure-tone threshold measurement of the former study. In the same way our present investigation clearly shows a slight sensorineural

hearing loss in the high frequency area. The calculation of the
mean hearing loss of the frequencies of 500, 1000 and 2000 Hz
according to Hearing Aid International Commission brought about
nearly normal hearing levels corresponding to the age whose mean
value was calculated with about 24 years of life. The speech
reception threshold was nearly normal as was the mean hearing loss
of pure tone hearing. The up-to-now demonstrated data correspond
to those of the former study of 1975 which means in general that
we found a small diminution of the pure-tone threshold in the high-
frequency area in cases of fronto-basal skull fractures without
measurable changes of the speech reception by the usual method
in our country, in our case the Freiburg speech test.

But if we tested the patients after fronto-basal skull fractures
with distorted speech, we have seen a clear increase of the
distorsion quotient in our investigations. The comparison of the
distorsion quotients of our patients with a normal hearing group
shows a distinct rise especially in lower intensity in spite of
the small number of adults.

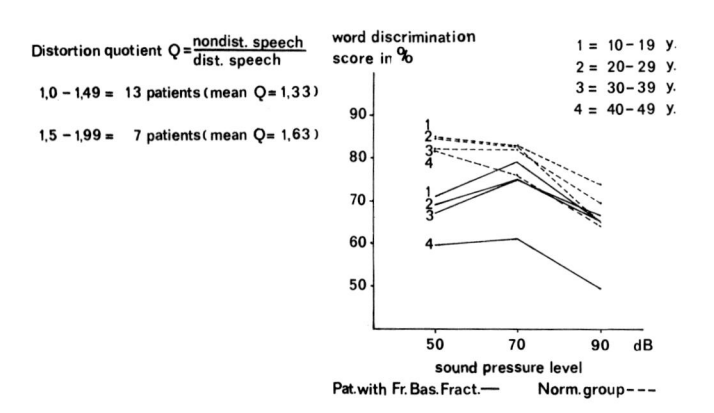

Distortion quotient $Q = \frac{\text{nondist. speech}}{\text{dist. speech}}$

1,0 – 1,49 = 13 patients (mean Q= 1,33)

1,5 – 1,99 = 7 patients (mean Q= 1,63)

word discrimination score in %

1 = 10 - 19 y.
2 = 20 - 29 y.
3 = 30 - 39 y.
4 = 40 - 49 y.

sound pressure level

Pat. with Fr. Bas. Fract.—   Norm. group - - -

As the growth of the distorsion quotient is caused either
by the process of degeneration in the hearing nerve itself or by
the central mechanism of the hearing system we have to ask, where
the damage may be localized. In our investigations in 1975 we
used the behaviour of the acoustically stimulated reflex of the
muscle stapedius by impedance measurement device, but we did not
found some hints of a presence of a degeneration in the hearing

nerve. According to the present knowledge about the pathophysiology of the inner ear it may be sure that such a small pure-tone hearing loss in the high frequency area cannot be caused in the inner ear cell layers or in the hearing nerve. The studies of Spoendlin, 1969, and especially of Hamernik and others, 1988, about the qualitative correlation between hair cell loss and hearing level makes clear that a diminution of the pure-tone hearing threshold up to about 30 dB hearing loss level may be caused only by a damage in the outer hair cell layer only as a sign of a contusio labyrinthi. In thus is in contrast to the destruction of the inner hair cell layer because there follows a process of degeneration in the hearing nerve according to Spoendlin. Therefore it may be sure that the rise of the distorsion quotient is the consequence of a central lesion which developed during the accident of the skull. Since we had measured an increase of the distorsion quotient after the 60th year of life we assume that adults with fronto-basal skull fracture may suffer more from speech discrimination difficulties in aging than other people.

REFERENCES

1. Dieroff, H.-G.: Zentrale Hörschäden bei frontobasalen Brüchen. Laryngo-Rhino-Otol. 54 (1975) 734-740

2. Dieroff, H.-G. u. W. Meißner: Verhallter Freiburger Sprachtest. Laryngo-Rhino-Otol. 64 (1985) 466-469

3. Dieroff, H.-G. u. W. Mangoldt: Erfahrungen mit dem verhallten Freiburger Sprachtest - Diagnostik und Rehabilitation von Hörstörungen.
Laryngo-Rhino-Otol. 68 (1989) 372-378

THE FUNCTION OF THE VESTIBULAR SYSTEM AFTER CRANIAL INJURY
A CRITICAL REVIEW

P. CHRIST, M. MEICHELBÖCK, W. GOERTZEN, S. WOLF, C.T. HAID
ENT-Clinic, University Erlangen-Nuremberg, Erlangen, F.R.G.

SUMMARY:

In a retrospective study, we compared the neurootological examination results of 123 patients, whose case history indicated a head trauma.
Different main symptoms are presented.
Answers are given to questions about the necessity of a vestibular examination after cranial injuries and the sensitivity of different parts of the investigation. The results of this critical review show, that central vestibular and combined vestibular lesions provide worse results and give dubious prognosis concerning the vestibular compensation.

INTRODUCTION:

Vertigo is a well known and frequent result following cranial injuries, but is it a cardinal symptom?
Which different characteristics of vertigo are patients complaining about and what kind of vestibular lesion appears most frequently?
How is a neurootological examination being able to give prognostic appraisal concerning the vestibular compensation and which significance show the different examination-parts?

MATERIAL AND METHOD:

To give an answer to these and other questions, 123 patients (76 male and 47 female) with cranial injuries between the years of 1982 and 1989 were subjected to a retrospective study.
All patients underwent a complete neurootological examination, consisting of an investigation for different nystagmus (spontaneous nystagmus, gaze nystagmus and positional- and positioning nystagmus, all under Frenzel's glasses and with the aid of electronystagmography), the tracing of pathological vestibulo-spinal reflexes, eye-tracking tests and the examination of the caloric excitability and the cranial nerves.

RESULTS:

Concussion and contusion of the brain were the most frequent diagnosis of our patients, but we also saw a relatively high number of petrous bone fractures, mostly of younger persons, as a frequent reason for cranial nerve lesions (Table 1; 3).
The positional test showed the most frequent pathological findings, followed by the caloric stimulation and the vestibulo-spinal reflexes. A spontaneous nystagmus was seen in only 23% of all patients (Table 2).

DIAGNOSIS OF PATIENTS AFTER CRANIAL INJURY
Examination period 1982 - 1989
(n = 123; 76 male, 47 female)

a) Concussion / Contusion of the brain	33 %
b) Concussion / Contusion of the labyrinth	24 %
c) Combination of a) and b)	13 %
d) Fracture of the petrous bone	21 %
e) Others	9 %

Table 1

PATHOLOGICAL VESTIBULAR RESULTS AFTER CRANIAL INJURY
(n = 123)

1. Spontaneous nystagmus	23 %
2. Gaze nystagmus	8 %
3. Positional/ Positioning nystagmus	50 %
4. Vestibulo-spinal reflexes	40 %
5. Eye tracking test	19 %
6. Caloric test	40 %
7. Cranial nerves	25 %

Table 2

At the time of the vestibular examination, 85 patients (respectively 69%) declared on inquiry, that they were still suffering from vertigo or dysequilibrium. Interestingly enough, only 30% did indicate vertigo as a main symptom. Hearingloss is the symptom with the highest incidence; together with vertigo, it was the reason for nearly two thirds of our patients, to come to a physical examination (Table 3).
More than half of the persons, who complained about equilibrium disturbance, reported a positional or positioning vertigo (Table 4).
Almost the same percentage of these patients showed abnormalities in the positional test. Very interesting is the fact, that the so-called benign paroxysmal positioning nystagmus occured only in 2% of our cases.
One third of the patients, who complained about unsystematic vertigo, reported of a continuous strange feeling (like being drunken or reeling), which increased under physical or psychical stress conditions (Table 4).

Table 3

MAIN SYMPTOMS AFTER CRANIAL INJURY (n = 123)	
Hearingloss	35 %
Vertigo	30 %
Disturbance of smell or taste	7 %
Ear bleeding	7 %
Facial paresis	3 %
Others	18 %

Table 4

CHARACTERISTICS OF VERTIGO AFTER CRANIAL INJURY (n = 85)	
1. Continous vertigo - acute	8 %
- chronical	6 %
2. Positional/ Positioning vertigo	55 %
3. Unsystematic vertigo	31 %

To find a more distinct differentiation in the vestibular findings, 85 patients suffering from vertigo, were confronted with a group of 27 patients, who actually had stated in their case history vertigo complaints immediately after the trauma and a certain period of time afterwards, but did not maintain any vertigo at the time of the vestibular examination (Table 5).

Group A, patients without vertigo, revealed a relatively high number of peripheral vestibular lesions.

On the contrary, group B, patients suffering from dizziness and dysequilibrium at the vestibular examination, showed a high incidence of central vestibular or combined (central and peripheral) vestibular lesions. A sign therefore was the higher incidence of gaze nystagmus and of disturbed eye trackings in this group.

In direct comparison, nearly all pathological vestibular findings in group B were more severe than in group A (Table 6).

Table 5

CLASSIFICATION OF THE VESTIBULAR LESION AFTER CRANIAL INJURY	Group A (no vertigo) n = 27	Group B (vertigo) n = 85
Peripheral vestibular lesion	44 %	20 %
Central vestibular lesion	15 %	34 %
Combined lesion	11 %	28 %
No vestibular lesion	30 %	18 %

Table 6

PATHOLOGICAL VESTIBULAR RESULTS AFTER CRANIAL INJURY	Group A (no vertigo) n = 27	Group B (vertigo) n = 85
1. Spontaneous nystagmus	11 %	28 %
2. Gaze nystagmus	4 %	11 %
3. Positional/ Positioning nystagmus	41 %	54 %
4. Vestibulo-spinal reflexes	37 %	44 %
5. Eye tracking test	7 %	24 %
6. Caloric test	37 %	44 %
7. Cranial nerves	33 %	19 %

Among the single examinations concerning vestibular findings, the positional test again is the most sensitive one.

DISCUSSION:

Only about one third of all patients complained of vertigo as a cardinal symptom spontaneously, but upon questioning, more than 80% stated, that they had experienced vertigo after the trauma (6).
This observation permits the conclusion, that with all patients, whose case history indicates a head trauma, a vestibular examination has to be recommended. The positional test showed the most frequent pathological findings (4).
Contrary to the caloric test, a maximal stimulus of the superior vestibular nerve, the positional test seems to be a threshold stimulus of the whole labyrinth and central vestibular pathways.
It presented itself as the most sensitive partial examination of all neurootological tests (4,5). We would like to emphasize, that in our opinion, this test must be performed in every vestibular examination, even if the patient does not complain of positioning or positional vertigo (2,6).
The fact, that nearly half of the patients of group A (i.e., patients without any subjective feeling of vertigo or dysequilibrium at the time of the vestibular examination) presented peripheral vestibular disturbances, shows the good prognosis, to compensate such lesions (11).
On the contrary, group B (i.e., patients with vertigo at the time of the neurootological testing) shows a high incidence of central and combined vestibular lesions. Nearly 40% of these patients came more than 1 year after the trauma to the vestibular examination, still suffering from vertigo.
The reason for this might be a prolonged or reduced vestibular compensation as a result of lesions of the central vestibular pathways or nuclei (11).

REFERENCES:

1. Baloh RW, et al (1985) Rotational testing in patients with bilateral peripheral vestibular disease. Laryngoscope 95: 85-88.

2. Barber HO (1964) Positional nystagmus, especially after head injury. Laryngoscope 74: 891-944.

3. Goertzen W, Christ P (1990) Diagnostik und Therapie von Läsionen des VII. Hirnnerven nach otobasalen Frakturen. Revue de laryngologie, otologie, rhinologie. In Druck.

4. Haid CT (1977) Das Positiogramm, eine Aufzeichnungsmethode der Lageprüfung in der Neurootologie. Laryng. Rhinol. 56, 1037-1045.

5. Haid CT, Graeff G (1983) Vertigo, a frequent symptom following cranial injury. In: Claussen CF (Hrsg.), Gesellschaft für Neurootologie und Äquilibriometrie, Band IX: 22.

6. Keim R (1985) The pitfalls of limiting ENG testing to patients with vertigo. Laryngoscope 95, 1208-1212.

7. Kornhuber H (1966) Physiologie und Klinik des zentral- vestibulären Systems. In: Berendes, Link, Zöllner, Handbuch der Hals-Nasen-Ohrenheilk., Bd. III. Thieme, Stuttgart.

8. Kumar A, Dale L (1984) Diagnostic value of vestibular function tests: An analysis of 200 consecutive cases. Laryngoscope 94, 1435-1442.

9. McClure JA, Lycett P (1983) Vestibular Asymetrie. Arch Otolaryngol-Vol 109.

10. Megighian D (1984) The physiopathological, clinical and theapeutic aspects of vertigo in peripheral vestibular lesions. Arch. Otorhinolayngol 241, 23-34.

11. Saito Y, et al (1983) Neurootological study of positional vertigo caused by head injury. Auris Nasus Larynx. 13 Suppl.1, 69-73.

12. Tuohimaa P (1978) Vestibular disturbance after acute mild head injury. Acta Otolaryngol. Suppl. 359, 3-59.

Dr. med. P. Christ
ENT-Clinic
University Erlangen-Nuremberg
Waldstr. 1
8520 Erlangen

OTONEUROLOGICAL PROFILE OF PATIENTS EXAMINED
FOR POSTTRAUMATIC SEQUELLAE

Marcel E. Norré, Dpt Otoneurology & Equilibriometry - University Hospitals - LEUVEN (Belgium).

Out of the patients, examined for otoneurological disorders and allied problems, a separate group concerns those where head trauma is considered the cause of the complaints.

METHODS AND PATIENTS

In a review of 1100 patients, examined in our department, we found 104 posttraumatic cases (9.45%). These patients can be subdivided into two groups. A first group (40%) includes the patients referred in order to make a statement of their complaints and dysfunctions in the scope of a legal report. A second group concerns those referred for treatment.

The trauma dated from more than 1 year in 53, between 6 weeks and 1 year in 42 and only in 9 cases from less than 6 weeks.

The patients were examined according to the usual scheme described elsewhere (1).

RESULTS

Complaints

Spontaneous vertigo with typical rotatory sensation was mentioned by only 5 cases, whereas atypical spontaneous dizziness was the complaint of 24 patients. Most patients complained of **instability and/or provoked vertigo**. In 7 a typical provoked rotatory vertigo (BPPV) was described, but the vast majority of patients described an atypical provoked dizziness (n=56). Instability (n=42) was mostly an accompanying complaint, in 5 it was the only complaint. In 6 patients no vertigo was present.

Functional evaluations

We compare two sets of examinations:
1/ the caloric and rotation tests for the vestibulo-ocular reflex (VOR), and 2/ the posturographic examinations (PG), for the vestibulospinal reflex (VSR) (3).

In 23 patients the findings were completely normal in VOR and VSR testing. Both test-sets indicated abnormal findings in 26. In only 12 the VOR tests alone showed abnormal results, whereas in 43 only the VSR tests were disturbed. This means that generally these patients showed more disturbance in the VSR than in the VOR tests (69 versus 38). Concordant findings are found in 49, discordant ones in 55 patients.

Concerning the VOR-tests (caloric and rotation tests), both were negative in 68 patients. The caloric tests were positive in only 14 cases, whereas the rotation tests in 24, whereof 22 with symmetrical caloric results. This means that out of the 14 cases with unilateral hypofunction, 12 were compensated in the rotation tests. Concordance is found in 70 cases.

VHT-testbattery

In only 24 patients (40%) a testing on the VHT-testbattery could be performed (2).
In 12 it was positive:
- 4 patients with atypical vertigo had no favorable effect of the proposed treatment.
- out of 4 patients with typical BPPV, three were completely cured by VHT - 1 typical case turned over to atypical dizziness.
- 4 patients showed a stereotypical pattern.

Such a **stereotypical pattern** means that for each maneuver the patient gives an identical response: the same intensity, the same duration and this in nearly all 19 maneuvers. This pattern could be attributed to "insurance disease".

DISCUSSION

Head trauma is a non-negligible cause of complaints in the otoneurological sphere. Generally, several structures and functions are involved. So is not only the labyrinth involved in the concussion of the head, but at the same time the endocranial content is shaked. This means that multiple foci of dysfunction may be present. Pure peripheral otovestibular lesion remains a rarity. In most of cases some central components are present. In this way, most of lesions are to be considered as **combined**. Peripheral loss of function, which must be centrally compensated, can have difficulties to reach a good compensation because of central components. Moreover, cortical and psychological involvement itself induces sensations of vague and atypical dizziness. So it occurs that such a dizziness complaint continues after correct and successful treatment of typical peripheral vertigo (cfr "stereotypical" pattern)

Furtheron it has to be noticed that the relationship with persons examined for legal report is very different from that with patients coming for medical help. The first group is mostly reticent and not cooperating. They consider the whole procedure as imposed and annoying, whereas they generally try to exaggerate their complaints.

In the patients we could examine for sequella of trauma, we found an increasing number of abnormal results, comparing caloric, rotation tests and posturography. In this way it appeared that the caloric test, fundamentally indicating a peripheral disturbance, had the least number of positive findings. The rotation tests were more frequently positive and this strikingly as a separate finding, i.e. in most cases with symmetrical caloric tests. This is likely to be rather correlated with central imbalance. In the same sense can be interpreted the still higher frequency of VSR disturbances and of separate PG abnormalities with normal VOR tests. These findings support the assumption that in these posttraumatic cases central components are dominatingly present.

As a general conclusion, we can say that in, our group of patients, the positive data are rather poor. This may be due to the fact that most patients were examined very late related to the time of trauma. Concerning the VOR, in 65% of the patients the classical tests remain negative. The complaints were dominatingly atypical. Complaints as well as findings point to rather vague central involvement, whereas typical peripheral pathology was rather rare.

REFERENCES

1. NORRÉ ME (1986): A concept of practical functional evaluation of a dizzy patient. In CLAUSSEN CF, KIRTANE MV (eds): Vertigo, nausea, tinnitus and hearing loss in cardiovascular diseases. Elsevier Science Publishers Amsterdam pp. 273-278.

2. NORRÉ ME, BECKERS A (1989): Vestibular habituation training: exercise treatment for vertigo based upon the habituation effect. Otolaryngol Head Neck Surg 101: 14-19.

3. NORRÉ ME: Posturographic findings in posttraumatic patients. Same volume.

THE NEUROOTOLOGICAL FINDINGS FOLLOWING MILD HEAD INJURY

AUGUSTO CASANI, PIERLUIGI GHILARDI, BRUNO FATTORI, ROBERTA VANNUCCHI
Institute of Otolaryngology, University of Pisa
via Savi, 10, 56100 Pisa (Italia)

INTRODUCTION

Vertigo and disorders of equilibrium can be considered as the most frequent sequaele of Head Injury (HI). Otherwise our knowledge of the mechanisms and the ethiopathogenesys of vestibular disturbances produced by HI is still not completely clear. From an otoneurological point of view, we can divide post-traumatic vertigo into two types : with temporal bone fracture and without temporal bone fracture (labyrinthine concussion). Vestibular disturbances following HI can be due to a central or a peripheral mechanism of lesion : vestibular damage can be produced by a post-traumatic pressure wave in the inner ear (1), or because of a vasomotoric damage (2) associated with microtrombs in the little vessels of the inner ear (3). Also ischemic and/or hemorragic damage in the brainstem (5) or functional lesions of the neurotrasmitters (4) were considered as possible causes of post-traumatic vestibular involvement.

A large controversy exists about the peripheral or central origin of post-traumatic vertigo (1,5,6,7,8). Also regarding the factors affecting the onset and the evolution of post-traumatic vertigo like the age of the patient, the severity of HI, the site of HI, there are a lot of different opinions (5,7,8).

In a great number of cases, post-traumatic vertigo can be due to a damage of the soft tissue of the neck, expecially in the case of the whiplash injury (WI). The mechanism of lesion was considered of vascular (9), propioceptive (10) or symphatetic origin (11).

MATERIAL AND METHODS

We have studied 514 patients (281 males and 233 females) aging from 9 to 74 years, complaining of post-traumatic dizziness and attending to the laboratory of Otoneurology of the ENT Clinic of the University of Pisa, in the period 1985-1988. 412 patients (80.2%) suffered from a mild HI and 102 (19.8%) suffered from WI. 279 of the patients suffering from HI had a period of unconsciousness whose duration was no longer than 2 hours. Patients suffering from intracranial hemorrages or temporal bone fractures were excluded. The vestibular function was assessed by a complete electronystagmographic recording comprehensive of the following tests : a saccadic test with the patient moving his eyes between 3 LEDs 10° apart; velocity and accuracy were evaluated semiquantitatively by direct ispection; PETT with the patient following a pendulum with a maximal velocity of 30°/s at a distance of 2 m ; a search for spontaneous, head shaking, positional and positioning nystagmus ; a search for cervical nystagmus as described by Greiner et al[12];a bithermal caloric test ; directional preponderance and canal paresis were manually evaluated resulting in a computation of the total number of the beats during the culmination ; a visual suppression test. By using the chi-square test, the results were compared with those obtained in the control group of 107 normal subjects in the same range of age. All the patients were previously evaluated from a neurological point of view.

RESULTS

202 (49%) out of the 412 patients suffering from HI showed pathological vestibular results, 141 (70%) of peripheral type and 61 (30%) of central type. The percentage of pathological results (in the whole and divided in central and peripheral) showed no significant difference regarding to the patients' age (Fig.1).

On the whole, the most frequent vestibular results following HI were canal paresis (92 cases, 22.8%) and paroxysmal positional vertigo (ppv)(77 cases, 18.6%). The incidence of ppv showed a clear increase with the raising of the patients'age (Fig.2). We also found a positional stationary ny (PSny) in 28 cases, an head shaking ny in 38 cases, a caloric hyperreactivity in 12 cases, an alteration of saccades in 25 cases and of the PETT in 47 cases. In 12 patients a rebound ny was discovered and in 2 cases a fixation nystagmus was registered.

We didn't find a statistical significant correlation between vestibular disturbances and site of HI (43% in frontal HI, 54% in parieto-temporal HI and 51% in occipital HI). The comparison between the site of HI and Canal Paresis put in evidence that a monolateral labyrinthine hypofunction was more frequent after a parieto-temporal HI (22.4%) than after a frontal (10%) or occipital (12%) HI, while no difference was found about the bilateral hypofunction (6% for frontal HI, 8% for parieto-temporal HI and 4% for occipital trauma).

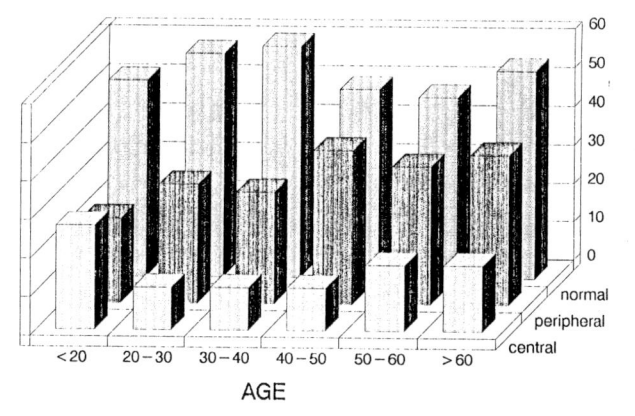

Fig. 1 : percentage of pathological results (divided in central and peripheral) in relation to the age of the patients.

PSny appeared more frequently after a frontal (7.6%) or parieto-temporal (6.4%) than after an occipital (1.2%) head trauma.

In the group of patients suffering from WI, 40 (39.2%) patients showed pathological vestibular lesions. The damage was considered of peripheral type in 27 cases (26.4%) and of central type in 13 cases (12.7%). Cervical nystagmus was the most common sign and it was found in 22 (21.5%) cases. This result was significantly different from the one of the control group (p 0.05). The incidence of cervical ny did not increase with the raising of the patients'age.Ppv was evident in 7 cases (6.8%) ; no correlation was found between cervical ny and PSny (p 0.001). PSny was found in 3 patients (3%).

DISCUSSION

Our results confirm the high incidence (49%) of the vestibular damage after mild HI, with a clear prevalence of the peripheral involvement (35% versus 14.8% of cases of central type of vestibular damage). The age of the patients doesn't

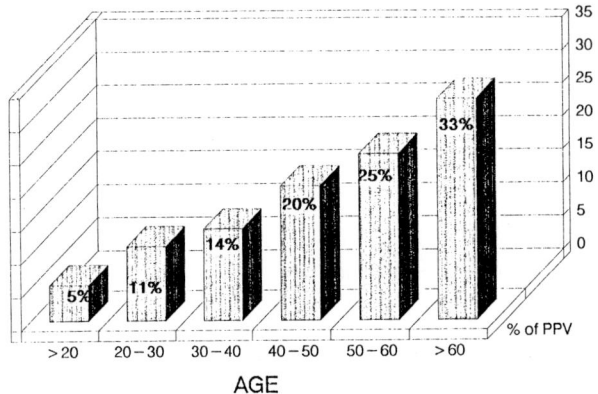

Fig 2 : percentage of post-traumatic ppv in relation to the age of the patients.

seem to have a great importance for producing a post-traumatic vestibular damage.

On the whole, the vestibular damage seems to have a poor correlation with the site of HI, while an evident correlation exists between the site of HI and the type of vestibular lesion, when it is present. So we can appreciate a great correlation between a lateral site of HI and the monolateral vestibular hypofunction; on the other hand, PSny is more frequent after a lateral or frontal than an occipital HI. Ppv and canal paresis were the most common vestibular results; the incidence of ppv showed an increase with the raising of the patients'age.

It must be stressed that an high percentage of the patients suffering from post-traumatic vertigo, showed a normal vestibular examination. In these cases psycological factors may play an important role, expecially if there is a medico-legal controversy (compensation neurosis).

In the group of the patients suffering from WI, the percentage of the subjects with vestibular disturbances was high (39%), but lower than the one encountered in the group of HI. Cervical ny was the commonest pathological sign; it was no age-related. So it is possible to consider cervical ny as the consequence of an irritative state of the spindles of the prevertebral and nucal muscles after WI (11), while no correlation seems to exist between cervical ny and cervical spondilosys. The absence of correlation among cervical ny and PSny indicates that PN ny should not be considered as a sign of pathological involvement of the C.O.R..

REFERENCES

1. Podoshin L, Fradis M (1975) Arch Otolaryngol 101 : 15
2. Brunner H (1925) Mschr Ohrenheilk 59 : 697
3. Axelsson A, Hallen C (1973) Acta Otolaryngol 76:136
4. Hyyppä MT, Vapalahti M (1977) Lancet 25:1367
5. Tuohimaa P (1978) Acta Otolaryngol Suppl 359
6. Kirtane MV, Medikeri SB, Karnik P (1982) J Laryngol Otol 96:521
7. Brancherau B, Hazan A, Sanson J, Peytral C, Toupet M (1988) Ann Otol 105:361
8. Schuknecht H, Davison R (1965) Arch Otolaryngol 63:513
9. Jongkees LBW (1969) Laryngoscope 79:1473
10. De Jong JMB, Bles W (1986) In : Disorders of posture and gait. Elsevier Publ.
11. Hinoki M (1985) Acta Otolaryngol Suppl 419:9
12. Greiner GF, Conraux C, Thiebaut MD (1967) Rev Neurol 117:677

VERTIGO AS A CAUSE OF ACUTE ADMISSION TO A NEUROLOGIC AND ENT DEPARTMENT

HANA KREJCOVA, RUDOLF CERNY, JAROSLAV JERABEK, JAROSLAV TOMAS
Medical Faculty Prague, Motol
Charles University,
Czechoslovakia

SUBJECTS AND METHODS :

Out of total of 10.299 patients admitted during last 5 years to the neurootologic and ENT departments of our medical faculty 301 suffered from vertigo causing the hospitalisation of these patients. Out of them 64 % complained of acute and 36 % of chronic vertiginous state. The mortality caused by consequences of acute vertigo reached 2.7 % at the neurologic department; none of the examined patients deceased at the ENT clinic. The age of the examined patients ranged between 15 - 83 years without any significant sex difference. All patients underwent otoneurologic examination, some of them also specialised examinations as spinal fluid, CT, MR, AG atc.

RESULTS :

From the total of admitted patients the incidence of vertigo did not exceed 2 %; true acute vertigo was present in 64 % of patients. Paroxysmal and sudden vertigo reached 38 % of patients, paroxysmal beeing in the majority of ENT and sudden vertigo in neurologic patients. Vertigo patients revealed stand and gait impairment in the whole of patients, nystagmus was present in 57 % of them, while other neurologic abnormalities were presented to a lesser degree, mostly in neurologic patients. More than 70 % of ENT patients suffered simultaneously from tinnitus and hypacusis, but accompanied vertigo only in a quarter of neurologic patients. BERA abnormalities did not reveal differences between either of these two groups of patients.

In 88 % present abnormality i X - ray pictures of cervical spine did not correspond with kinesiologic disorder found only in 31 % of patients.

22 % of patients revealed laboratory abnormalities in high blood sugar, cholesterol and triglycidaemia. In indicated cases spinal fluid examinations was performed and evaluated together with serological findings. We proved pathological findings in 40 % of examined patients, in 21 % of them the herpetic origin, in 19 % influenza, and in 9 % either CMV or Borrelia Burgdorferi were assessed; other cases remained unspecified.

As for the ethiopathogenetic parameters, the most numerous were inflamatory and vascular groups, each consisting of 43 patients. The inflammatory group revealed the neccessity to examine the cerebrospinal fluid and serum with antibodies to detect the cause of the inflammatory origin of vertigo. In the high percentage the vascular origin revealed the symptomatology of VBI. Among patients with plurifactorial origin of vertiginous states again most often clinical pattern of VBI was presented, caused by combination of cervical and vascular factors. " Cervicogennous " group of patients with kinesiological pathology of acute vertigo revealed peripheral vestibular syndrome and cochleovestibular disorder as the clinical pattern of this impairment, while unspecified cause of vertigo manifested itself mostly with the clinical picture of central syndrome. Other ethiopathogenetic groups with clinical pattern of acute vertigo as intoxication, truma, tumours, degenerative, psychogen and epileptic disorders consisted of small number of patients. The therapeutic efficacy in favour of amelioration of the vertiginous state prevailed in neurologic patients, especially in those with known diagnosis.

DISKUSSION :

In our group of patients a small amount of traumatic disorders is caused by admitting them to the traumatologic department where they are followed during acute hospitalisation.

The high incidence of X - ray pathologies of cervical spine is not congruent to kinesiological abnormalities so that it does not contribute substantially to the ethiopathogenesis of vertigo. Beside severe findings, it reflects only the structural changes accompanying the age and load of spinal cord. The functional blockage with its proprioceptive afferent influence seems to be the very reason of " cervicogenous " vertigo, not dependent upon the extent of structural vertebrogenous abnormalities.

In comparison to other vertigo studies (Aschoff 1978, Bloom and Katsarkas 1989, Harker 1988, Mizukoshi et al. 1988 and Ojala et al. 1989) our group differs in several ways : it consist not only of ENT but also neurologic patients and only of hospitalised pacients. There is no significant difference between the number of hospitalised patients at both departments and between the sexes. We found the highest peak of acute vertigo incidence between 54 and 66 years of age, then as the cause of acute admission the incidence of vertigo steeply decreases. Frequent incidence of benign paroxysmal vertigo in the elderly above 70 years of age described by Bloom and Katsarkas was not the cause of acute admission of our patients.

CONCLUSIONS :

1. Catamnest emphasizes the neccessity of close neurologic and ENT cooperation in evaluation of vertigo using
2. simple but complex otoneurologic examination and in indicated cases
3. specialised examinations to assess the
4. causal diagnosis and administering the proper
5. treatment

REFERENCES :

1. Aschoff, J. C.: Differentialdiagnostische Überlegungen zur Schwindelsymptomatik.
HNO, 1978:26(5), 149-154.

2. Bloom, J., Katsarkas, A.: Paroxysmal positional vertigo in elderly.
J. Otolaryngol. 1989, 18 (3), 96-8.

3. Blessing, R., Mann, W., Beck, C.: Differential diagnosis of benign paroxysmal positional vertigo in Meniere´s Disease.
HNO, 1986, :34 (9), 372-5.

4. Harker, L. A., Rassekh, C. H.: Episodic vertigo in basilar artery migraine.
Otolaryngology Head and Neck Surgery, 1987, 96, 239-250.

5. Mizukoshi, K., Watanabe, Y., Shojaku, H., Okubo, J., Watanabe, I.: Epidemiological Studies on Benign Paroxysmal Positional Vertigo in Japan.
Acta Otolaryngol. Suppl. (Stockh.), 1988, 447, 67-72.

DISBARISM AND OTO-BARO TRAUMATISM: CLASSIFICATION, CLINICAL PICTURE AND MECHANISMS

KOLCHEV Chr., UZUNOV N.
Neurology Clinic, Medical Academy, Sofia

INTRODUCTION

The hearing disturbances are among the earliest and most prevaled medical problems appearing in high pressure environment, both in simulated barochamber axposures, or in the real underwater dives (9, 12, 13).

This type of disorders have been encountered during all phases of the hyperbaric exprosition: during compression, at stable deep depths and during dezompression. Moreover, they are the leading symptoms of the High Pressure Nervois Syndrome, HPNS (6).

For the present there is no a comprehensive classification of the High Presure-related Hearing disorders (HPHD). Some aspects of their hathophysiology are still not enough clarificate or a lot of contrabictions exist.

In this report we are seeking to summarize the types of HPHD and to provide some knoledge on the clinics and mechanisms of the so called Hyperbaric-associated Neurosensorial Deafness syndrome (HaNSeD syndrome) (14).

MATERIAL AND METHODS

Altogether 18 aquanauts and 36 divers were investigated during series of long lasting saturation exposures (15 up to 32 days) in barochambers, or in non-saturated real inderwater dives. The ambient pressure was from 6.0 up to 46.0 ATA. A total of 933 measurments, registrations and examinattions were done, including: acoustic measurment, tonal threshold and suprathreshold audiometry, EEG audiometry, registration of cortical and brainstem AERs, Blink reflex, speesh audiometry and spectral speech analysis, psychophysiological tests (Event-Related Potentials), vestibular tests, neurologic and otonejrological examinations.

COMPREHENSIVE CLASSIFICATION
OF HING PRESSURE-related HEARING DISORDERS (H.P.H.D.)

N	1. Phase of H.P. exposition	2. Mode of the Onset of HPHD	3. Duration of HPHD - Sympt.	4. Topics of the Damages	5. Mechanisms of H.P. influences
1.	Compression "C" - phase	Acute	Difinitive	Conductive	Difficulties of Pressure equalization between both sides of Tympanic Membane (Oto - Barotrauma)
2.	H.P.-exposition "Stable" - phase	Subacute	Reversible	Sensorbineural (in air atm)	Nitrogen narcosis
				Conductive (in Helium atm)	Increased Acoustic Jmpendanse of Tympano-ossicular chain, H.P.N.S.
3.	Decompression "D" - phase	Acute	Definitive	Conductive	Oto - Barotrauma
		Subacute	Reversible	Sensorineural	Decompression Sickness of babyrinth and related Brain structures
4.	Post-efposition "Post-E" - phase	Subacute	Reversible	Sensorineural	Hearing fatiguability (Temporary Threshold Shift)
5.	Background Period	Insidious	Definitive	Sensorineural (for 4000 and 6000 Hz)	Para-hyperbaric factors (Noise from life-supporting installations)

RESULTS

There are numerous types of HPHD syndromes. The basic classification criteria are acording to the Phase of the hyperbaric exposition, mode of oncet of the HPHD symtoms, Duration, Topics and Pathogenetic Mechanisms. (Table I).

Diving injures to the inner ear can be the major or only manifestation of diving pathology; during compression they are considered as an inner ear barotrauma due to round window ruptures occuring with straining, or Valsalva's manuever during inadequate middle ear pressure equilibration. During decompression they are considered as an otoneurological manifestation of the Decompression sickness. Usually, these kind of injures are resulting from transient intralabyrinthine osmotic pressure differences, or from bubble formations at labyrinthine tissue interfaces occuring with the counter-diffusion of the two dissolved inert gases at high partial pressures (12, 13).

Especial interes represent the cases with High Tone Hearing loss of neurosensorial character, which we called Hyperbaric-associated Neuro-Sensorial Deafness Syndrome (HaNSeD syndrome).

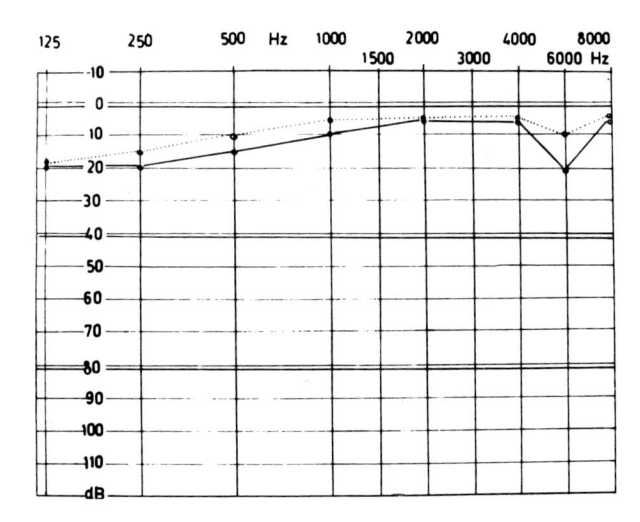

Fig.1. Audiogram of a 32 years old diver with initial sings of HaNSeD syndrome.

It is concerning a syndrome of insidiously developing High Frequency Deafness among the aquanauts and divers, who have inderwent repetetive hyperbaric exposures. This type of hyperbaris-associated hearing loss possesses neurosensorial character and lead to definitive high frequensy hearing loss.

There are discrepancies about the existance of the HaNSeD syndrome. Some authors reject the existance of the this syndrome (3, 5, 7, 19), other assume the existance of such of syndrome, but they consider it as a presbiacusis manifestation in experiences divers (4, 8, 9, 10). The majority of autohors believed that the HaNSeD syndrome probabaly exists, but there is no enough evidences about its causes and mechanisms (2, 11, 12, 13, 14, 17, 18).

In our groupe of aquanauts there was established statistically significant impairment of 6000 Hz tone thres-Lold value for the group of 13 (out of 18) auditory damaged aquanauts in compearance to non-diving general population of corresponding age (Tabl.II).

Tabl.II. Mean data for hearing thresholds (air and bone conduction) with their level of significanse (P) for the group of auditory damaged aquanauts (HaNSeD syndrome)

N	Frequency, Hz	Hearing Thresholds, dB $\bar{X} \pm$ S.D.	N	P
1.	4000 Hz	44.16 $\pm$ 19.66	(6)	$P < 0.10$
		(26.67 $\pm$ 7.99)	(6)	$P < 0.10$
2.	6000 Hz	40.26 $\pm$ 13,71	(19)	$P < 0.001$
		(30.52 $\pm$ 10.11)	(19)	$P < 0.001$
3.	8000 Hz	45.10 $\pm$ 10.0	(5)	$P < 0.10$
		(39.00 $\pm$ 6,63)	(5)	$P < 0.10$

Probably, the intimate mechanisms of the hyperbaric noise effect upon the hearing funciotn is similar to that in noise industrial workers, in which a Noise-induced Permanent Threshold Shift (NIPTS) can occur. There is a lot of considerations for the High Freqency tone affection during hyperbaric exhositions.

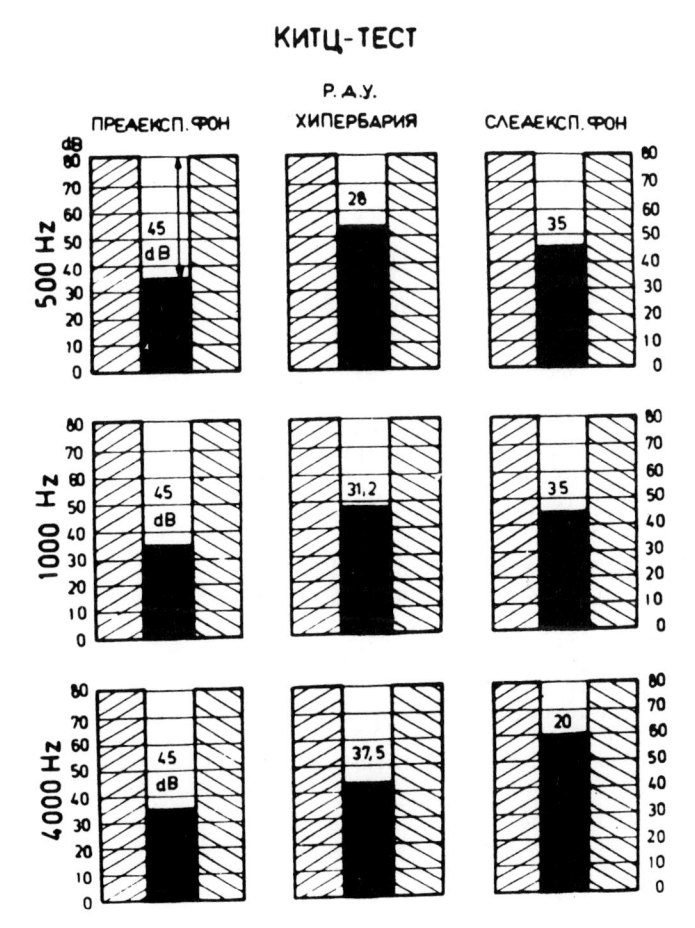

Fig.1. Kitz test measurment of an aquanaut during the pre-expositional period (left column), hyperbaric exposition up to 36.0 ATA (middle column), and posteqpositional state (right column)

REFERENCES:

1. Alberti PW (1979) Noise and the Ear.In: Scott Brown's Diseases of the Ear.Nose and Throat (J.Ballanthine and J.Groves, Eds), Fousth edition, vol.2, Butterworths, pp. 551-622.
2. Appaix A, Demard F (1972) Etude audiometrique et electronistragmorgraphique chez l'home normal en prongees tres profonde. Acta Otolaryng, (Stockholm), 73:141-147.
3. Barnini C, Gilardi G. (1977) Alanni aspetti della funzionalita otovestibulare nella saturatione iperbarica Minerva Med., 68 (20), 1357-1360.
4. Benson AJ, King PF (1979). The ear and nasal sinuses in the aerospace environment. In: Scott Brown's Diseases of the Ear, Nose and Throat. (J.Ballanthine and J.Groves, Eds), Fourth edition, vol.2, Butterworths, pp.205-245.
5. Brady JL, Jr, Smith JK, Berghage TE (1976). An audiometric survey of Navy divers. Undersea Biomed.Res., 3:41-47.
6. Brauer RW, Dimov S, Fructus X, Gosset A, Naquet R. Syndrome neurologique et electrographique des hautes pressions. Rev.Neurol., 1969, 121:265.
7. Brown CV (1977) Aquatic first aid. Skin Diver, 26:20, 23, 30-31, 1977.
8. Coles RRA (1976) Cochelo-vestibular disturbances in diving. Audiology, 15:273-278.
9. Edmonds C (1973) Round window ruptre in diving. In: Proc. of the first ann.Sci. Meeting of the European Undersea Biomed.Soc., (C.M.Hesser and D.Linnarson, Eds).
10. Edmond C, Thomas RL (1972) Medical aspects of diving. Med.J.Aust., part 3, 2:1300-1304.
11. Eichel BS, Landes B. (1970). Sensorineural hearing loss caused by skin diving. Archiv. Otolaryng., 92:182-187.
12. Farmer JC. (1977) Diving injures to the inner ear. Ann. Otol.Rhinol.Laryngol., Suppl.36, 1pt.3; 56; 1-20.
13. Farmar JC. (1981) Inner ear injures in diving; differential diagnosis of inner ear decompression sickness and inner ear barotrauma. In: Proc. of the VII th Symp. on Underwater Phusiol., (A.I.Bachard and M.Matsen, Eds), Bethesda, pp.805-810.
14. Kolchev Chr. (1989) Hearing and speech communication in Hing Pressure Environment (Otoneurological and Electrophysiological aspects), Dissertation for Sci. Degree "Doctor of Medical Scinces", Sofia, 1989.
15. Smidt RP, Thews G. (1983) Handbook of Physiology.
16. Shilling CW, Beckett MW (1981) Underwater Physiology, Proc. of the VI th Symp. on Underwater Physiology, FASEB, Bethesd

17. Schmitt HP (1983) Die physikalischen Schaden des ZNS und seiner Hullen. Schäden durch anderung des Umdebungsdruckers (Barotrauma, Dysbarinmus). In: Pathologie des Nervensystems, II. (H.Berlot, H.Noetzil, G.Quadbeck, W.Schlote, H.P.Schtitt, O.Ule, Eds), Band 13 III, Springer Verlag, pp.867-893.
18. Soss SL (1971) Senzorineural hearing loss with diving. Arch. Otolaryng., 93:501-504.
19. Zannini D, Odaglie G, Sperati G. (1976) Auditory changes in proffessional divers. In: Underwater Physiology, Proc. of the V ih Symp. on Underwater Physiology (C.J.Lambertsen, Ed), Bethesda, Med.Feder, Amer, Soc.Exper.Biol., pp-675-684.

PROGNOSIS OF VERTIGO IN TEMPORAL BONE FRACTURES

CARSTEN WENNMO
Dept of Otolaryngology, Hospital of Helsingborg, S-251 87 Helsingborg, Sweden.

INTRODUCTION

Secondary effects of trauma to the temporal bone are vertigo of the continous or positional type, hematotympanon, cerebrospinal fluid otorrhea, facial paralysis or persistent hearing loss of the conductive or sensorineural type. Immediately after trauma to the pyramid, a nystagmus reaction changes in direction when the position of the head is altered[1]. After some time the direction of the nystagmus changes to the opposite side.

In the period immediately after trauma the observed nystagmic reaction depends on irritation of the inner ear, vestibular nerve or vestibular centra in the brainstem. Sometimes the presence of nystagmus is only observed with careful examination because of other masking circumstances when injuries are multiple. Vertigo is sometimes the symptom which prevents the patient from returning to work in the long run. Usually, however, it disappears within a couple of months[2]. In an investigation by Ghorayeb and coworkers (1987) involving patients with fractures of the temporal bone, 23 patients (70 per cent) presented with vestibular symptoms.

This material comprises forty-one patients admitted to the ENT-clinic because of petrosal fractures.

PATIENTS AND METHODS

We analyzed and examined data from forty-one patients with fractures of the temporal bone received during the period 1978-1987. Twenty-seven men and 14 women with mean age of 48 years (range 10-90) were investigated at the time of trauma and at follow-up. The drum membrane and ear canal was inspected and occurrences of nystagmus and of dizziness were recorded. All patients except one were investigated with x-ray and were later examined oto-neurologically and with audiometry. In some cases electronystagmography was performed.

Vestibular examination

At clinical examination the presence of spontaneous nystagmus or positional nystagmus was noted. A caloric test or computerized electronystagmography was performed in 29 of the patients. Corneo-retinal signals were collected by Tracoustics electronystagmographic recorder (ENR-200) d.c. coupled with an upper cut-off filter of 30 Hz. Signals were analyzed on line by an IBM XT computer equipped with a 64 kb memory and a Winchester disc of 10 Mb.

Audiometric examination

Audiometry was performed twice or, more commonly, pure tone audiometry but in those cases which were intended for surgery (4) speech audiometry was also performed.

Chain incongruence

Surgery of the middle ear was performed in four patients (10 per cent) where a conductive hearing loss persisted.

RESULTS

Eighteen patients (43 per cent) received their fractures from falls, ten (24 per cent) from car accidents, five (12 per cent) from occupational accidents and four (10 per cent) from biking accidents. In four patients (10 per cent) the circumstances behind the trauma were not completely known.

Dizziness

At the time of examination immediately after the accident vestibular symptoms were noted in 15 patients (37 per cent), who complained of dizziness. Furthermore a spontaneous nystagmus was noted in 3 patients, positional nystagmus in 2 and vertical in one patient. In most of the patients the vertigo or dizziness had completely disappeared within some months; twenty-seven patients experienced no dizziness at all. In two of the patients, however, the dizziness persisted for several years.

Chain incongruence

Conductive hearing loss may result from an ossicular lesion, filling of the ear with blood or rupture of the tympanic membrane. A conductive hearing loss exceeding 30 dB is strongly suggestive of an ossicular incongruency.

The four patients with chain incongruence have been operated with good hearing results (Table 1). In one patient the incongruence consisted of a pseudarthrosis of the malleus handle while in the other three the distal end of the incus had been fractured.

Sensorineural hearing loss

Partial sensorineural hearing loss may improve slightly during the first week but after longer periods no further improvement can be expected. According to Schuknecht (1974) such improvements are more likely if the hearing loss is most marked in the low frequencies or with a flat sensorineural hearing loss. In the present investigation improvements were mainly noted in patients with a combined sensorineural-conductive hearing loss, and this better hearing depended, in these cases, on absorption of blood in the middle ear. However, in four patients with sensorineural hearing loss a slight recovery was noted.

DISCUSSION

As a rule the impairment of vestibular function is also associated with decreased cochlear function. According to Tos (1973) the incidence of apparent inner ear damage gives a moderate high tone loss up to 25 dB in 20 per cent, severe high tone loss in 6 per cent and total cochlear loss in 4 per cent of cases. With severe trauma the vertigo is frequently more long lasting due to dizziness of the central type. These patients frequently complain of a sensation of disequilibrium rather than a sensation of rotation. The most common dizziness of the peripheral vestibular kind is vertigo of the positional type. Fractures of the labytinthine capsule provoke more symptoms of vertigo, nausea and vomiting, persisting for days to weeks.

The fractured ear is usually deaf and associated with tinnitus. If one labyrinth is left normal the remaining labyrinth and the vestibular system are only severely challenged, for example, by walking in darkness, standing on one leg with eyes closed or other extraordinary loadings.

TABLE
Change of air-bone conduction treshholds before and after surgery (averaged for 1000, 1500 and 2000 Hz).

Case 1	Case 2	Case 3	Case 4
bone 15-10	bone 11-3	bone 8-6	bone 15-12
air 63-26	air 40-11	air 40-10	air 45-21

REFERENCES

1. Belluci R (1983) Traumatic injuries of the middle ear. Otolaryngol Clin N Am 16(3) pp 633-650
2. Cannon R, Jahrsdoerfer R (1983) Temporal bone fractures. Arch Otolaryngol 109 pp 285-288
3. Ghorayeb B, Yeakley J, Hall J, Jones E (1987) Unusial complications of temporal bone fractures. Arch otolaryngol Head Neck Surg 113 pp 749-753
4. Schuknecht H (1974) Pathology of the Ear. Cambridge Harvard University Press
5. Tos M (1973) Course of and sequele to 248 petrosal fractures. Acta Otolaryngol 75 pp 353-354

INNER EAR TRAUMA

VECTORNYSTAGMOGRAPHIC STUDY OF PATIENTS WITH MENIERE'S DISEASE

CARLOS AUGUSTO ANADÃO
MAURÍCIO MALAVASI GANANÇA
HELOISA HELENA CAOVILLA
PEDRO LUIZ MANGABEIRA ALBERNAZ

DEPARTMENT OF VESTIBULOMETRY
EAR, NOSE AND THROAT CLINIC
ESCOLA PAULISTA DE MEDICINA
SÃO PAULO - BRAZIL

INTRODUCTION

Since PROSPER MENIERE's report of january 8th, 1861, a great number od reports and reseach has been presented about this disease of great importance.

On the other hand, several aspects aren't totally known yet.

Vectornystagmography (VENG), presented by PANSINI & PADOVAN (1969), is a method of labyrinthine examination that allows study of oblique movements of the eyes, by the observation of the vertical and horizontal movements of the eyes.

MANGABEIRA ALBERNAZ et alii (1980) reported the presence of spontaneous nystagmus and signs of alterations of the vertical semicircular canal in patients with Meniere's Disease.

MATERIAL AND METHOD

We examined 90 patients : 52 male, 38 female
                          Age : 34 - 63 years old.
Diagnose according MANGABEIRA ALBERNAZ report (1982).

The Neurootological Examination was made by the Technique of MANGABEIRA ALBERNAZ & GANANÇA (1977) and MANGABEIRA ALBERNAZ et alii (1984) , in the inter-critical period (out of crisis):
 A - Anamnesis
 B - Ear, Nose and Throat Examination
 C - Audiological Examination : Pure tone audiogram, Speech
       discrimination score and Impedanciometry
 D - Vestibular Examination :

1 - Balance Tests
2 - Vectornystagmography :
    a - Eye Movement Calibration
    b - Study of Spontaneous Nystagmus
    c - Stugy of Semi-Spontaneous Nystagmus
    d - Study of Positional Nystagmus
    e - Study of Optokinetic Nystagmus
    f - Pendular Eyetracking
    g - Torsion Swing Test
    h - Caloric Test (Fitzgerald & Hallpike)

RESULTS

Symptomatology - All patients complained of vertigo, tinnitus an ear fullness. Hearing loss ocurred in 97,8%; nausea in 71,1%; loudness sensitivity in 67,8%; dizziness in 51,1%.

TABLE I

SYMPTOMS IN 90 PATIENTS WITH MENIERE'S DISEASE

SYMPTOM	PATIENTS	%
Vertigo	90	1oo,o
Tinnitus	90	100,0
Ear Fullness	90	100,0
Hearing Loss	88	97,8
Nausea	64	71,1
Loudness Sensitivity	61	67,8
Dizziness	46	51,1
Disturb of Speech Discrimination	40	44,4
Mental Depression	39	43,3
Headache	29	32,2
Vomiting	28	31,1
Anxiety	28	31,1
Pallor	24	26,7
Sleeplessness disturbance	19	21,1
Phobyas	14	15,5
Tachycardia	13	14,4
Falls	11	12,2
Sensation of liquid in the ear	3	3,3
Otalgy	3	3,3
Diplacusis	1	1,1

Audiological Findings - The 66 patients with sensory-neural hea loss presented the following graph :

High Tones (Descendent) : 24 Patients - 35,45 %
Flat Curve (Horizontal) : 16 Patients - 24,24 %
Low and High Tones (Inversed "U"):14 Patients-21,21%
Low Tones (Ascendent) : 12 patients - 18,18 %

TABLE II
AUDIOLOGICAL FINDINGS IN 90 PATIENTS WITH MENIERE'S DISEASE

FINDINGS	PATIENTS	%
Pure Tone Audiogram		
Normal	24	26,7
Sensory-neural Hearig Loss	66	73,3
Speech Discrimination		
Normal	52	57,8
Abnormal	38	42,2
Impedanciometry		
Normal	46	51,1
Abnormal	44	48,9
Vestibular Findings -The principal findings were :		
- Positional Vertigo	24	26,7
- Positional Nystagmus	5	5,5
- Horizontal Spontaneous Nystagmus	28	31,1
- Torsion Swing Test : Directional Preponderance		
lateral semicircular canal	34	37,8
vertical semicircular canal	13	14,4
- Caloric Test		
Symmetrical	30	33,3
Directional Preponderance	22	24,4
Unilateral Weakness	17	18,9
Hyperreflexy	16	17,8
Bilateral Weakness	3	3,3
Unilateral Arreflexy	2	2,2

CONCLUSIONS
- Most of the patients complained of vertigo, tinnitus, ear fullness and hearing loss.
- Less than 50% of the patients complained of hearing loss or tinnitus during the attacks of Meniere's Disease.
- The auditory and/or vestibular symptoms were predominantly unilateral.
- Most of patients showed sensory-neural hearing loss, disturb of speech discrimination and presence of recruitment at the

Impedanciometry.
- Most of the cases presented alterations of the vestibular activity at the Vectornystagmography in the Torsion Swing Test and in the Caloric Test; Spontaneous Nystagmus with closed eye and Positional Vertigo.
- Some cases presented only disturbs of the vertical semicircular canal at the Rotatory Test.
- At the Vectornystagmography, half of the patients showed unila teral alterations and half, bilateral alterations.

REFERENCES

Caovilla,HH,Ganança,MM, Mangabeira Albernaz,PL Optovestibular exercises in the therapy of vertigo. In: CONGRESS OF THE INTER-NATIONAL NEUROOTOLOGICAL & EQUILIBRIOMETRIC SOCIETY, XVI, KRETE/GREECE, 17-22 April 1989.

Capella,G & Garcia Piris,A Hallasgos electronistagmograficos en la enfermedad de Meniere. In: CLAUSSEN,CF Equilibriometria y audiologia clinica.Hamburg, Verlag, 1976. p. 47-58.

Ganança,MM, Mangabeira Albernaz,PL, Ito,YI, Caovilla,HH, Castro,H Optokinetic habituation training in the treatment of vestibular diseases. Annals of the XIX Pan Am Congr Otorhinolaryngol and Broncho-Esophagol. Quebec, 1984. p.41.

Mangabeira Albernaz,PL & Ganança,MM Atlas de electronistagmografia São Paulo, Editamed, 1977. 21p.

Mangabeira Albernaz,PL, Fukuda,Y, Ganança,MM Ménière's disease. ORL (Basel), 42:91-100,1980.

Mangabeira Albernaz,PL, Doença de Ménière. J.Bras.Med.42:22-30, 1982.

Mangabeira Albernaz,PL, Ganança,MM, Caovilla,HH, Ito,YI,Castro,HD Atlas de vecto-electronistagmografia. SãoPaulo,Aché,1984. 60p.

Menière,P Mémoire sur des lésions de l'oreille interne donnant lieu a des symptômes de congestion cérébrale apoplectiforme. Gazette Médicale de Paris. 16:597-601, 1861.

Pansini,M & Padovan,I Three derivation in electronystagmography. Acta Oto-Laryngol. (Stockh), 67:303-9, 1969.

THE DIFFERENT TYPES OF PERILYMPHATIC FISTULE

GEORGE BODO, LORANT HEID

Central Military Hospital, ENT Department,
Pf. 1, 1553 Budapest, Hungary

The Cavital system of the inner ear may open from different reasons and perilymph may leak to the tympanic cavity. Sudden decrease of hearing and vertigo are characteristic. Valvular type of perilymph leakage causes undulating hearing loss. The disease was put down by *Politzer* (1) already in 1908 in his book in connection with the imflammation of the middle ear. The different causes of perilymphatic fistule are published in the latest literature are as follows: stapedectomy - *House* (2), blunt .skulltrauma - *Fee* (3), barotrauma - *Freeman* and *Edmond* (4), shot injury - *Emmett* et al.(5). *Kaufman Arenberg* et al. (6) publishes a case of labyrinth fistule imitating Ménière´s disease. Many studies have appeared during the past years.

We would like to introduce some of our cases.

1. H.K. 49 y.o. pilote after landing with his plane the hearing in his left ear suddenly decreased, had strong tinnitus and vertigo. He received vascular dilating infusion without any effect. Then he got admitted to our department. Where tympanotomy was performed on his left ear during which perilymphatic leakage could be seen from the round window. The surrounding mucosa was preparated and turned towards the cavity and the opening was blocked by fascia pieces. The vertigo and the vestibular symptoms ceased but there was a slight increase in hearing.
2. G.F. 21 y.o. male fell down from the stairs, became deaf on his right ear and dizzied. He got admitted to our department only one and a half months later. During tympanotomy perilymphatic flow could be seen from the oval window. The operational solution was similar as at the previous case only the incus and the stapes made the manipulation difficult. Hearing returned on this completely deaf ear, but on to a very low level, and the vestibular complaints completely ceased.
3. Sz.Z. 21 y.o. male whose head was injured by a truck door. The hearing on his left ear decreased, he had vertigo and vomited. He was transported to our department immediately where after the examinations tympanotomy was performed. The perilymph was leaking from the oval window. The fistule was blocked by the usual way. The patient´s hearing increased 30 minutes after the operation but he was dizzying strongly again, and his vestibular symptoms were of opposite directional compared to that before operation. The

phenomenon was considered as operational Lermoyez syndrome. The vestibular symptoms ceased by the following day. The hearing that was 30 - 70 dB before operation after one month returned to normal.

4. F.Gy. 68 y.o. male got admitted to our department because of bilateral chronic otitis. The discharging right ear was operated on, attico-antrotomy and tympanoplasty of type 3 was performed with succesful anatomical and functional results. There was a large rear perforation on his left eardrum. We planned to close this perforation by conservative method, by trichloride acetic acid treatment. Lidocaine spray was used for local anaestetic the pressure of which caused perilymphatic fistule on the round window. The patient´s hearing decreased to deafness, he had strong vertigo and vegetative symptoms for which i.v. Torecan was administered. After calming down perilymphatic flow was seen from round window, which we tried to block by fibrin sponge, but this was unsuccessful. After the normalisation of the tympanic mucosa the round window was blocked by fascia piece during the usual tympanotomy. Slight increase in hearing and the cease of vestibular symptoms were resulting.

On basis of studying our cases our experiences can be summarised as follows:
- Barotrauma and the pressure of spraying or washing the ear can cause the fistule of the round window.
- Blunt skulltrauma deformes the oval window for a second and the *anulus fibrosus* is torn which holds the foot of the stapes.
- We consider the turning of the mucosa into the recess of the windows and stabilising by pieces of fascia a suitable methode for blocking the windows
- The success of blockage is indicated by the appearing Lermoyez syndrome short after operation.

REFERENCES
1. Politzer A: Lehrbuch der Ohrenheilkunde. ENKE VERL. STUTTGART (1908)
2. House HP: The fistule problem in otosclerotic surgery. Laryngoscope 77, 1410 (1967)
3. Fee GA: Traumatic perilymphatic fistulas. Arch. Otolaryngol. 88, 477 (1968)
4. Freeman P, Edmonds C: Inner ear Barotrauma. Arch. Otolaryngol. 95, 556 (1972)
5. Emmett JR, Staab EW, Fischer ND: Perilymph fistulas secondary to gunshot wound. Arch. Otolaryngol. 103, 98 (1977)
6. Kaufman Arenberg I, May M, Stround MH: Perilymphatic fistula: an unusual cause of Ménière´s syndrome in a prepubertal child. The Laryngoscope 84, 243 (1974)

DOES DELAYED LABYRINTHINE HYDROPS DEVELOP IN CONSEQUENCE OF HEAD TRAUMA?

JENŐ CZIGNER and ÉVA SZABADOS
Oto-rhino-laryngology Department, Albert Szent-Györgyi Medical University, Szeged, P.O.Box: 422. (Hungary)

INTRODUCTION

Méniere symptoms have been described by several authors after lesion of the endolymphatic duct in association with a temporal bone fracture[1,4,5]. Ylikoski et al[6]. Paparella and Mancini[3] and Hicks and Wright[2] reported Méniere disease in cases involving earlier skull traumas, but without fractures of the petrous bone. On the basis of a retrospective analysis of the anamnestic data and cochleovestibular findings on Méniere patients, we have investigated a presumed causal connection between Méniere disease and preceding head traumas.

PATIENTS

Data on 76 subjects were evaluated. The patients were classified into two groups (Table I).

TABLE I
AETIOLOGIC CLASSIFICATION OF MÉNIERE PATIENTS

	Méniere's disease		
(n = 76)	unilateral	bilateral	total
UNKNOWN ORIGIN	29	3	32
PRESUMED CAUSES	29	15	44
TRAUMA	7	2	
Virus infection in childhood	14	6	
Hyperlipidaemia	5	2	
Hypothyroidism	–	1	
Otitis media in childhood	1	2	
Arnold-Chiari Syndrome	1	–	
Diabetes mellitus	1	–	
Contraceptive	–	1	
Prematurity	–	1	
TOTAL	58	18	76

Thirty-two Méniere patients in whom the aetiology was unknown were excluded from further analysis.

Nine distinct possible aetiologic factors were revealed in 44 cases, with highest incidences of childhood virus-infections and previous head traumas. In the present study, the main interest was focused on 9 patients with head injuries in their histories, followed by Méniere symptoms mostly after a long time-period.

RESULTS

All the 9 patients (20-68 years of age) complained of tinnitus, fluctuating hearing loss, sensations of fullness and pressure in the affected ear. The physical state of the ears was found to be normal when the diagnosis of Méniere disease was established; no signs of previous fractures of the temporal bone could be detected by means of X-ray or computed tomography. The head injuries were consequences of traffic accidents in 3 cases, falling from an appreciable height in 3, and sport accidents in 2; the head of one patient was kicked by a horse. Six patients suffered cerebral concussion on the occasion of the injury. In 2 cases, traumas preceded the first Méniere features by 6 months, whereas the interval was longer than a year (average: 16.5 years) in all the others. The Méniere-type complaints of the patients started 2 months to 8 years before the initiation of their otoneurological observations. Neurological, EEG and cerebrospinal fluid (CSF) examinations revealed no pathognomic alterations in 8 subjects, while signs of multifocal superficial and deep destruction were registered electroencephalographically in 1 without concomitant CSF changes. (Table II)

As concerns the total Méniere patient material, audiograms of four main types were obtained on pure tone threshold audiometry:
type 1: apicocohlear hearing loss, "up-sloping" audiogram;
type 2: hearing loss with relatively maintained perception of
2000 Hz frquency;
type 3: "flat" audiogram of pancochlear deafness;
type 4: basocochlear hearing loss, "down-sloping" audiogram.
The type 4 audiogram was rare among all these Méniere patients and it did not occur at all after head traumas. The "up-sloping" audiogram was the most general form. Suprathreshold audiometry revealed the recruitment phenomenon, bearing witness to the lesion of Corti's organ; the latter was also demonstrated by BERA investigations.

As far as the vestibular system is concerned (Table III), 5 patients complained of vertigo and 4 of uncertain dizziness.

TABLE II
AUDIOLOGIC FINDINGS OF MÉNIERE PATIENTS WITH PREVIOUS HEAD TRAUMAS
(n = 9)

Sex	Age (y)	Concussion	Time between Trauma and first Symptoms	Duration of Symptoms	Type of Audiogram[x]
♀	37	−	L 9 y	1 y	1
♂	37	−	L 6 m	1.5 y	1
♂	20	−	R 6 m	1 y	1
♀	55	+	R 1 y	7 y	1
			L 6 y	2 m	1
♀	37	+	L 12 y	3 y	1
			R Mumps in childhood	∅	∅
♀	54	+	L 24 y	1 y	3
♂	38	+	R 23 y	2 y	2
♂	49	+	L 26 y	3 y	1
♂	68	+	R 47 y	8 y	3

x Types of Audiogram   1 ⟍   2 ⟋   3 —   4 ⟍   R = right ear   L = left ear   y = year   m = month

Harmonic spontaneous vestibular symptoms were found in 5 cases. From among the 3 individuals who underwent head traumas without cerebral concussion, vestibular hypaesthesia was detected in 1 and a directional preponderance of the nystagmus in 2.

TABLE III
VESTIBULAR FINDINGS OF MÉNIERE PATIENTS WITH PREVIOUS HEAD TRAUMAS
(n = 9)

Sex	Age (y)	Concussion	Time between Trauma and first Symptoms	Duration of Symptoms	Spont. nystagmus	Vestibular functions(ENG) Normal↓ — ↑	DP
♀	37	−	L 9 y	1 y	−	+ − − −	+
♂	37	−	L 6 m	1.5 y	−	+ − − −	+
♂	20	−	R 6 m	1 y	+	− + − −	+
♀	55	+	R 1 y	7 y	+	− + − −	−
			L 6 y	2 m		+	
♀	37	+	L 12 y	3 y	+	− − + −	+
			R Mumps	∅		+	
♀	54	+	L 24 y	1 y	−	− − + −	−
♂	38	+	R 23 y	2 y	+	− + − −	+
♂	49	+	L 26 y	3 y	−	− − − +	−
♂	68	+	R 47 y	8 y	+	− + − −	−

DP = direction preponderance of nystagmus

In 5 out of 6 patients with cerebral concussion in their histories, vestibular hypaesthesia was recorded, whereas a total vestibular anaesthesia was found in 1, and hyperaesthesia associated with a deficient inhibition of ocular fixation in further case.

DISCUSSION

In a retrospective analysis of the cochleovestibular functions of 67 unselected Méniere patients and 9 with previous head traumas, no special features could be discovered in the latter subgroup. The averaged audiograms of these cases showed a hearing loss similar to that of Méniere disease in general: impairment predominantly at lower tone frequencies; "up-sloping" type (Figure 1). Figure 2 shows the individual audiogram of a patient immediately after head injury: the "deep notch" hearing loss at around 4000 Hz can be considered characteristic of a post-traumatic inner ear lesion that has not been followed by the development of Méniere disease so far.

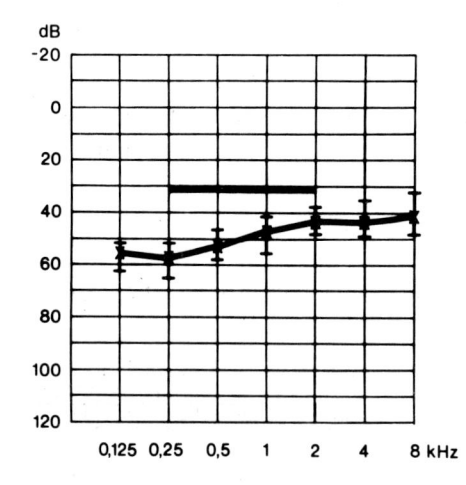

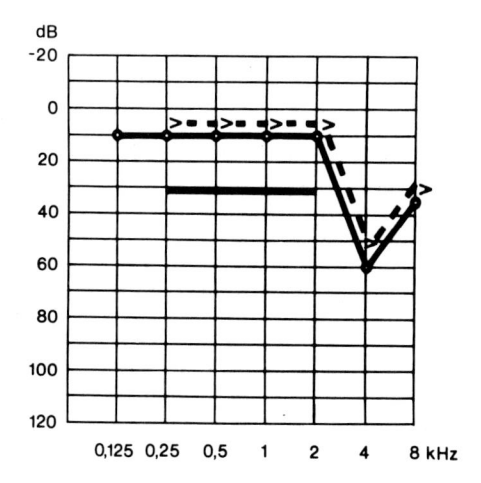

Fig. 1. Averaged pure tone threshold audiogram of Méniere patients with previous head traumas (n=9; $\bar{x}$+SEM).

Fig. 2. Audiogram of a patient immediately after head injury.

The spontaneous or provoked vestibular signs in the 9 patients with earlier traumas corresponded to the usual Méniere symptoms rather than to the trauma. Since Méniere disease sometimes commences very late after cranial injury, the verification of a causal connection between the two events hardly seems possible.

REFERENCES
1. Clark SK, Rees TS (1977) Arch Otolaryngol 103:725-726
2. Hicks GW, Wright JW (1988) Laryngoscope 98:840-845
3. Paparella MM, Mancini F (1983) Laryngoscope 93:1004-1012
4. Rizvi SS, Gibbin KP (1979) Ann Otol Rhinol Laryngol 88:741-748
5. Schuknecht HF (1978) Ann Otol 87:743-748
6. Ylikoski J, Palva T, Sanna M (1982) Am J Otolaryngol 3:343-352

TRAUMATIC PERILYMPH FISTULA

W. G. HEMENWAY, M.D., F. OWEN BLACK, M.D., R. GRIMM, M.D. & S. PESZNECKER, R.N.

INTRODUCTION

Traumatic perilymph fistulas were first reported by Fee [1] in 1968. Other significant papers published on this subject are as follows: 2, 3, 4, 5, 6 and 7. This report is on 94 patients with perilymph fistulas and other inner ear injuries caused by motor vehicle accidents and work-related injuries. The head injury was mild in 63 patients (36 whiplash, 27 head strike without loss of consciousness). In a majority of patients the diagnosis was significantly delayed; 65 cases were diagnosed between six months and six years. Furthermore, in 22 cases the onset of symptoms was delayed from eight days to more than one year.

TEST RESULTS

Eighty-Five percent of the patients had a positive platform fistula test [8]. BPPN was recorded in 33 patients. Electronystagmography testing revealed positional nystagmus in 66 patients and caloric tests on 47 patients were normal in 36 and showed a reduced function in 11. Rotation tests were done on 93 patients; they were normal in 77 and showed reduced function in 16. The moving platform posturography test (Black et al [9]) was performed on 93 patients, and was abnormal in 76, normal in 16 and non-organic in one. Electrocochleography was positive in 53 patients.

Patients with inner ear injuries were monitored frequently with audiometric testing. Thirty-three out of 94 patients with traumatic perilymph fistula developed a sensorineural hearing loss (usually mild). Thus, in the majority of patients (61), hearing remained within normal limits during the period of treatment.

SYMPTOMS

Vestibular symptoms were common; chronic disequilibrium, positional vertigo and attacks of spontaneous vertigo were often reported. Tinnitus was frequent and about one-third had sensorineural hearing loss. Cognitive problems, such as memory loss and inability to concentrate, were often noted. Chronic motion sickness

was common and very disturbing. Symptoms of visual dependency
frequently occurred. Psychological problems and domestic difficulties often developed if diagnosis and treatment were delayed.

CONSERVATIVE MANAGEMENT OF PLF

Conservative treatment (sixs weeks' bed rest) as an alternative
to surgery pre-operatively is not widely practiced. We have used it
for several years with generally satisfactory results. Traumatic
fistulas are bilateral in at least 50% of cases. Usually both
fistulas heal with bed rest, or neither heals. Occasionally one
heals and the other remains open and must be treated surgically.
Grimm [10] et al report slightly less than one-half (47%) of the
patients studied had healed their fistulas on bed rest. Of the 76
patients who were treated with bed rest in this study, 43 (57%)
closed their fistulas. (All are now back at work and their level of
activity is almost the same as before their injury.) We have had no
serious complications from bed rest in several hundred patients. The
majority of these patients who respond to conservative treatment
need vestibular physical therapy treatment for abnormal postural
strategies and for positional vertigo [11]. This treatment lasts
six weeks and consists of weekly sessions supplemented by prescribed
exercises done at home.

Fifty of these patients developed post-traumatic hydrops.
Sometimes hydrops seems to develop after the fistula closes (post-
closure hydrops). In others it comes prior to closure months or
years later. In our experience, most cases of hydrops respond to
medical therapy.

SURGICAL TREATMENT

The 33 patients who failed bed rest, and the 18 patients with
progressive sensorineural hearing loss, were treated surgically.
Tympanotomy was performed under monitored local anesthesia with a
neurolept supplement. A PLF was said to be present if one or both
of the following criteria was met: 1) An active leak of crystal
clear fluid versus the thicker, more viscous mucosal transudate seen
emanating from the depths of the oval or round window, and the fluid
rapidly re-accumulated when suctioned away; or 2) an actual hole or
defect seen in the structures of one or both windows. Prior to
grafting, the area around both windows was prepared using a hand-

held argon laser and angled sharp picks and hooks. Both windows were grafted regardless of whether or not a PLF was identified. Multiple small (0.25 mm) bits of areolar graft bits soaked with autologous cryoprecipitated fibrinogen were packed in both windowed and then congealed or "flashed" with the laser probe.

DISCUSSION

We have thoroughly studied 94 cases of traumatic perilymph fistulas that have been diagnosed and treated in our facility and followed for at least one year after definitive treatment. Usually several months had elapsed between the accident and diagnosis. These chronic inner ear injuries are often devastating to patients. In addition to disabling symptoms, they often develop psychological and financial problems which complicate their condition. Patients diagnosed two or more years post trauma rarely make a complete recovery, although there are some exceptions. Other ear injuries besides fistulas were frequently identified. Eighty patients had some form of positional nystagmus, 58 had post-traumatic endolymphatic hydrops, 27 had a vestibular deficit and 33 sustained some degree of sensorineural hearing loss.

Both medical and surgical treatments were employed. Medical management was successful in 43 out of 76 patients. Fifty-one cases were treated surgically. Of the surgical patients, 33 had a very good or good result, while 18 were listed as being in fair to poor condition. Many of the poor results had other severe injuries that interfered with recovery. Combining the surgical and conservative treatments, very good or good results were obtained in 76 patients (82%). Surgical patients sometimes required more than one operation to stabilize the fistulas. Our hydrops patients are usually controlled by medical treatment consisting of a low salt diet and a diuretic. If this fails, surgery is performed, usually an endolymphatic shunt. None of these 94 patients have had a shunt.

Bilateral fistulas occurred in over 50% of these patients. Bilateral fistulas were first reported by Tonkin and Fagan [12] in 1975 and recently by our group [10].

After closure of the fistulas, the patient's condition usually improves dramatically. Fatigue and seasick symptoms improve or disappear. Balance problems, dizziness and vertigo improve or disappear. Positional nystagmus is treated successfully in about 90% of cases by vestibular physical therapy. Many of our patients (34 in this series) needed psychological diagnosis and counseling.

As there is no epidemiological data known in the U.S.A. for any type of vestibular disturbance, it is impossible to say how commonly perilymph fistulas occur after head injuries. Most probably heal rapidly and are never diagnosed. The few which do not heal become chronic and disabling and their numbers accumulate over time (as they are often not diagnosed).

REFERENCES

1. Fee, G.A. Traumatic perilymph fistulas, *Arch Otolaryngol*, 88:477-480, 1968.

2. Healy, G.B., Strong, M.S., Sampagna, D. Ataxia, vertigo, and hearing loss: a result of rupture of inner ear window. *Arch Otolaryngol*, 100:130-135, 1974.

3. Singleton, G., Post, K.N., Karlan, M.S., and Bock, D.G. Perilymph fistulas, diagnostic criteria and therapy. *Annals of Otology Rhinology and Laryngology*, 87:797, Nov-Dec, 1978.

4. Thompson, J.N., Kohut, R.I. Perilymph fistulas: variability of symptoms and results of surgery. *Otolaryngol Head and Neck Surgery*, 87:898-903, 1979.

5. Kohut, R.I., Waldorf, R.A., Haenel, J.L., and Thompson, J.N. Minute perilymph fistulas: vertigo and Hennebert's sign without hearing loss. *Ann Otol*, 88:153-159, 1979.

6. Lehrer, J.J., Rubin, R.C., Poole, D.C., Hubbard, J.H., Wille, R., and Jacobs, J.B. *West J Med*: 57-60, 1984.

7. Seltzer, S., and McCabe, B.F. Perilymph fistula: the Iowan experience. *Laryngoscope*, 94:37-49, 1986.

8. Black, F.O., Lilly, D.J., Nashner, L.M., Peterka, R., and Pesznecker, S.C. Quantitative diagnostic test for perilymph fistulas. *Otolaryngol Head and Neck Surgery*, 96:125-134, 1987.

9. Black, F.O. Vestibulospinal function assessment by moving platform posturography. *Amer J. Otol* (supplement issue), 39-46, Nov 1985.

10. Grimm, R.J., Hemenway, W.G., LeBray, B.P., and Black, F.O. The perilymph fistula syndrome defined in mild head trauma. *Acta Oto Laryngol* (Supplement 46), 1989.

11. Shumway-Cook, A., and Horak, F.B. Vestibular rehabilitation: an exercise approach to managing symptoms of vestibular dysfunction. *Seminars in Hearing*, Vol #2, 196-209, 1989. Thiema Medical Publishers, Inc., 387 Park Ave. South, New York, N.Y. 10016.

12. Tonkin, J.P. and Fagan, P. Rupture of the round window membrane. *J. Laryngol* 80:733-756. 1975.

VESTIBULAR TRAUMATIC ACTION OF THE DIFFERENT LOADINGS

TRINUS K.F., OLEINIK V.S., CHERNIUK V.I., LASTOVCHENKO V.B., MESHCHERIAKOV G.V., NIKOLENKO V.Y.
BCA, Lukianivsky Str. 27, Apt.47, Kiev-71, Ukraina, GSP252601

INTRODUCTION

Loadings in the laboratory experiment are used for the evaluation of the factor action on the organism. Combination of the loading laboratory experiments with the examination of the occupational groups exposed to the principal factor studied allows us to light out the mechanisms of the traumatic action of the occupational factors (1). From this point of view the vestibular function of the tractor drivers who are exposed to the whole-body vibration and mental loading is poorly studied (2).

That is why the main aim of the paper presented is the studies of the action of the short-lasting loadings on the vestibular function and the evaluation of the latter in the tractor drivers with the experience of about 20 years.

MATERIAL AND METHODS

99 persons are examined: 60 of them being healthy persons, 29 of which are used as a control group, and the other 31 have taken part in the loading tests as paid volunteers, some of them have taken part in two tests. In the Coriolis accelerations test the 13 persons are examined, visual informational loading - 14, whole-body vibration - 6. 39 persons are tractor drivers with the established vibration disease diagnosis.

In the control group of the healthy persons and in patients the vestibular evoked potentials (VestEPs) are recorded once. The recording method is already described elsewhere (3). In the loading tests first the control VestEP is recorded, then the loading is presented, and again the VestEPs are monitored with the intervals of 15-30 minutes up to the moment of the reaching the initial parameters.

The data proceeding is made with the Basic statistics for the Macintosh: Descriptive Statistics and Dependent t-test. The changes are considered to be significant if p is not more than 0.05.

RESULTS
Loading tests

Coriolis accelerations. After this test used as the loading the latent times of the VestEP peaks in the 3 persons with high level of the vestibular tolerance are increased. The other 10 persons examined, who are susceptable to motion sickness have demonstrated the decrease of the peak latencies (P_1 not significant) for: P_1 - 2.4±4.8 ms, N_1 - 11.6±4.2, and P_2 - 9.0±6.4 ms. Earlier, we have noted that the return to the initial values passes through the period of the increased latencies and is highly individual.

Informational loading. As the Coriolis acceleration is the powerful stimulus, we also examine the low intensity stimulation action on the VestEP parameters. We have chosen the informational loading as such a stimulus. In this case the peak latencies are increased. The standard deviation levels are also increased. The absolute figures of the latencies increase are almost the same - about 11 ms. In relative units the greatest increase factor (ratio of the increase to the mean initial value) for P_1 is 27.5%, the lowest is for P_2 - 9.6%. The greatest increase is also typical for N_1 standard deviation with the increase factor - 74%, P_1 and P_2 have lower values, 37% and 36% - respectively.

The analysis of the individual particularities have shown that in 75% of the persons examined the increase of all the peak latencies is noted, in 17% - decrease of one peak latency, while the others increase, and in 8% - decrease of all the peak latencies.

Vibration. Studies of this factor action are conducted in the 1 hour and 2 hours exposures. In the course of the 1 hour exposure the latencies increase for P_1 from 23.2±3.0 ms to 45.6±14.9, N_1 from 68.0±22.2 to 104.0±23.5 and P_2 from 140.8±24.3 to 165.6±19.9 ms. The change for N_1 is significant for P_2 - reflects the tendency, and for P_1 - is not significant.

Individual analysis have shown that in all but one person the latencies increase. In one person they decrease moderatelly: P_1 from 28 to 20 ms, N_1 from 64 to 60, and P_2 - from 140 to 128 ms. It is interesting that the return to the initial level for N_1 and P_2 have passed through the time of the increased latencies as compared with the initial figures:
N_1 - before loading 64 ms, and after with 15 minutes interval: 60, 108, 64, 68 ms;

P_2 - before 140 ms and after: 128, 180, 136, 132 ms.

The return time of all the parameters is in the range between 0.5 and 1.0 hour. The prominent feature is that the most exact return is for the N_1 peak, and the least - for P_1 (the differences of the alpha coefficients of the two-tailed t-test for the control versus the last values9.

After the 2 hours of the vibration exposure the increase of the absolute values of the latencies are also noted. They are: for P_1 from 28.0±16.2 ms to 34.4±21.7, N_1 from 74.4±28.7 to 91.2±34.1, and P_2 from 126.4±14.9 to 149.6±45.0 ms. But these increases appeare to be not significant. The detailed analysis have shown that out of the 5 persons examined in 2 ones the latencies increase, in the other 2 ones - decrease, and in 1 person the latencies of the P_1 and N_1 are not changed, and P_2 latency is decreased. The peak latent times in this person decrease after 0.5 hour of loading cessation and have remained decreased during 1.0 hour. For example: N_1 - before loading 128 ms, and after the loading with 15 minutes interval: 128, 72, 68, 60 ms.

Analysis of the latent time dynamics after the loading in two persons who are prominent for the peak latencies decrease have shown that during 1 hour the data for P_1 and N_1 appear to be decreased and for P_2 they moved to the initial level through the period of the increased latencies. It is important to note the absence of the vegetative symptomatics in the persons with the decreased latencies, in the contrary to the Coriolis accelerations exposure test. The latter finding may become a basis for the creation of the test for the professional selection of the operators, in the activities of which the motion sickness susceptibility plays an important role. In the volunteers with the latencies increase the return to the initial level is noted to occur in about 0.5 hour, the time shorter then for those with the latencies decreased.

Occupational group

In 27 tractor drivers VestEPs are studied, while recorded in the threshold range. Only in 9 of them the VestEPs have been recorded satisfactory, in the others - only the averaged EEG have been obtained. The latencies of the peaks in this group are: P_1 - 39.5±13.0 ms, N_1 - 82.7±13.2, and P_2 - 168.0±

31.1 ms, which are clearly different from the normal data.

In the other 12 tractor drivers VestEPs are studied in the suprathreshold range. In 2 of them almost normal VestEPs are recorded, in 5 - the transitory potential in which both the components of the vestibular and somatosensory potentials are clearly seen. In the last 5 persons - only the somatosensory evoked potentials are recorded. We suppose that the ratio of the vestibular and somatosensory components in this accelerations area may indicate the degree of the vestibular lesion, and also be the basis for the express-diagnostics of the vestibular function.

All the data presented indicates the possibility of the accumulation of the vestibular function damage in the case of the occupational vestibular loadings. These changes may be irreversible.

CONCLUSIONS

1. Moderate loadings result in the temporary increase of the VestEPs peak latencies.
2. Havy loadings, perhaps in the persons with high vestibular susceptibility, cause temporary decrease of the latencies.
3. Vibration, as an occupational factor, results in the stable latencies increase, which may reflect the decrease of the vestibular sensitivity.

REFERENCES

1. Hamernik RP, Ahroon WA, Davis RA (1988) In: Manninen O (ed) Recent Advances in Research on the Combined Effects of Environmental Factors. ISCES,Tampere, pp 223-238
2. Cherniuk VI, Tashker ID (1989) In: Hygiena Truda: Republ. Interdiscipl. Recueil. Kiev, Zdorovia 25:64-67
3. Trinus KF (1988) In: Manninen O (ed) Recent Advances in Research on the Combined Effects of Environmental Factors. ISCES, Tampere, pp 143-152

MULTIVARIATE STATISTICAL PROCEDURES FOR THE DIFFERENTIATION OF COCHLEAR AND RETROCOCHLEAR HEARING IMPAIRMENTS

J. KLUBA[1], S. KROPF[2], and H. DEIKE[3]

[1]Klinik für HNO-Krankheiten, [2]Abteilung für Biomathematik und Medizinische Informatik, [3]Klinik für Neurologie und Psychiatrie, Medizinische Akademie Magdeburg, Leipziger Str. 44, DDR-3090 Magdeburg,

Differential diagnosis of cochlear and retrocochlear hearing disorders ranks among the most complex problems in audiology. To this end, use is made of conventional and objective audiometry in function diagnosis to make a functional analysis of the actual status. The findings are classed with the aim of detecting impairments and assigning them in topodiagnostic terms to pathological events in the auditory pathway. In this context, it is desirable to know to which extent multivariate statistical methods can contribute towards achieving this target [1,2].

Therefore, an audiologic study involving 203 males and females was conducted from 1985 to 1989. The tone threshold audiogram, the speech audiogram, and the CARHART test were employed for subjective investigations. Fast and middle latency auditory evoked potentials at four intensity levels each were used as objective procedures. The five methods yielded 159 single parameters. Of these, 12 to 40 per analysis were selected in view of relevant criteria and evaluated by means of multivariate discriminant analysis, adopting a program given by LAEUTER and HERMANN [3]. Discriminant analysis is advantageous in that new discriminant features can be calculated from the original data and less efficient data can be disregarded.

In addition to 60 normal-hearing subjects, the analysis involved 51 patients with cochlear hearing impairments and 27 patients with neural muscular atrophy. It is known that neural muscular atrophy can give rise to polyneuropathies with delays in nerve conduction velocity, i.e. a typical retrocochlear lesion [4]. Moreover, 65 lead-exposed patients with suspected polyneuropathies were included in the study. Since the group of lead-exposed subjects did not exhibit any substantial signs of polyneuropathy and, thus, met the criteria of the group of normal-hearing subjects it was disregarded for further analysis.

Resulting from the computations, the combination of variables of three or four methods and six to eight single parameters was found to be most appropriate in accomplishing the task. This combination of variables yielded correct topodiagnostic information for about 75% of the cases. This estimate was made by means of a cross validation procedure.

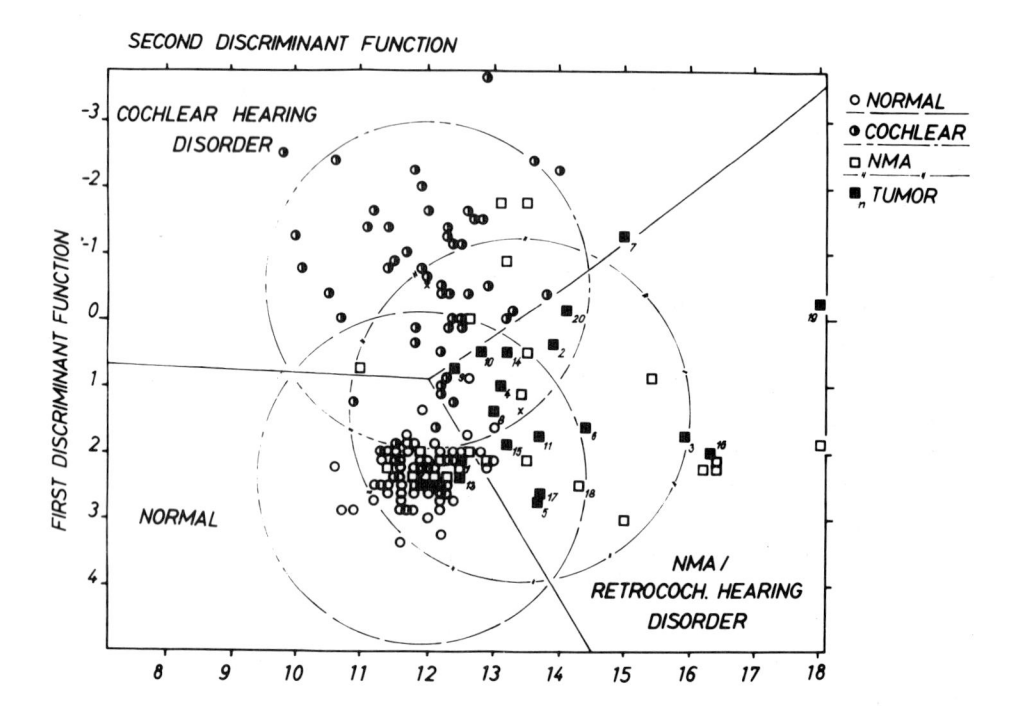

Fig. 1. Results of discriminant analysis for differentiation of normal-hearing subjects, cochlear and retrocochlear hearing impairments, referred to eight features. Borderlines of discrimination by maximum probability. Circles: Spread of groups.

In a next stage, the analysis involved 20 patients with cerebral tumours which, demonstrated by computed tomography, surgery and/or histologically, had also affected the auditory pathway. They were classed by adopting the discriminant rule derived from the above groups. Of those 20 patients, 18 were classed correctly into retrocochlear hearing disorders, and two with cerebral tumours localized remote from the auditory pathway (one olfactory nerve neurinoma and one astrocytoma) were classed into the group of normal-hearing subjects (Fig. 1).

The diagnostic algorithm so determined proved to be adequate in assessing the auditory pathway such that patients can be classed into sufficient topodiagnosis with little discomfort and in an economic approach [5,6]. In this respect, the CAHART test and the speech audiogram did not provide any substantial gain in information.

REFERENCES

1. Krause B, Metzler P (1988) Angewandte Statistik. Deutscher Verlag der Wissenschaften, Berlin
2. Ahrens H, Läuter J (1981) Mehrdimensionale Varianzanalyse. Akademie-Verlag, Berlin.
3. Läuter J, Hermann K (1983) Anwendungsbeschreibung PS MDV. Programmsystem Mehrdimensionale Varianzanalyse OS/ES. Akademie der Wissenschaften der DDR, Institut für Mathematik, Berlin.
4. Bekeny G (1987) Klinik der Muskelkrankheiten. Thieme, Leipzig.
5. Kropf S (1984) Zur Schätzung der Fehlklassifikationswahrscheinlichkeit bei der linearen Diskriminanzanalyse unter besonderer Berücksichtigung parametrischer Verfahren. Dissertation, Technische Hochschule "Otto von Guericke", Magdeburg.
6. Wernecke K-D, Kalb G, Stürzebecher E (1980) Biomed J 22: 639-649

PATHOLOGICAL NYSTAGMUS FINDINGS AFTER HEAD TRAUMA

OBLIQUE PURSUIT EYE MOVEMENTS IN NORMAL ADULTS AND IN CASES WITH VESTIBULAR DISTURBANCES

ARNE W.SCHOLTZ, HEINZ J.SCHOLTZ, UWE SIEVERT
Dept. of ORL, University of Rostock, Doberaner Str. 137, 2500 Rostock (DDR)

The examination of the horizontal pursuit eye movements has a fixed place in the neuro-otological diagnostics. After examinations by Aantaa, Bousseljot and others, this method is very sensitive to disorders of the opto-vestibulo-spinal system, but less sensitive to topodiagnostic findings.

The vertical pursuit eye movements were also included in the equilibriometry since according to Claussen and others a complex analysis of the horizontal and vertical movements, allows extended conclusions.

The problems of oblique eye movements however are dealt with only by a few neuro-otologists, as for instand by Bender and coworkers. Gabersek, who predominatly examined the oblique optokinetic nystagmus in the electrooculographic registration, found out 3 different curve patterns in normal adults, which seem to be entailed by different periocular electrical fields. In our previons investigations of oblique saccades the horizontal components showed higher velocities than the vertical, among which, in turn, the upward movement is carried out slowest.

This means, that the oblique saccades present themselves as curves as can be seen in the figure.

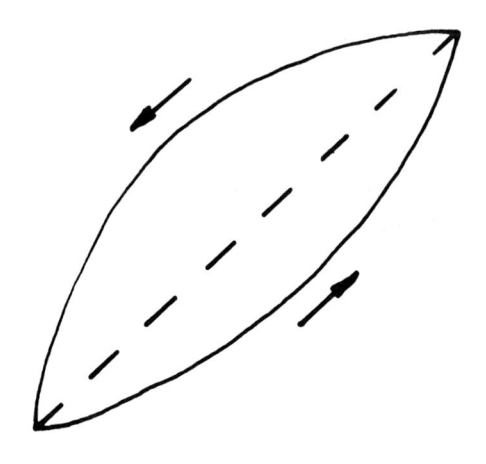

Fig. 1.
Orbit of oblique saccades

The curve for the upward movements is higher than for the downward movement.

Since the pursuit eye movements are largely caused by the same neural structures, but can be carried out with different velocities, we intended to examine, firstly, up to which velocities the eyes are able to follow the stimulus linearly, secondly, what course is taken by the horizontal and vertical components of these movements during high stimulation velocities, and thirdly, are there differences between normal subjects and patients with disorders of the opto-vestibulo-spinal system.

MATERIAL AND METHODS

The examinations were carried out with 40 healthy subjects aged between 18 and 61 years, who had never suffered from ear or nervous diseases, Visual discorders were excluded. In addition, 17 patients with peripher al and central disturbances of the vestibular function participated in our examinations.

They sat on a chair with a head-rest and had a 100 cm long row of light-emitting diodes before their eyes. At first, the row was bent by 45°, and in the second test series bent by 135°. Light-emitting diodes were used as a stimulus performing sinusoidal, pendular movements, seen by the test person under an amplitude of 30° at the most.

The eye movements were recorded by means of PENG according to Gestewitz and, at the same time, represented on an oscillograph screen and recorded on a xy-plotter.

At first, each test person performed oblique saccades of 30° in both oblique planes. This was followed by 11 individual examinations of the eye tracking test in the frequency range between 0,2 an 1,2 Hz for each subject, where at least 6 pendular eye movements were performed.

RESULTS

In healthy persons the examinations of the oblique saccades resulted in bent eye movement recordings, corresponding to the findings by Nakazawa and other of our department.

When performing the pursuit eye movements it was recorded that the movement from left-up to right-down and backward was performed safer and with fewer saccades. However, from right up to left down such decay phenomena occurred already at lower frequencies.

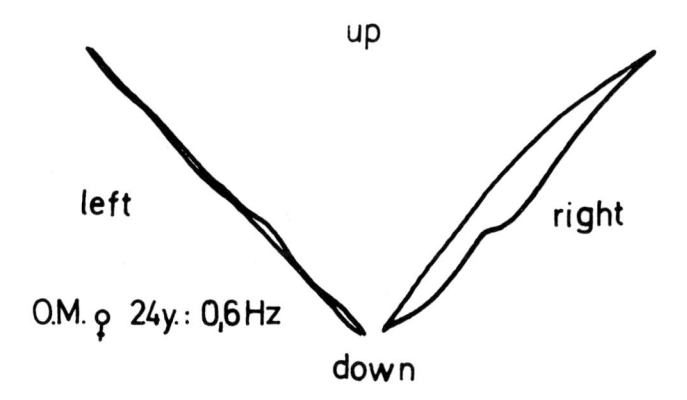

Fig. 2. Oblique pursuit eye movements in healthy persons with frequency of 0,6 Hz.

Only in 2 test subjects no difference was recorded.

The average stimulus frequency, up to which a linear pursuit eye movement was possible, amounts to 0,9 Hz for the plane left-up to right-down and 0,6 Hz in the other plane.

From this, an eye velocity of the maximum linear pursuit of $57,8°/s$ or $38,4°/s$, is calculated. The difference is statistically significant.

In a two-dimensional recording the eye movement behaves at higher stimulus velocities in the same way as in the saccade test, apart from the appearance of saccades there will be a higher velocity of the horizontal movement component.

In 5 patients with unilateral loss of the vestibular function the pursuit eye movements is interrupted by the spontaneous nystagmus. The limit values of the linear pursuit movements amount to 0,8 Hz or 0,6 Hz, respectively, and do not differ significantly from the normal values.

12 patients with post-commotio-vertigo without spontaneous nystagmus demonstrated a more intensive saccadation already from 0,2 or 0,3 Hz, respectively, and showed a non-linearity of the oblique eye movement already at 0,45 or 0,38 Hz, respectively.

DISKUSSION

In the diagnoses of the vertical pursuit eye movement the PENG method offers advantages, since it permits, within its limits, so far open influences of the upper eyelid movements in the EOG to be avoided.

Based on the results of our determinations of the oblique saccades and the oblique OKN, we extended this programme and determined those eye velocities, at which the oblique linear pursuit eye movement changes into an arched one, showing an initial prevalence of the horizontal component- This phenomenon could be explained by the general preponderance of the horizontal eye movements in adults. As frequently confirmed, eye movements can be faster in horizontal plane than in vertical one.

Gabersek also found difference between both oblique eye movements.

It was made sure in the PENG examinations that in correspondance with the principle of the binocular community according to Trendelburg, both eyes show the same behaviour. Therefore, a connection with the training of eye movements in learning and performing of reading and writing should be discussed. An examination of Arabian people could contribute to a clarification.

Since the performance of the oblique pursuit eye movements represent complex reflexes, it is not surprising that different cerebral disturbances become evident Whereas a labyrinth disorder despite of a spontaneous nystagmus does not result in a fundamental change compared with the normal behaviour.

Our results support the demand to use pursuit eye movement tests for proving central neurootological disorders.

REFERENCES

1. Bender MB (1960) Comments on the physiology and pathology of eye movements in the vertical plane. J.nervous and mental diseases 130: 456-466
2. Bousseljot W (1977) Die diagnostische Wertigkeit von Störungen der Blickfolgebewegung. Greifswald, Diss. (B)
3. Claussen CF (1983) Optokinetische Tests. In: Claussen CF (ed) Verhandlungen der GNA EV Bd. IX Edition m + p, Hamburg, pp 123-144
4. Gabersek V (1987) Some aspects of Purkyne's in fluence on recent studies of oblique eye movements. Physiologia Bohemoslavica, Prag 36: 269-282
5. Gestewitz HR (1975) Methoden zur Untersuchung des Gleichgewichtsapparates anhand des funktionellen Zusammenwirkens seiner einzelnen anatomischen Abschnitte. Das opto-vestibulo-spinale System. Militärmed, Berlin 16: 301-307
6. Grenman R, Aantaa S, Aantaa E (1983) OKN, PETT and voluntary saccadic eye-movements in 36 multiple sclerosis patients. In: Claussen, CF (ed): Verhandlungen der GNA EVm Bd, IX Edition m + p, Hamburg, pp 183-191
7. Nakazawa H, Scholtz HJ, Sievert U, Käcker N, Sakata E (1989) Der diagonale Sakkadentest. 36. Gemeinschaftstagung HNO Greifswald, Rostock, Magdeburg, Stralsund (im Druck)
8. Scholtz HJ, Pyykkö L, Henriksson HG (1983) Electrooculography of vertical saccades. Adv. Oto-Rhino-Laryng. - Basel 30:
9. Scholtz HJ, Sievert U, Scholtz AW, Nakazawa H (1989) Influence of head position on optokinetic nystagmus. IV.Symposium für Neuro-Otologie Berlin (im Druck)
10. Trendelenburg W (1961) Der Gesichtssinn. Springer, Berlin

DETECTION AND LOCALIZATION OF VESTIBULAR LESION DUE TO HEAD AND NECK TRAUMA. A VECTOR-NYSTAGMOGRAPHIC STUDY.

HELOISA HELENA CAOVILLA, YASUKO IMASATO ITO, TEOTONIO T. COSTA NETO, FABIO AKIRA SUZUKI, CARLOS AUGUSTO ANADÃO, FERNANDO FREITAS GANANÇA, MAURICIO M. GANANÇA

Department of Otoneurology, Escola Paulista de Medicina, Rua Botucatú 834 - 04023 São Paulo - Brazil.

INTRODUCTION

Audio-vestibular disturbances as a consequence of head and neck injury are commonly observed. Vertigo happens in the majority of individuals who have had a head and neck trauma.

Trauma to vestibular - auditory system may follow direct blows to the head, penetrating wounds to the head, sudden severe changes of atmosphere, surgery in or about the ear, etc.(1).

The pathology of traumatic vestibular disorders may involve the labyrinth, VIIIth nerve or Central Nervous System pathways.

Head injury generally damages the fragile labyrinthine membranes with or without associated bone fracture. Fractures of temporal bone are divided into two types: longitudinal and transverse (2). Combination of these fractures and concomitant Central Nervous System damages to the auditory and vestibular systems may give different clinical pictures.

Sensorineural hearing loss and vertigo characteristics of inner ear concussion frequently accompany a longitudinal temporal bone fracture. Nevertheless, the bone labyrinth is seldom fractured. Transverse fractures often pass through the labyrinth and VIIIth nerve, producing a total loss of vestibular and cochlear functions (3).

Vertigo, nausea and vomiting are usually present for several days after the transverse fracture.

In the other cases, positional vertigo is the most common symptom (4). Headache, irritability, insomnia, forgetfulness, mental obtusiness and loss of initiative are also other symptoms observed.

The disequilibrium reported differs from true spontaneous vertigo to postural dizziness or further a giddiness. The patient could develop sudden brief attacks of vertigo on changing head position which varies in intensity with gradual improvement. The persistence of symptoms and signs, however, seems to be related to the severity of the injury.

Any kind of dizziness, nausea and vomiting usually subside within two or three weeks. However, feelings of unsteadiness may persist for months.

Lack of response to caloric stimulation occured only in patients who had skull fractures.

The onset of hearing loss is tipically acute. However, on rare occasions, it may be postponed according to the damage extension. The initial degree of loss may be variable. Fluctuation, recovery or deterioration of pure tone sensitivity may occur (5).

As a general rule, recovery of auditory function occurs during the first three weeks after the injury. However, improvement in hearing sensitivity has been observed for as long as six months after the trauma (6).

Tinnitus may be also present in many of these patients (3).

MATERIAL AND METHODS

We have studied 50 patients with head and neck trauma. Their age varied from 20 to 61 years. Twenty-six were males and twenty-four females. Twenty-nine cases had direct blows to the head as the cause of trauma. Twenty-eight of them without fracture of the temporal bone and just one had a longitudinal fracture. Underwater diving caused labyrinthine trauma in nine patients. Airplane flights determined labyrinthine trauma in five patients. Penetrating wounds were observed in only one case.

The patients were evaluated from 2 to 30 days after the head and neck trauma.

All the patients were submitted to a complete neurootological examination including anamnesis, audiological and vestibular tests. The eye movements were recorded through a Nystar Plus nystagmography computarized system and a three-channel Berger vectornystagmograph.

Vestibulo-oculomotor tests included recordings of saccades, spontaneous and gaze nystagmus, positional and positioning nystagmus, smooth pursuit, optokinetic nystagmus, torsion swing stimulation and bithermal caloric tests (7).

RESULTS AND COMMENTS

We have verified high incidence of vertigo and other kinds of dizziness (72 % of the cases) and nausea (26 %), tinnitus (18 %), noise intolerance (18 %), hearing loss (18 %) and fulness in the ear (14 %) were also frequently reported.

It is interesting to emphazise the presence of psychological symptoms such as depression, anxiety and phobias in 24 % of the patients.

Unilateral sensorineural hearing loss was noticed in 24 % of the cases. Only one patient with normal audiogram presented an abnormal horizontal configuration in the impedanciometry: reflexes on both ears are consistently absent to crossed stimulation and consistently present to uncrossed stimulation. In this patient the auditory brain stem evoked response audiometry showed a considerably delayed waves III and V, characterizing a brain stem lesion. In spite of this, no neurological findings were found in this patient.

Abnormal speech intelligibility scores were verified in 2 % of the patients who presented sensorineural hearing loss.

An important spontaneous recovering of hearing loss was observed in one patient within 30 days after the trauma.

Abnormal vestibular findings were noted in 64 % of the patients.

Pathological spontaneous nystagmus occurred in 28 % of the cases. Positional vertigo or positional nystagmus were found in 26 % of the patients. Perrotatory nystagmus directional preponderance was seen in 24 % of the cases , 22 % of the patients presented post-caloric nystagmus directional preponderance and 4 % showed unilateral vestibular hypo-reflexia.

CONCLUSIONS

Concerning patients with head and neck trauma we have found that:
1) Audio-vestibular impairment was frequently observed without any neurological findings;
2) Vestibular disturbances were more frequent than the audiological ones;
3) Abnormal spontaneous, positional, perrotatory and post-caloric nystagmus were commonly verified in these patients.

REFERENCES

1. Alberti P, Jerger J (1974) Arch Otolaryngol 99:206
2. Barber H (1969) Ann Otol Rhinol Laryngol 78:239
3. Jerger S, Jerger J (1981) Auditory Disorders. Little Brown, Boston
4. Barber H (1964) Laryngoscope 74:891
5. Hough J (1973) In: Papparella M, Schumrick D Otolaryngology. Sauders, Philadelphia, pp 241-262
6. Schulman J (1979) In: Goodhill V Ear Diseases, Deafness and Dizzines. Harper & Row, New York, pp 504-516
7. Mangabeira Albernaz PL, Ganança MM, Caovilla HH, Ito YI, Castro HD (1984) An Atlas of Vector-nystagmography. Aché, São Paulo.

THE INFLUENCE OF POSTCONTUSIONAL OCULAR DISTURBANCES UPON THE ENG

W. D. SCHÄFER, C.-F. CLAUSSEN

University Eye Hospital Wuerzburg and Neurootological Research Center Bad Kissingen (West Germany)

DEFINITION

In anglo-american literature brain-injuries are called concussions of the brain[11]. The severity of the disease is stated by using the terms slight, moderate and severe. In German language doctors further on are using the terms commotio and contusio cerebri. Thereby mistakes concerning the judgement of patients complaints may occur by sticking to a formerly made diagnosis. In the same way the sequels of a brain concussion are described as postconcussion-syndrome or postconcussional state [2,5,12].

MECHANICS OF BRAIN CONCUSSIONS

In contusions of the skull in general the principle of the coup- and contre-coup-focus are well known. The smaller contusional focus on the position of the impact at the head has a larger injury at the opposite side of the brain.-The effect of the liquor-space in this matter is not completely known. In function as a kind of a shock absorber after slight concussions it might however alterate the brain tissue strongly in severe trauma.

There is a certain shifting of the liquor in the third and the two side ventricles. The fourth ventricle is narrowed to the spinal cord like the neck of a bottle, so that high velocity movements hit the liquor against the brainstem or/and against the cerebellum. Damages like falling on water from a great height may occur. Additionally the effect of the tentorium cerebelli, being situated between brain and cerebellum commonly is neglected. In the slot of the tentorium tissue of the brain may be pushed in as it may happen at the foramen occipitale magnum. Thereby strains of the oculomotoric nerve may be caused too [7].

Severe contusions of the brain mostly affect the brain-stem with the nuclei of the eye muscles and the supranuclear centres. In a rostral position the nuclei of the nerves III, IV and VI are located as well as the paramedian pontine reticular formation (PPRF) controlling the horizontal movements of view and the rostral interstitial fasciculus longitudinalis medialis (ri MLF), which controls the vertical eye movements [8]. Beside the nuclei of neighboured organs of the eye in the brainstem the neuronal centres of convergence, accommodation and fusion are supposed to be located in the same area.

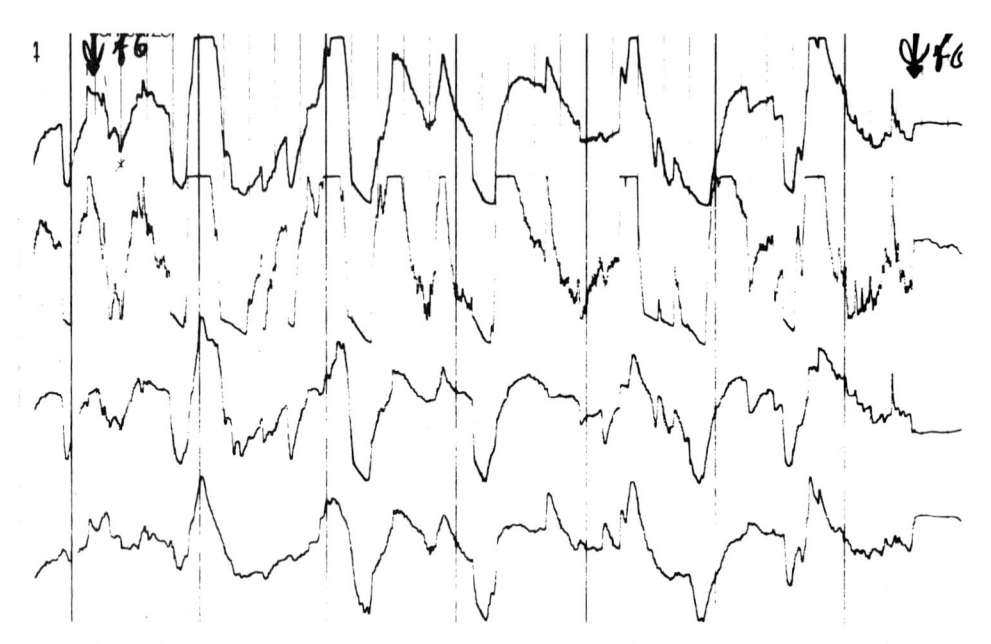

Fig. 1 General dysrhythmics in horizontal registration of the spontaneous nystagmus. (from up to down:1. tracing : both eyes, time-constant 0,6 sec.; 2. tracing : both eyes, time constant 0,01 sec; 3. tracing : right eye; 4. tracing : left eye)

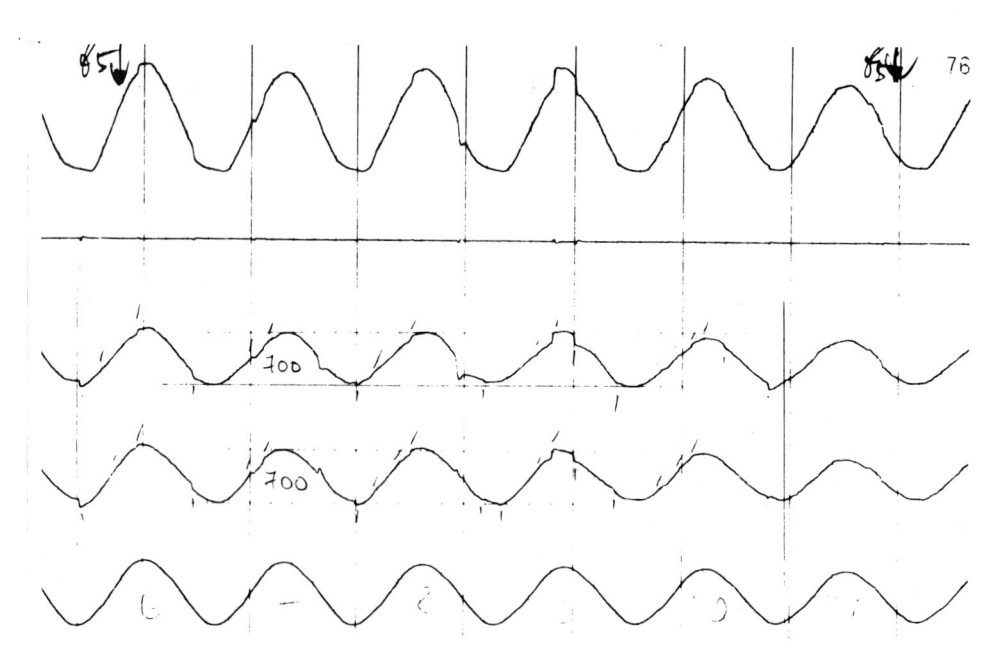

Fig. 2 Horizontal ocular tracking over 30 degrees. (1. tracing : right eye; 2. tracing : left eye; 3. tracing : stimulus)

COMPLAINTS OF PATIENTS

Missing paresis of the eyes or supranuclear disturbances the complaints of the patients are often very unspecific as far as the eyes are affected [10]. These patients generally complain of visual disturbances, hazy vision or blurred vision. These statements may be interpreted as retino-vascular problems. More specific complains concern problems in short distance viewing, changing diplopia, vertically and horizontally with changing distance of two images. Vertigo, headache, disturbing of cognition and memory and alterated concentration are general complaints in a post concussional state. In this case these patients are noticed as changed in personality and state of emotion.

OPHTHALMOLOGICAL AND NEUROOTOLOGICAL FINDINGS

Both, ocular findings and cases of brain contusion reveal wide ranges of clinical aspects. Nuclear and supranuclear pareses of different intensities are to be found. Pareses of convergence, accommodation and fusion are striking at a quite low, in many cases unnoticable level. All three functions may be completely or partially affected. Paresis of convergence is most frequent followed by paresis of accommodation and fusion [6].

Testing convergence is the easiest clinical method. Instead of fixating an object opposite to the eye, moving towards the face, the patient sometimes reveals a short impulse to fixation. Then one or both eyes may be deviating quickly. In this cases we consider an intermittant divergent squint of the type of convergence weakness. Most of those cases do not reveal specific neurological findings and changes in the ENG. Applying a horizontally 30 dgr. swinging pendulum dysrhythmic movements of the eyes (Fig. 1) might be seen, sometimes interposed by square waves. Similar effects due to central disorders of coordination may appear during the ENG-registration of spontaneous nystagmus [3] (Fig. 2).

THERAPY

As spontaneous improvements are registered up to about three years after a concussion of brain and functional changes may arise due to rehabilitation events therapy should be started cautiously [1,4,9]. As some patients are showing a deep change in personality, ophthalmologic therapy by spectacles, prisms or eye-surgery is strictly refused. In other cases the correction of even small anomalities of refraction has prooved to be helpful. In purpose of curing pareses of accommodation reading glasses or bifocals are applicable. Surgery of the eye muscles has to be planned carefully. Weakness of fusion and differences between the angle of squint for far distance and short distance viewing are the main reasons for restraining surgical interventions. If there is additionally a latent eye-deviation, decompensated by an accident surgery can be applied.

In some cases small areas free of double vision might be mentioned as a result of an intervention leading to a better ability of spatial orientation. General advice on managing the own life after head injuries is necessary. Patients should be advised in any matters of private life, profession and behaviour in traffic and sports.

SUMMARY

The sequels of concussions of the brain are commonly disregarded especially concerning cases with unveiled paresis. These cases occur due to brain damaging in the region of the fourth ventricle. The patients complaints are very unspecific. The ophthalmologist may detect combinations of paresis of convergence, accommodation and fusion differing in intensity. Dysaequilibriometric states are detectable as well. Eye motility testing and applying electronystagmography provides complete diagnosis. Respecting therapy patients should behave entirely forebearing, as noticable improvements have been registrated more than three years after an accident. Ophthalmologists can provide aid by correcting anomalies of refraction with eye glasses. In some cases bifocals and eye-muscle surgery are indicated.

REFERENCES

1. Albert HH v (1988) Fortschr Med 106: (20)10
2. Becker DP, Miller JD, Greenberg RP(1982) In: Youmans JR (ed.) Neurological Surgery, Vol. 4, Saunders, Philadelphia, p 2137
3. Claussen CF, Aust G, Schäfer WD (1986) : Atlas der Elektronystagmographie, edition medizin + pharmazie, Hamburg
4. Dikmen S et al. (1987) J Neurol Neurosurg Psychol, 50 : 1613
5. Duke-Elder St, Mac Faul PA (1972) In : Duke-Elder St (ed.) System of Ophthalmology Vol. XIV, Part 1, Kimpton, London, p. 66
6. Flick H (1976) In : Ehrich W, Remler, O (Hrsg.) : Das Kopftrauma aus augenärztlicher Sicht, Enke, Stuttgart, S. 36
7. Hermann HD (1976) In : Ehrich W, Remler, O (Hrsg.) Das Kopftrauma aus augenärztlicher Sicht, Enke, Stuttgart, S.1
8. Kömpf D (1984) In: Marx, P(Hrsg.) Augenbewegungsstörungen in Neurologie und Ophthalmologie, Springer, Berlin, S. 1
9. McLaurin RL (1975) In : Farmer TW (ed.) Pediatric Neurology, Harper & Row, Hagerstown, p. 303
10. Schäfer WD(1989) Z prakt Augenheilkd. 10 , 243
11. Verjaal A, Van't Hooft F(1975) In : Vinken PJ, Bruyn GW (eds.) Handbook of Clinical Neurology, Vol. 23, , North Holland Publishing Co., Amsterdam, p. 417
12. Young B (1985) In : Wilkins RH, Rengachary SS (eds.) Neurosurgery, Vol 2, McGraw Hill, New York, p. 1688

RATIONALE FOR ROUTINE EVALUATION OF PROVOKED NY IN CNS DISEASES

ALPINI D., CESARANI A°, CAPUTO D*, GHEZZI A**, ZAFFARONI M** MINI M*
ENG Laboratory Busto Arsizio Hospital
Institute of Audiology University of Milan
Institute Don Carlo Gnocchi Multiple Sclerosis Center
Gallarate Hospital Multiple Sclerosis Center

INTRODUCTION
A pt. with a lesion, suspected or defined, of the central nervous system (CNS) is usually studied by the mean of a lot of morphological and functional tests.
In this field the aim of neurotological examination is to evaluate the functional involvement of the disease.
The problem is the choice of the tests to perform in this spite in order to evaluate the patient(pt) in a way that is as complete and as quick as possible.
The goal of the paper is to report our experience regarding routine evaluation of pt with CNS diseases.

MATERIALS AND METHODS
The tests of choice to study vestibular-ocular-reflex(VOR) in a routine clinical point of view must answer to the following criteria:
- evaluation of peripheral labyrinth lesion
- evaluation of central vestibular pathways
- simple execution
- quick execution in order to not cause stress in a variously and extendly studied pt.

In this spite we avoided liminar methods such as Montandon rotatory stimulation.
Spontaneous ny was studied with and without fixation, in primary and lateral positions of gaze.
Provoked ny was differentely studied in 4 groups of omogenous pt.
To simplify the analisys of the results we studied only pt. affected with probable and defined Multiple Sclerosis. The pt. were studied by the mean of different vestibular stimulation according random criteria.
Group A) 70 pt(43 females and 27 males, mean age 38 yy)
The following tests were performed:
- bithermal Veits caloric stimulations
- visual supprression test during warm stimulation responses
- pendular sinusoidal Greiner stimulation

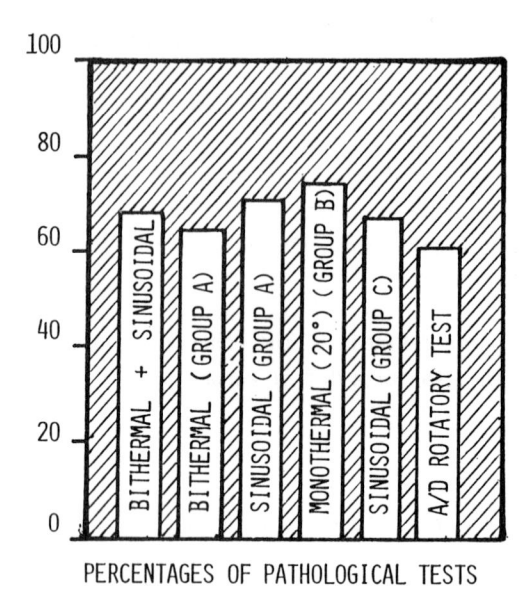

Figure 1.

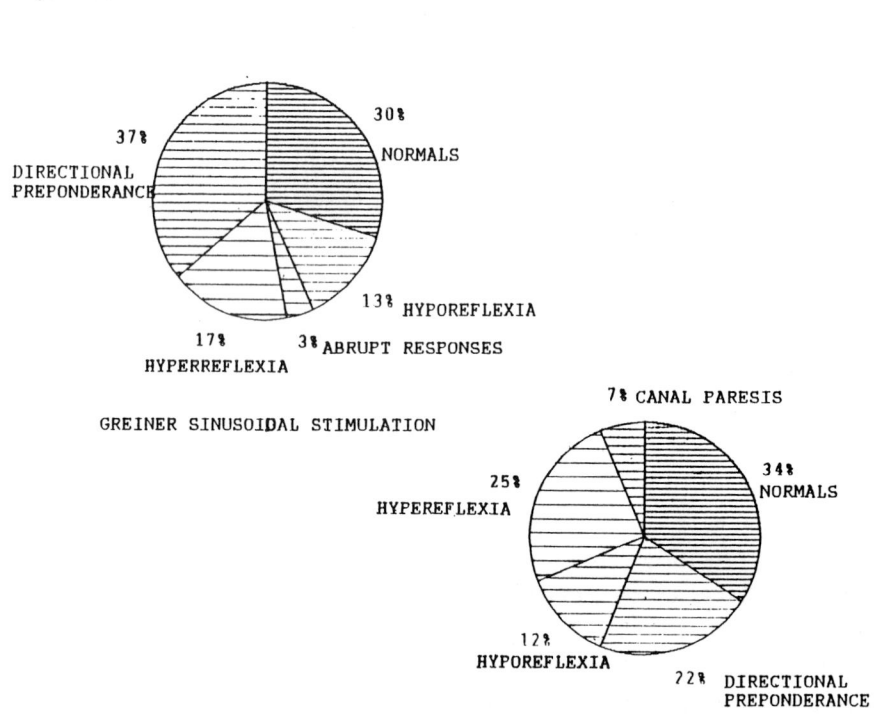

PERCENTAGES OF PATHOLOGICAL TESTS

(bars: BITHERMAL + SINUSOIDAL, BITHERMAL (GROUP A), SINUSOIDAL (GROUP A), MONOTHERMAL (20°) (GROUP B), SINUSOIDAL (GROUP C), A/D ROTATORY TEST)

GREINER SINUSOIDAL STIMULATION
- 30% NORMALS
- 37% DIRECTIONAL PREPONDERANCE
- 17% HYPERREFLEXIA
- 3% ABRUPT RESPONSES
- 13% HYPOREFLEXIA

BITHERMAL CALORIC STIMULATIONS (20' - 47')
- 7% CANAL PARESIS
- 34% NORMALS
- 25% HYPEREFLEXIA
- 12% HYPOREFLEXIA
- 22% DIRECTIONAL PREPONDERANCE

Figure 2.

- visual suppression test during the second pendular stimulation
  A Beckman dynograph was employed
Group B) 32 pt(15 females and 17 males) in which only cold (20°, 10cc in
5 sec) stimulations and VST were performed.
A Nicolet Nystar computerized electronystagmograph was used.
Group C) 30 pt(20 famales and 10 males) in which only pendular Greiner
stimulation and VST were performed.
Group D) 20 pt(9 females and 11 males) in which only rotatory A/D
(Sthale modified by Pirodda) stimulation was performed.
Directional preponderance and canal paresis were calculated on slow phase
velocities according to Jongkeess' formulae.
For roto-acceleratory tests the following formula was adopted to calculate
directional preponderance:
left SPV-right SPV/left SPV+right SPV

RESULTS
Group A) In figure 1 the results of bithermal caloric stimulations are
summed:
Normal responses have been found in 34%, Bilateral hyforeflexia in 12%;
bilateral Hyperreflexia in 25%; canalparesis in 7% and directional
preponderance in 22%
In fig. 2 the results obtained by pendular stimulation is summed:
30% normal resposes; 37% directional preponderance; 17% bilateral
hyperreflexia; 13% bilateral hyporeflexia.
15% out of this group had an abnormal visual supprression test during
caloric stimulations while one pt had normal sinusoidal VST and abnormal
caloric VST.
 Group B) cold stimulations were alterated in 72%
Group C) sinusoidal stimulation was alterated in 67%
Group D) In fig. 3 the results of A/D rotatory test are summed:
37% normal responses; 19% bilateral hypereflexia; 5% canal paresis.
In order to simplify the comparison of different tests performed in fig.4
we summed the percentages of pathological results indepentely from the
kind of alteration. The kind of alteration in fact, is too much strictly
depending on the site of neurological lesion that are not omogeneous in
the different groups and into each group.

CONCLUSION
In our experience the different provokative tests performed gave the same
results. The percentage of pathological examination are around 60%. The
differences among the tests are not significative .

We think that Multiple Sclerosis may be a good example of utilization of otoneurological investigation in routine functional evaluation.
The test to choice is depending on the experience of the neurotologist and the technical structures.
A simple method of vestibular stimulation followed, if necessary, from more precise tests is our operative proposal.

REFERENCES

1. Arslan M.: On the renewing of the methodology for the stimulation of the vestibular apparatus. Acta Oto-Laryng. 1955, Suppl., 122, 7-92
2. Claussen C.F., Schilachia I.: Butterfly chart for caloric nystagmus evaluation. Arch. Otolaryng. 1972, 96, 371.
3. Greiner G.F., Conraux C., Collard M.: Vestibulomètrie clinique. Doin ed., Paris 1969.
4. Hallpike C.S.: The caloric test. J. Laryngol., 1956, 70,15.
5. Hart C.W.: Ocular fixation and the caloric test. Laryngosc., 77, 2103-2113, 1967.
6. Hennebert P.: La nystagmographie dans les épreuves thermiques. Acta Otolaryng., Belg. 14, 5-88, 1960.
7. Henrikosson N.G.: The correlation between the speed of the eye in the slow phase and vestibular stimulus. Acta Oto-Laryng.,1955, 45, 120-136
8. Jongkees L.B.W.: Value of the caloric test of the labyrinth. Arch. of Otolaryng. 1948, 48, 402.
9. Montandon A., Huguenin S., Lehmann W., John F.: Aspects quantitatifs de l'èpreuve rotatoire. Vè symposium de nystagmographie de langue française, Arnette Edit., Paris 1971, 87.
10. Mulch G., Leonardy B., Petermann W.: Which are the parameters of choice for the evaluation of caloric nystagmus? Arch. Oto-Rhino-Laryng. 1978, 221, 23-25.
11. Mulch G.: Criteria for the evaluation of nystagmus. ORL 1978, 40, 263-277
12. Norrè M.E.: The unilateral vestibular hypofunction. Acta Oto-Rhino-laryngol. belgica 5, 1978
13. Torok N.: The culmination phenomenon and the frequence pattern of thermic nystagmus. Acta Oto-Laryng., 1957, 48, 530-535.
14. Veits C.: Neue untersuchungen Uber die Kalorischen vestibularisreaktionen. Acta Oto-Laryng., 1928, 13, 94-115.

LATE ELECTRONYSTAGMOGRAPHIC FINDINGS IN PATIENTS WITH HEAD TRAUMA.

JOSÉ CARLOS RAMOS FERNANDES; ANTONIO CARLOS CEDIN; VERA HELENA GUIMARÃES
Dept. of Otorrinolaringology, Hospital Servidor Público Municipal e Hospital São Joaquim, Beneficência Portuguêsa, São Paulo, Brazil.

INTRODUCTION

Different kinds of vestibular disturbances may result from head and neck trauma. Labyrinthine disorders of traumatic origin are very frequent and very important in Medicine.

The purpose of the present study was to investigate the occurrence of late vector-electronystagmography abnormalities in patients with moderate or severe head trauma.

TOGLIA and EGYED (1972) studied 333 patients with head injury and found 83% of abnormalities in electronystagmography.

MATERIAL AND METHOD

This study was carried out in 27 patients with moderate or severe head injury due to car crashes or in door accidents. By means of anamnesis we could measure the intensity of the trauma. The trauma could classyfied as severe when the patients had unconciousness for at last one hour and as moderate whe the patients had not conciousness disturbances.

In our study 60% of the patients had severe head trauma.

Twenty-three were males and 4 females. Their age varied from 28 to 69 years.

All patients were submitted to a neurotological examination including: ear, nose and throat examinations, pure tone audiogram, discrimination scores, impedanciometry and vector-electronystagmography recordings of spontaneous, gaze and positional nystagmus; eye-tracking and optokinetic tests, torsion swing stimulation and caloric test[6].

RESULTS AND COMMENTS

The findings obtained from 27 patients with head trauma are shown in tables I to IV.

Table I shows the audiometric findings in these patients. Only two presented high frequencel hearing loss.

TABLE I
AUDIOMETRIC FINDINGS IN 27 PATIENTS WITH HEAD TRAUMA.

Pure tone audiometry	Nº Patients	%
Normal	25	92,4
High frequency hearing loss	2	7,6
Total	27	100,0

Electronystagmography must be used in all patients with head trauma, because 66,6% had some kind of electronystagmography (ENG) abnormalities (Table II). Only nine patients presented normal electronystagmography finding.

TABLE II
VECTOR-ELECTRONYSTAGMOGRAPHY FINDINGS IN 27 PATIENTS WITH HEAD TRAUMA.

Vector-electronystagmography	Nº Patients	%
Normal	9	33,3
Vestibular abnormalities	18	66,7
Total	27	100,0

In this study the more prevalent electronystagmography finding was hypo-reflexia that occurred in 33,3% of patients (Table III).

The other ENG abnormal sign was directional preponderance (11,1% of the cases) and labyrinthine preponderance (22,2% of the cases) as we can see in tables III and IV.

TABLE III

VECTOR-ELECTRONYSTAGMOGRAPHY FINDINGS IN 18 PATIENTS WITH HEAD TRAUMA.

Vector-electronystagmography abnormalities	Nº Patients	%
Hypo-reflexia	9	33,3
Labyrinthine preponderance	6	22,0
Directional preponderance	3	11,3
Total	18	66,6

TABLE IV

VECTOR-ELECTRONYSTAGMOGRAPHY VESTIBULAR IN PATIENTS WITH HEAD TRAUMA.

Case	Age	Findings
1	28	Bilateral hipo-reflexia
3	31	Direcional preponderance
4	33	Direcional preponderance
8	38	Directional preponderance
12	45	Unilateral hypo-reflexia
13	46	Unilateral hypo-reflexia
15	47	Unilateral hypo-reflexia
16	47	Labyrinthine preponderance
17	53	Bilateral hypo-reflexia
18	54	Labyrinthine preponderance
19	55	Labyrinthine preponderance
21	55	Unilateral hypo-reflexia
22	58	Labyrinthine preponderance
23	60	Bilateral hypo-reflexia
24	60	Labyrinthine preponderance
25	60	Bilateral hypo-reflexia
26	64	Unilateral hypo-reflexia
27	69	Labyrinthine preponderance

Dizziness was complained by all the patients.

CONCLUSION

The majority of the patients with head trauma, complaning of vertigo, presented vector-electronystagmography abnormalities corresponding to peripheral vestibular disorders. No central vestibular impairement was observed in these patients.

These results suggested that vector-electronystagmography must be sistematically used in all patients with head trauma.

SUMMARY

On our study the results obtained through the use of electronystagmography in 27 vertiginous patients, who were examined at least 180 days after the occurrence of moderate or severe head trauma, has shown 66,6% of vestibular abnormalities.

The most frequence electronystagmography sign that occurred in 33,3% of the patients was hypo-reflexia.

REFERENCES

1. Toglia, J.U. and Egyed, J. (1972) Disturbios vestibulares en el traumatismo cráneo-encefálico. Otorrinolaringológica X: 216-222.

VISUAL-VESTIBULAR INTERACTION AND OPTOKINETIC MODIFICATIONS IN THE POST CONCUSSIONAL SYNDROME

JOSE LUIS CARDENAS N.
Department of Neurology.Barros Luco-Trudeau Hospital.
School of Medicine.University of Chile.Santiago de Chile.

INTRODUCTION
It is feasible to stablish a relationship between the polimorfism of the post concussional syndrome after head injury and the hypothesis of an uncompensated peripheral vestibular lesion owing to a brainstem disfunction of the mechanisms of the vestibular central compensation.(1-2).The most frequent symptoms of this syndrome are generalized or localized headache,vertigo,vague dizzines , imbalance , tinnitus, loss of concentration, irritability and somnolence.In a previous experience with a selected sample of 150 patients with post concussional syndrome, have been demonstrated the existence of vestibular disturbances in 85% of the group. The audiological disturbances were 47% of the sample(2).
The vestibular nuclei encode the labyrinthine inputs.These informations can be modified by the visual input and modulated by the floccular Purkinje cells of the cerebellum.(3).
Optokinetic nystagmus(OKN) is a visual-oculomotor reflex with a direct component(visual-oculomotor pathways=rapid initial rise in slow phase velocity) related to smooth pursuit eye movement and an indirect component (velocity storage component=slower rise in slow phase velocity to a steady state level and optokinetic after-nystagmus OKAN) related to activity in vestibular system.(4)
In humans and in monkeys , a predominant portion of the direct visual-oculomotor pathways mediating the rapid initial rise in slow phase eye velocity OKN as well as pursuit eye movements are mediated through the flocculus and probably paraflocculus(5).

MATERIAL AND METHODS
Thirty patients(age=18-40 yrs) with post concussional syndrome and **without demonstrable peripheral vestibular disfunction** were submitted to optokinetic tests. The subjects were seated in a Barany chair and the OKN was elicited using an internally illuminated motorized striped drum projecting 8 alternating black and white vertical stripes, each subtending $7,5°$ of the visual angle. 1,5 m in front of the subjects there was placed

a half cylindrical projection screen on which vertical black
and white stripes were projected. The subjects were asked to
perform active visual fixation during the optokinetic stimulation.
OKN was induced by constant positive acceleration($3^0/s^2$) from
0^0 to 80^0/s.(right and left horizontal ;up and down vertical)
followed by constant negative acceleration ($3^0/s^2$).
As control group, thirty healthy volunteers of similar average
age have been tested.
PARAMETERS:1.) slow phase velocity (SPV)of OKN promediated during stimulation at 10-20- 40- 60-80 ^{0}/s. in positive and negative acceleration. The significance of differences between SPV
of the experimental and control groups was tested applying Mann-
Whitney U and Kruskal Wallis H test.
2)Qualitative modifications of OKN in form of deviation towards
the slow phase, dysrhythmia and inversion of the direction of
the fast phase were investigated in each period of the optokinetic responses.

RESULTS

The difference between SPV of experimental and control groups
was significantly at velocity stimulation of 40- 60- 80^0/s.
right(Fig.1) and left (Fig.2) horizontal and up and down vertical(Fig.3) .($p<0.05$) with lower slow phase velocity of OKN in
100% of the experimental group.

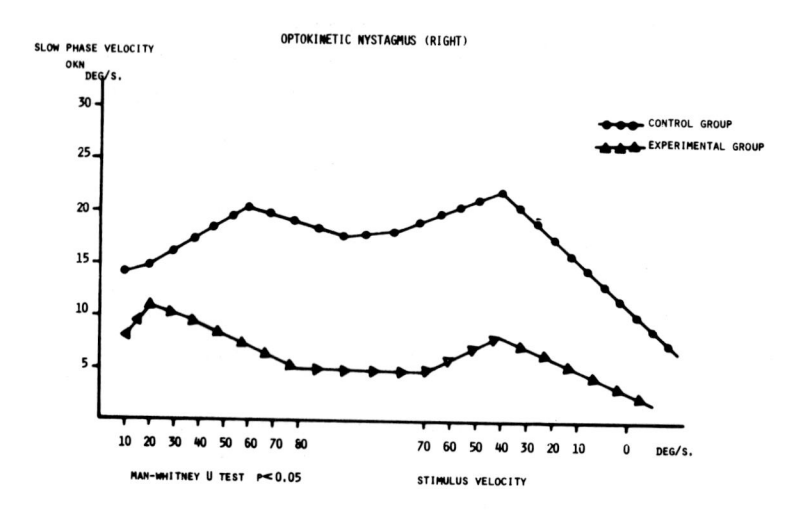

Fig.1. SPV OKN responses (right).

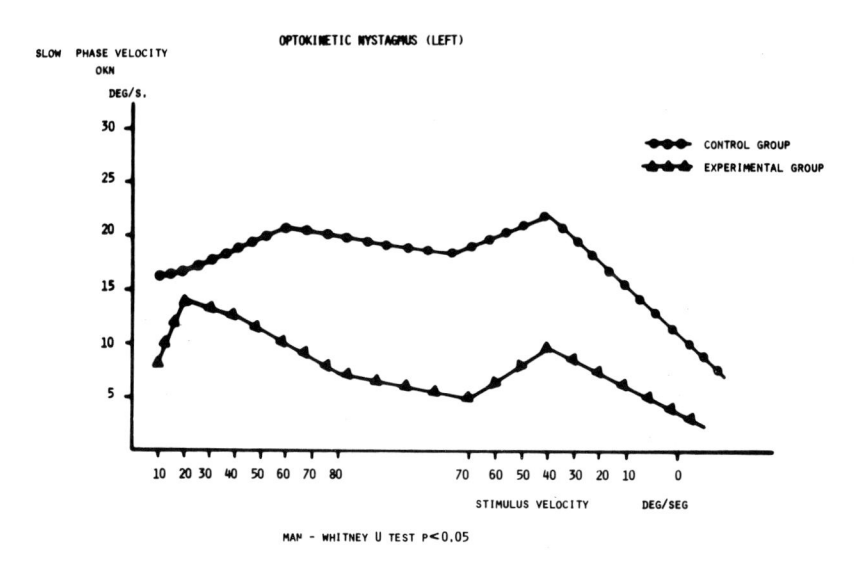

Fig.2. SPV OKN responses(left)

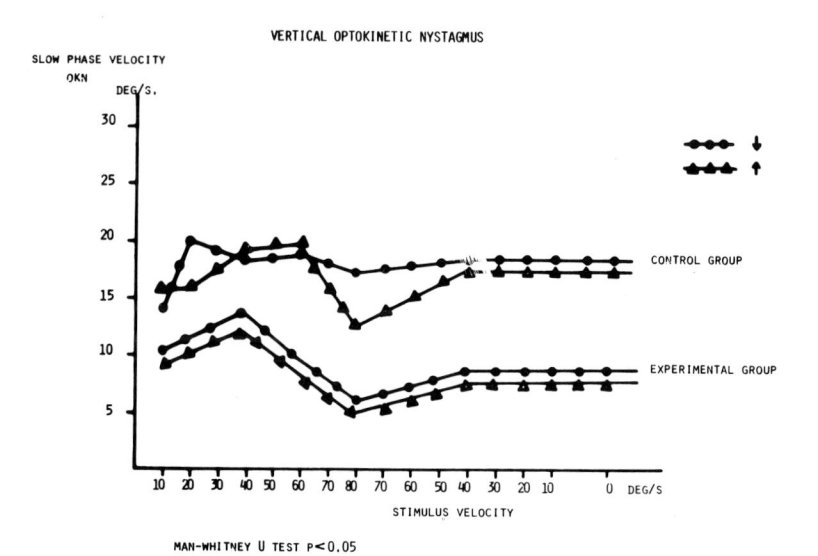

Fig.3. SPV OKN responses(vertical)

TABLE I

QUALITATIVE OKN MODIFICATIONS	horiz.	vert.
Tonic deviation towards the slow phase	73%	85%
Dysrhythmia	66%	78%
Inversion of the direction of the fast phase	7%	11%

DISCUSSION.

The qualitative and quantitative modifications in a selected sample of post concussional patients suggests that the visual-vestibular interaction presents a disfunction of the input-output modulation of the supranuclear vestibular activity.Experimentally it is known that this visual-vestibular transfer mechanism is interdependent of the signal integration between the paramedian pontine reticular formation, nucleus reticularis tegmentis pontis, intersticial nucleus of Cajal and nucleus prepositus hypoglossi. (6-9). The modifications of the OKN morphology associated with disfunction of the visual-vestibular transfer signal at 40-60-80°/s are results of a disturbance in the supranuclear vestibular modulation.

ACKNOWLEDGEMENTS

Supported by a grant from SANDOZ Foundation for Gerontological Research (Basel) and a grant from D.I.B M-2156(Universidad de Chile).

REFERENCES.

1. Rudge P(1983) In : Clinical Neuro-otology (Part Three:Specific diseases and the Auditory and Vestibular Systems).Churchill Livingstone,Edinburgh,London, Melbourne,New York.

2. Cárdenas JL,Morales-García C, Valladares H,Arriagada C,Otte J, García A,Lay-Son L, Certanec B, Díaz F, Carrasco J,PosadaJ,GómezJ (1987) Otoneurological symptoms after head injury. ACTA AWHO. Vol.VI.,2:101-102.

3. Waespe W,HennV.(1981) Visual-vestibular interaction in the flocculus of the alert monkey. Exp.Brain Res.43:349-360.

4. Cohen B,Matsuo V, Raphan T.(1977) Quantitative analysis of the velocity characteristics of optokinetic nystagmus and optokinetic after-nystagmus.J.Physiol.270:321-344.

5. Waespe W,Cohen B,Raphan T(1983) Role of the flocculus and paraflocculus in optokinetic nystagmus and visual-vestibular interactions:effects of lesions. Exp.Brain Res. 50:9-33.

6. Cazin L,Magnin M,Lannou J(1982)Non-cerebellar visual afferents to the vestibular nuclei involving the prepositus hypoglossal complex.Exp.Brain Res 48:309-313.

7. Gerrits NM,Voogd J (1986) The nucleus reticularis tegmenti pontis and the adjacent rostral paramedian reticular formation;differential projections to the cerebellum and the caudal brain stem. Exp Brain Res,

8. Hess BJM,Blanks RHI,Lannou J.Precht W(1989)Effects of kainic acid lesions of the nucleus reticularis tegmenti pontis on fast and slow phases of vestibulo-ocular and optokinetic reflexes in the pigmented rat. Exp.Brain Res. 74:63-79.

9. Mc Crea RA.(1988)The nucleus prepositus.In:Büttner-Ennever(ed) Neuroanatomy of the oculomotor system.Elsevier Science Publishers B.V,Amsterdam,pp203-223.

COMPUTERIZED CALORIC RESPONSES IN CHRONIC OTITIS MEDIA

CARSTEN WENNMO

Dept of Otolaryngology, Hospital of Helsingborg,
S-251 87 Helsingborg, Sweden

ABSTRACT

Caloric responses to water have been compared in 16 ears (8 patients) of which 8 were normal ears, 6 were radical mastoid cavities and two were ears with preserved canal wall but with central drum perforations. Radical cavity ears presented with hyperactive responses and shorter time constants whereas ears with central drum perforations showed no difference in variability as compared to normal ears.

INTRODUCTION

The most common method for examining the function of the labyrinth is the alternate binaural bithermal caloric test with water as stimulus[1]. To assess an abnormal caloric reaction it is important to know the value for each side as well as the difference, as these values supplement each other. Time of irrigation and water temperature may be varied. The end organs of hearing and equilibrium are closely asociated within the bony labyrinth. Cochlear and vestibular function are, for this reason, generally disturbed together by labyrinthine disease. In patients with chronic otitis media, including those treated by surgery the inner ear function as regards hearing, however, is frequently less well preserved than labyrinthine function. The disadvantage of using water as a vestibular stimulus is that it is contraindicated in patients with radical mastoid cavities or in patients with tympanic membrane defects. If the ear is protected, however, for example with a "latex thimble" covering the ear canal, water can be used. Using a "latex thimble" provides an alternative to the closed loop water system[2] where probe tips resembling deflated ballons are filled with circulating water.

NYSTAGMUS   0 - 10 s :   C(hange), A(uto), S(tart): S
Code: 44L   STATUS: ANALYSIS ENABLED   SCREEN: 50 deg

SLOW PHASE

34 accepted

Vel: 57 deg/s
Amp: 7 deg
Dur: 133 ms

FAST PHASE

34 accepted

Vel: -117 deg/s
Amp: -7 deg
Dur: 66 ms

Fast ph, Min vel: 75 deg/s Min dur: 30 ms   ACCEPT
Slow ph, Min vel: 2 deg/s Min dur: 150 ms Noise: 0.5 deg   (Y,N,S,R,Q) : _

NYSTAGMUS 10 - 20 s :   C(hange), A(uto), S(tart): S
Code: 44R   STATUS: ANALYSIS ENABLED   SCREEN: 50 deg

SLOW PHASE

20 accepted

Vel: -8 deg/s
Amp: -2 deg
Dur: 289 ms

FAST PHASE

13 accepted

Vel: 79 deg/s
Amp: 2 deg
Dur: 29 ms

Fast ph, Min vel: 75 deg/s Min dur: 30 ms   ACCEPT
Slow ph, Min vel: 2 deg/s Min dur: 150 ms Noise: 0.5 deg   (Y,N,S,R,Q) : _

Comparison of nystagmic reactions in a female patient with radical cavity on the left side and healthy ear on the right.

This report will deal with the vestibular function in
patients with chronic otitis media sequelae due to
cholesteatoma or inflammatory disorders.

MATERIAL

Eight patients, 4 men and 4 women, aged 54-69 years, (16
ears, altogether) participated in the investigation. All
patients suffered from chronic otitis media in one ear, 5 on
the right and 3 on the left side, with the contralateral ear
being normal. Six of the patients were operated with a
radical mastoid cavity due to previous disease and the other
two had a chronic otitis media with central perforation of
the ear drum.

METHODS

The ears of the patients were carefully investigated
clinically under magnification of a microscope, as well as
audiologically. Each subject was tested using
electronystagmography. As stimulus in the caloric test, water
at $44°$ and $30\ °C$ was used bilaterally and the duration of
irrigation was 30 seconds at each temperature. To protect the
diseased ear a "latex thimble" was placed in the ear with
chronic otitis media and to make comparison possible an
identical thimble was placed in the healthy ear. The "latex
thimble" was placed with the help of a microscope to permit
the stimulus to reach all parts of the ear outside the ear
drum. Nystagmus was analyzed online by an IBM XT computer
with a 64 kb memory and a Winchester disc of 10 Mb. Signals
were recorded by a two-channel electronystagmographic
recorder (ENR-200, Tracoustics, Stockholm, Sweden) with an
upper cut-off filter at 30 Hz.

RESULTS

Ears with radical mastoid cavities

Five of the six radical mastoid patients reacted more
intensively to bithermal water stimulus on the radical cavity
side, whereas another failed to show any vestibular reaction

at all on the cavity side. In this latter patient the absence of reaction was due to a cholesteatoma having grown into the labyrinth with invasion of the anterior and lateral canal; there was also deafness in that ear. The slow phase velocities on the radical side were thus 16-150 degr/sec, with mean 66 s, compared to 4,5-50, with mean 34 s on the healthy side, with exception of the patient whose reaction was absent. As a rule time constants were also shorter on the cavity side, range 32-120 s with mean 55 compared to 40-112 s with mean 75 on the healthy side. There was no difference, however, in time constants with cold stimulus versus warm water stimulus, which has been noted by other investigators[2].

Ears with drum perforations and intact canal wall

In these two patients alternating warm and cold water bithermal stimulus produced caloric reactions without significant difference between sides as far as slow phase velocity and time constants were concerned.

DISCUSSION

As shown in the present investigation the time constant is shorter when using a strong thermal stimulus, when for example a radical mastoid cavity is stimulated with 44 or 30 degr water[3]. The time constant is defined as the time in which the reaction (slow phase velocity) declines to 37 per cent of its maximum. The thermal stimulus of a radical cavity is much stronger than the corresponding stimulus for a healthy ear or an ear with perforated ear drum but with intact posterior canal wall. It also appeared from the present data that cold water responses were almost equivalent to hot water responses. Another method is to use air[4]; when air is used as stimulus instead of water an inverse nystagmic reaction is sometimes seen at the beginning. This is due to a vaporisation from the middle ear mucosa, which causes a cooling of the canals when warm water is used. In contrast to the observations of hyperactive caloric responses of radical cavities, the reactivity of a chronic ear with preserved canal wall does not differ from that of a normal ear. Another disadvantage of using air[1] is the lower heat carrying capacity compared to water, while the placement of the irrigating tip is much more critical in air caloric stimulation. On the other hand, the "latex thimble" used in water calorics has to be placed carefully, covering the cavity so that the water temperature is transformed to the labyrinth. Our observations are in agreement with other investigations of hyperactive responses occurring in patients with radical mastoid cavities on the operated side[2].

REFERENCES

1. Wetmore S (1986) Extended caloric tests. Ear and Hearing 7, pp 186-190
2. Brookler K, Baker A, Grams G (1979) Closed loop water irrigator system. Otolaryngol Head Neck Surg 87:364-365
3. Reker and Müller-Diehle J (1989) Time constants of the vestibular thermal reaction. Acta Otolaryngol suppl 468, pp 333-336
4. Fiebach A, Heilmann-Jedanick Ch (1987) Die Intensität des vestibulo-occulären reflexes als antwort auf die thermische Labyrinthreizung mit Wasser und Luft. Laryngol Rhinol Otol 66 pp 428-432

**VESTIBULO-SPINAL DISTURBANCES
DUE TO HEAD TRAUMA**

POSTUROGRAPHIC FINDINGS IN POSTTRAUMATIC PATIENTS

Marcel E. Norré, Dpt Otoneurology & Equilibriometry - University Hospitals - LEUVEN (Belgium).

As was demonstrated in the former paper (5), posturographic (PG) abnormalities were the most frequent findings in our series of 104 posttraumatic cases.

METHODS

This study concerns the same patients as in the former one. The posturography (PG) applied comprises two test-procedures: Static Posturography (SPG), which is the recording of the postural sway in standing position on a stable platform and Kinetic Posturography (KPG), which is the photographic recording of the stepping test (2). In the evaluation of the KPG two parameters are used: 1/ width of the sway and 2/ angle of rotation/deviation (rot/dev) (4).

In these patients two types of SPG-examination have been used.
<u>Type 1</u>: the postural sway was recorded for 60s, test 1 = eyes open (EO), test 2 = eyes closed (ECl) and test 3= eyes closed head in retroflexion (retro). Parameters S(surface) and L(length) were computed and the degree of abnormality was estimated related to the SD (2).
<u>Type 2</u> is a simplified Equi-test (1-6): the sway was recorded for 30s with EO, ECl and StV (stabilized vision) on stable platform (tests 1,2 and 3) and once again on interposed foam rubber (tests 4,5 and 6). The same parameters were used as for type 1 (6).

RESULTS

SPG AND KPG COMPARED

Out of the 104 patients, both tests (SPG and KPG) were positive in 25 cases and both negative in 37 cases. In 40 cases only one of both tests was positive and this in nearly an equal percentage (19 SPG+, 21 KPG+). The positivity of the KPG consisted of too a large sway (n=34) or a dev/rot (above 45°) (n=12).

SPG - TYPE 1

Comparison of parameters S and L

In 10 cases S indicated a higher degree of abnormality, whereas L did it for only 1 case.

EO/EC1

Most of the positive cases (n=22) had abnormal values for EO and EC1, only one case was normal with EO and abnormal with EC1. In a number of cases EC1-recordings indicated a lower degree of abnormality than did the EO-testing. This non-expected relationship was found in 9 cases (40%) for L and in 10 cases (45%) for S.

Head in retroflexion (test 3)

In 2 cases the values were normal for EO and ECL, but abnormal for test 3. In 4 cases a higher degree of abnormality was found in test 3 (retro) compared to test 2 (EC1) for parameter L and in 5 for parameter S. This formula can be interpreted as an indication for a cervical component.

SPG TYPE 2

No typical formula, as has been described e.g. for vestibular deficiency (1-6), could be found.

S/L

Parameter S showed higher degree of abnormality in nearly all cases. In only 3 cases L had a higher degree.

EO/EC1

In only one case the test with EO was normal, whereas with EC1 the value was abnormal. In the other cases all measurements were abnormal. In 4 cases recording with EC1 gave a lower degree of abnormality than with EO for parameter L, in 5 for S and in 2 for both.

Stabilized vision

On the contrary to some statements in the literature (1), stabilized vision (StV) did not indicate more abnormalities than did EC1-testing.

Comparing test 2 and 3:

In 3 cases EC1 indicated abnormal values, whereas StV was normal. In only 3 cases for L and in 5 cases for S, StV gave a higher degree of abnormality, whereas ECL did it in 10 cases for L and in 12 cases for S.

Comparing test 5 and 6:

The same remarks are valuable. EC1 (test 5) indicated a higher degree of abnormality in 14 cases for L and in 11 cases for S. In one case StV was normal and EC1 abnormal.

COMMENTS

As already pointed out in former studies, KPG and SPG indicate two different types of dysfunction of the VSR (4-6). In this way each test can be positive separately. In the posttraumatic cases examined, KPG was mostly positive by a broadening of the sway, which has been considered as central sign (2). Deviation/rotation was never linked to an asymmetrical caloric test, which is also rather suggestive for a central disturbance.

There was no specific formula of sensory interaction in SPG type 2 (1-6). We find here a rather over-all instability, with even some contradictory formulae. Indeed in 40% of the cases the EC1 condition showed less disturbed performance than did the EO condition. This inversed relationship means a destabilising effect of the visual input, which has been described as postural blindness (3). The cases with more disturbed values in test 3 of type 1 may suggest concomitant cervical involvement, as a whiplash injury.

Generally parameter S showed higher degrees of abnormality, which indicated an increased lack of precision in the postural working rather than an increased activity. As for other groups of patients (6), also in these patients StV appeared to be a weaker indicator of abnormality than is EC1.

A final remark is that, for these posttraumatic cases, PG could be a less reliable test, as the patient may easily exaggerate his instability deliberately.

REFERENCES
1. BLACK FO, WALL C, NASHNER LM (1983): Effects of visual and support surface orientation references upon postural control in vestibular deficient subjects. Acta Otolaryngol (Stockh) 95: 199-210.

2. CLAUSSEN CF (1981): Die objecktive Aufzeichnung und quantitative Auswertung von Raum-orientierungsaufgaben mittels eines photooptischen Schnelltests, der Cranio-Corpographie. In CLAUSSEN CF (ed): Gleichgewichtsprufungen un Arbeitsmedizin. Proc Neurootological and Equilibriometric Society vol VIII pp 107-150

3. GAGEY PM (1986): Huit leçons de Posturologie. Association française de Posturologie Paris.

4. NORRÉ ME, FORREZ G, BECKERS A (1987): Static and kinetic posturography compared in peripheral vestibular pathology. Acta AWHO 6: 144-145.

5. NORRÉ ME : Otoneurological profile of patients examined for posttraumatic sequellae. In this volume.

6. NORRÉ ME (1990): Posture in Otoneurology. Acta Otorhinolaryng Belg (in press).

CRANIAL TRAUMA AND POSTUROGRAPHY PERFORMED WITHOUT AND WITH CALORIC TESTS.
ANDREE M.T.HADJ-DJILANI, ENT, University Hospital, 1011 Lausanne/Switzerland

INTRODUCTION :
Cranial trauma signifies head injury and central disorders of diverse degrees in severity and duration. Osseous and neurological lesions were usually documented by neurological and X-ray assessments. To the otoneurologist will be mainly asked to determine if vestibular lesion(s) may be responsible for patients' complaints. The aim of the present paper is to precise if posturographical recordings performed in frame of a complete otoneurological examination (including nystagmography) may bring additional informations to the diagnosis on patients examined after a cranial trauma. Among the recordings on the platform we differenciated between recordings without specific vestibular stimulation, and recordings after caloric tests.

MATERIAL AND METHODS :
Tested subjects: This study concerns 50 patients, 37 men and 13 women, aged 16 to 75 (mean age 39 years). All had complaints of "vestibular type" they reported historically to a cranial trauma which had occured 3 months to 30 years before our examination. According to the severity of the suffered trauma patients were divided into 3 groups: (i) single labyrinthine concussion (20 patients, follow-up time 3 months to 18 years); (ii) single petrous bone fracture (19 patients, follow-up time 6 months to 30 years); (iii) complex cranial fracture(s) and/or neurological lesions (11 patients, follow-up time 6 months to 25 years). The otoneurological examinations were performed either in frame of insurance evaluation or because of persisting complaints pointing to vestibular possible lesions. The complaints noticed at time of examination are represented on the following table with regard to the degree of severity (see the 3 groups above) of trauma.

COMPLAINTS:	(i) 20 patients /	(ii) 19 patients /	(iii) 11 patients
VANISHED	1x	1x	
DEAFNESS ALONE	1x	1x	
BPPN	4x	2x	1x
CONTINUOUS VERTIGO-UNBALANCE	4x	4x	3x
IMPROVING VERTIGO	2x	6x	2x
SPELLS VERTIGO-TINNITUS-HEARING LOSS	6x	3x	
VERTIGO SPELLS	1x	1x	1x
PROGRESSIVE UNSTEADINESS	1x	1x	4x

Performed tests and evaluation: All patients had complete otoneurological examination in addition to the posturographical recordings. The latter were performed according to devices and methods we have elsewhere described (1). We recorded statokinesigraphically the tramping tests (tramping 20 paths on the place, eyes open and eyes closed). Results of <u>standing tests at rest</u> with opened eyes (REO) and with closed eyes (REC) were appreciated by means of a computer program; the quantitative measured parameters were areas (A) and 1Hz-smoothed lengths (Ls1). A same computerized evaluation was used with the caloric tests (CALT) recorded while standing with closed eyes. According to the normal range of vestibular responsiveness to CALT on the platform soon published (1), based on calculation of quotients of results measured after CALT versus results measured with REC, we were able to determine normal, unsufficient (lesional) or hyperactive responses on the patients. Unsufficient lesional responses allowed then to diagnose vestibular lesion(s) with vestibulo-spinal reflex (VSR). On each patient we had then a possible diagnosis of vestibular lesion evidenced either with nystagmography (vestibulo-ocular reflex, VOR), or with VSR, or by both VOR and VSR. Such results allowed us to divide the patients into groups according to the kind of vestibular lesion(s): no vestibular lesion (group 1), dissociated vestibular lesion evidenced only with VSR (group 2), whole vestibular lesion evidenced by both VOR and VSR (group 3).

RESULTS :

1) RESULTS WITH TRAMPING TESTS (EYES OPEN/EYES CLOSED)
Recordings obtained while tramping are represented as normal or abnormal into 2 tables, with regard to different parameters. The first table represents results with regard to the complaints and to the kind of vestibular lesion.

TRAMPING-TESTS (20 PATHS) EYES OPEN / EYES CLOSED   Normal ●   Deviation ♂
                                                     Ataxic-enlarged ○   Spin ⚥

COMPLAINTS	Gr.1 / 13 patients ∅ vest.lesion	Gr.2 / 14 patients VSR-lesion(s)	Gr.3 / 23 patients VOR+VSR lesion(s)
Vanished	●● | ●●		
Hearing loss alone	○ | ♂ ● | ○		
BPPN		⚥♂ | ⚥♂ ●● | ●●♂	●○ | ○♂ ●● | ●●
Continuous vertigo-Unsteadiness	○♂ | ○♂ ●● | ●○	○ | ○ ●○ | ●○	○♂ | ○♂ ●● | ●○
Improving vertigo-unsteadiness	● | ⚥♂	○⚥♂ | ⚥⚥♂ ●●○ | ●○●	○ | ○ ●● | ●●
Spells of tinnitus - hearing loss- vertigo	● | ●	● | ●	●⚥○ | ●⚥○ ●●● | ●●●
Vertigo spells alone			●●⚥ | ●○⚥
Progressive worsening unsteadiness	●○♂ | ●○♂	○ | ○	●○ | ●○

The following table represents results with the same tramping tests but as a relationship with severity of cranial trauma and neurological lesions in addition to the relationship with the kind of diagnosed vestibular lesion (see following page).

| TRAMPING 20 PATHS | EYES OPEN / EYES CLOSED | Normal ● Enlarged-ataxic ○ Spin ⟲ Deviation ♂ |

	LABYRINTHINE CONCUSSION 20 patients	"SINGLE PETROUS BONE FRACTURE" 19 patients	PETROUS B.FRACT. + NEUROLOGICAL LESIONS 11 patients
Group 1 (13 pat.) ∅ Vestib.lesion	●♂● ●♂♂ ○●● ○○● ○ ○	●○● ●♂♂ ●● ●⟲	○ │ ○
Group 2 (14 pat.) VSR-lesion(s)	●○ ●○ ●⟲⟲ ●⟲⟲♂	●○⟲○ ●○⟲○ ●♂● ⟲●●♂	●●○ │ ●⟲○
Group 3 (23 pat.) VOR + VSR lesion(s)	●●○● ●●○○ ●●●● ●●●○	●●●● ○○⟲⟲ ●●●♂ ●●♂♂	○⟲○ ○⟲● ○○●○ ●○●●

2) <u>RESULTS OF STANDING TESTS AT REST (EYES OPEN REO / EYES CLOSED REC)</u>.
<u>Qualitatively</u> we observed no constant findings, especially no constant body sway toward side of a vestibular lesion (if present unilaterally).
<u>Quantitatively</u> results were normal or raised, could be with REO, with REC, or with the quotients calculated with REC/REO. On the following table are illustrated the measured results represented with regard to the degree of vestibular lesion and with regard to the severity of central accompanying lesions.

| STANDING AT REST | EYES OPEN / EYES CLOSED / QUOTIENTS EC/EO | Normal ● all variables ○ Abnormal lengths alone Ⓛ |

	LABYRINTH.CONCUSSION 20 patients	"SINGLE" PETROUS BONE FRACTURE 19 patients	PETR.B.FRACTURE + NEUROLOGICAL LESIONS 11 patients
Group 1: ∅ Vestib.lesion 13 patients	ⓁⓁ ●● ●○ ●○ ○ ○ ⓁO ●●	●Ⓛ ⓁⓁ Ⓛ● ● Ⓛ ● ○Ⓛ ●Ⓛ ●●	○ │ ○ │ ●
Group 2: VSR-lesions(s) 14 patients	○○ ○○ ● ● ⓁO ⓁO	●○ ●○ ● ● ○○ ●○	○ ○ ○ Ⓛ Ⓛ ● Ⓛ* ○ Ⓛ**
Group 3: VOR + VSR les. 23 patients	●● Ⓛ● Ⓛ● ○○ ○○ ○Ⓛ ●● ●● ●● ●Ⓛ ●Ⓛ ●Ⓛ	●● ○● ○○ ●○ ○○ ○○ ●○ ●○ ●○ ●● ●● ●●	○Ⓛ ○○ ○○ ●○ Ⓛ● Ⓛ● ●○ ○Ⓛ ○Ⓛ ○ ○ ○

*: Lt   **: Lsl

Abnormal results with standing test appreciated with regard to the patients' complaints gave no more constant findings than as represented above with tramping tests. Even patients with vanished complaints gave any abnormal results while standing at rest, and among the 6 patients impaired by a progressive unsteadiness one patient had normal results at rest while standing.

3) CALORIC TESTS (CALT).
By use of CALT performed on the platform, 37 patients had a vestibular lesion evidenced at vestibulo-spinal level. Among them 14 patients (28%) had normal results with nystagmography (VOR-CALT). However the lesional results with VSR were always in accordance with the clinical background, located at the side of petrous bone fracture or of labyrinthine concussion, accompanying often a unilateral hearing loss: such findings corroborate our previous observations on divergences between vestibular lesions at VOR- and at VSR-levels, the latter being often more sensitive (3). On patients with benign peripheral positional nystagmus we found as previously published (2) a constant relative vestibular weakness at the ear contralateral to the side of undermost ear when BPPN occured, regardless to the presence or not of a vestibular lesion at VOR-level. Normal results with CALT performed on the platform were most often noticed on patients with vanished complaints or with extra-vestibular impairments of neurological or orthopaedical type.

CONCLUSIONS :
Recordings obtained on a passive force platform without specific vestibular stimulation, i.e. while tramping or standing at rest, could be interesting as documents for impaired walking or standing but in an otoneurological point of view these tests did not allow to diagnose involvement of vestibular lesion(s) in the patients' complaints. Specific vestibular stimulations are necessary: results of caloric tests performed on the platform gave useful informations on lesions which could not be diagnosed by means of nystagmography, corresponding possibly to "dissociated" vestibular peripheral lesions, sparing any of the vestibular endorgans.

REFERENCES :
1. A.M.T.HADJ-DJILANI. Multiparametrical Study of Posturography using Force Platform: Recordings with and without Vestibular Caloric Stimulation.
   Neuro-Orthopedics 6: 93-100, 1988

2. A.M.T.HADJ-DJILANI. Peripheral Positional Nystagmus and Responses to Caloric Tests on Force Platform.
   Acta N.E.S. under press

3. A.M.T.HADJ-DJILANI. Vestibular Lesion Revealed by Caloric Testing. Relationship Between Vestibulo-Ocular and Vestibulo-Spinal Reflexes.
   Neuro-Orthopedics, under press

ADDRESS OF THE AUTHOR :
Andrée M.T.HADJ-DJILANI, M.D., ENT-Outclinic, University Hospital 07,
1011 LAUSANNE, SWITZERLAND.

MOTOR CONTROL AFTER HEAD TRAUMA

MANOL GOSPODINOV
Institute of Neurology, Psychiatry and Neurosurgery
Blvd. Lenin 4km, 1113 Sofia (Bulgaria)

INTRODUCTION

It is a well known fact that the motor coordinations are the highest form of expression of the systematics in the nervous system function, being the direct consequence of the refinement with which the complex time-dimension schemes of dynamic control occur. With regards to this, the present study was carried out precisely for the purpose of quantitative defining of the equilibrium function and symetrical motor coordination in patients after head trauma. This would enable a more intimate penetration into the Head Trauma mechanism of action referring to the complex hierarchic system, ensuring static and dynamic motor regulation. On the other hand, this can supply additional criteria for estimating the neuro- and pathophysiological reflection of head trauma in a given patient, for the individualization of therapy and the assessment of the effect of its application.

METHODS AND CONTINGENTS

Investigations were carried out with 10 patients who had undergone head trauma for a perion ranging from 1 month to 4 years prior to the examination moment (3 men and 7 women), right handed, at average age of 44 years. The standard methods for investigation of the equilibrium and motor coordination included stabilometry and symmetrical sensor coordinatometry (B.Polnarev et al, 1983). In the case of stabilometry ($x1-x7$) is studied and the equilibrium stability of the body in standing position, for a period of 40 sec., with open eyes, and for the same duration of time - with closed eyes. By means of an original platform is assessed the quantitative amplitude of oscillation in sagital ($x1$ - with open eyes, $x4$ - with closed eyes) and frontal ($x2$ - eyes open, $x5$ - eyes closed) direction, by projection of the gravity center of the body upon the platform. The quotiont of the digital indication with closed eyes ($x6=x4+x5$), and with open eyes ($x3=x1+x2$) is the so called coefficient of Romberg ($x7$).

The symmetric coordinometry enables the carrying out of a quantitative evaluation of the dynamic motor coordination of the hands. The method is relized by means of simple touch with maximum possible velocity of the sensory platforms, in a determined order, that switches the digital indicator on or off (at sec.$^{-2}$). The interhemispheric balance of the brain is estimated by means of the coefficient of functional assymetry, equal to the fraction of time required for the performing of a definite movement task of the dominant /right(d) and left(s) hand/. For the purpose of the study the following programs have been adopted:

1. Ballistic movement (open loop): "central" time -x8/d/ and x10/S/; motor time - x9/d/ and x11/S/.

2. Controllable movement (closed loop): x12/d/, x14/S/ and x13/d/, x15/S/.

3. Complex movement: x16/d/, x18/S/, and x17/d/, x19/S/. This type of movement requires preliminary planning of a more complex time-dimensional model.

The ascend complex programs mentioned so far are based upon audio-motor reaction.

4. Serial movement: x20/d/, x21/S/.
5. Alternating movement Ist degree: x22/d/, x23/S/.
6. Alternating movement II degree: x24/d/, x25/S/.
7. Tremorometry.

   a) static tremor: amplitude - x28/d/, x32/S/; frequency - x30/d/, x34/S/.

   b) dynamic tremor: x29/d/, x31/S/ and x33/d/, x35/S/.

8. Dynamometry: x26/d/, x27/S/.
9. Stabilometry (x1-x7): x1, x2, x3, x4, x5, x6, x7.
10. Pulse frequency before (x27) and after (x38) complete investigation.

As control groups served 10 clinically healthy individuals, at an average age of 31 years, and 10 patients with neurological syndromes on a functional basis (average age - 30 years).

The data obtained was analyzed utilizing neurocybernetic approach towards extreme clinical conditions, on the basis of personal computer stato-coordinatory analysis.

RESULTS AND DISCUSSION

Our investigation shows the statistically relevant deviations in the dynamic and static motor coordination indices in patients with Head Trauma.

Of greatest significance as to the differential-diagnostic information regarding class Head Trauma and class "clinically healthy individuals" proved to be the following indices (ranging according) to the degree of adequateness (F) for identification of the above mentioned classes): x35 (F=2.78), x34(2.36), x30(2.18), etc.

Of lowest differentiating capacity concerning the aforementioned classes, proved to be the symptoms: x23(0.00), x37(0.01), etc.

The analogical ranging of the examined motor coordinatory indices relating to the remaining couples of classes studied, showed the following results:

1. Head Trauma - Neurosis -
    a) most informative indices x35(0.96), x31(0.62), etc.
    b) informative indices - x27(0.00), x24(0.00), x37(0.00), etc.
2. Neurosis - Clinically healthy individuals:
    a) x29(1.12), x38(0.96), x35(0.90), etc.
    b) x15(0.00), x36(0.00), x37(0.00), etc.

Likewise, disorganized appear to be both the superior regulatory levels of psychomotorics, as well as the rudimentary formations of the neuro-motor complex.

CONCLUSION

1. The differential hierarchic-constellation stato-coordinatory analysis performed by us, when compared to normal control groups, enables the complex participation assessment (and its vegetative "cost"), of the static, serial, ballistic, controllable, anticipational and biorhythmological components of the movement in patients undergone Head Trauma.

REFERENCE

1. Polnarev BL, et al (1983) In: Apparatus Complex for Investigation of the Static and Dynamic Coordinations. Industrial Model No 901

SCOLIOSIS: A MODEL TO EVALUATE SPINO-VESTIBULAR INTERACTIONS

P. SIBILLA, A. CESARANI, S. BAROZZI, D. ALPINI, G. RAINERO

Centro Scoliosi Institute Don Gnocchi (Mi); Institute of Audiology University of Milan; Neurophysiology Laboratory Institute Don Gnocchi (Mi)

INTRODUCTION

Vestibular-spinal reflexes can modify the activity of the longitudinal paravertebral muscles and they can control or modify the position of the spine.

The main problem of the specialist who study the scoliosis is how to treat these spine modification especially at the onset of the disease.

The aim of this paper is to clarify the correlations between scoliosis and vestibular system in order to help the treatment planning of the disease.

MATERIAL AND METHODS

27 females and 13 males (mean age 13 yy) affected with idiopathic scoliosis were investigated.

The neurotological examination comprehended both postural and vestibular-oculormotor evaluation:
- Romberg and Fukuda tests
- evaluation of the convergence
- evaluation, by the mean of palpation-inspection and Fukuda-modified test, of the prevalence of paravertebral muscles
- evaluation of the bipupillaris, shoulder and pelvis axis
- spontaneous, positional and positioning ny
- caloric and rotatory ny
- optokinetic ny (40 and 20°/s)
- smooth pursuit and saccadic eye movements in the horizontal and in the vertical plane
- posturography.

All the vestibular-ocularmotor and ocular motor tests were recorded by the mean of electronistagmography (ENG).

DESCENDING SCOLIOSIS

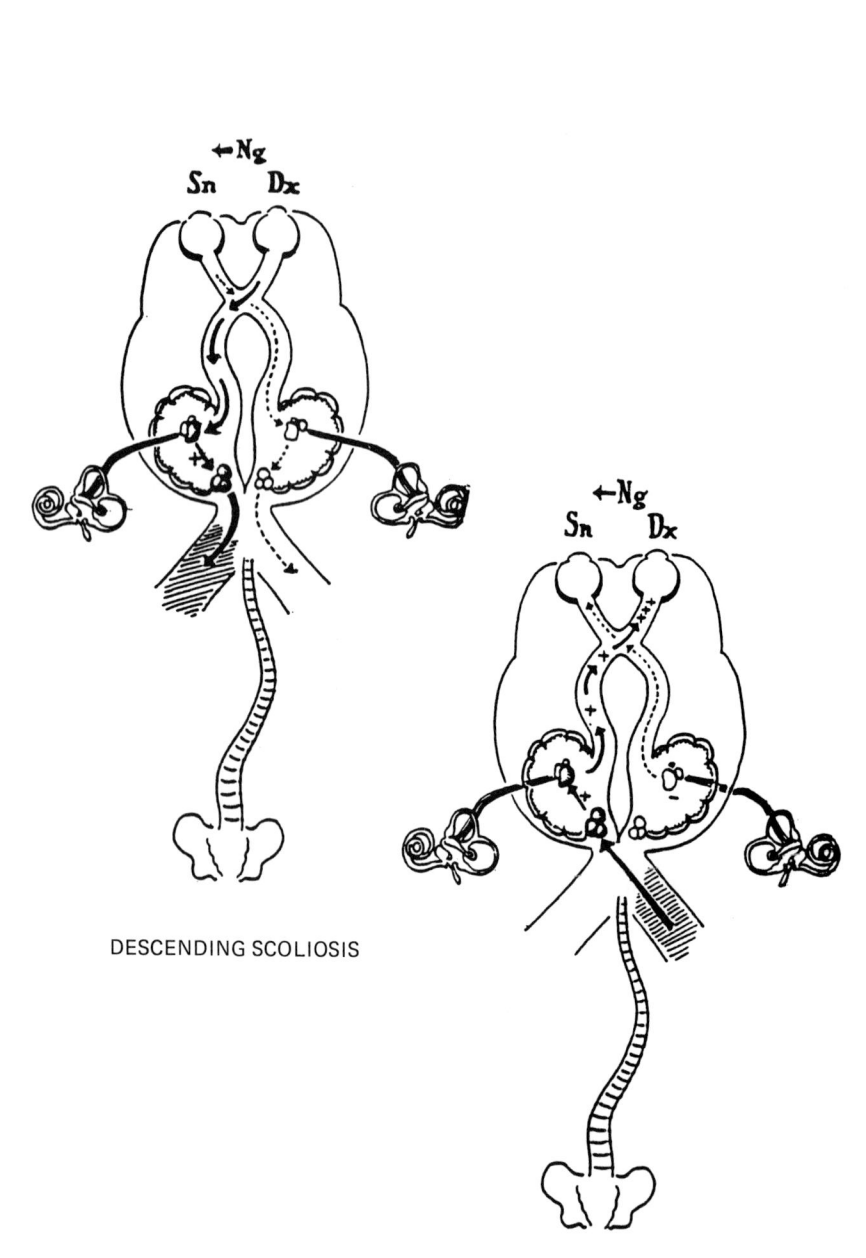

ASCENDING SCOLIOSIS

CORRELATION BETWEEN PARAVERTEBRAL
PREVALENCE AND FOR DIRECTIONAL
PREPONDERANCE

RESULTS

In all the patients we found either a prevalence of a site of paravertebral muscles or a ny directional preponderance (not always significative according to Jongkees's formula).

In some pt the qualitative alterations of provoked ny were mild, while in other pt they were very frequent and important.

Also the gain of horizontal smooth pursuit was different among the children: in a group it was 0.9-1, in an another group it was lower (0.6-0.8). Saccades were similar in every pt.

We found that the examined scoliostic children could be devided into two groups, on the basis of the neurotological examination:
A) a group with caloric and rotatory normoreflexia; a mild directional preponderance of ny toward the opposite side of paravertebral muscles prevalence; normal OKN and higher pursuit gain.
B) a group with hyporeflexia of provoked ny; directional preponderance of ny toward the same side of paravertebral muscles prevalence; abnormal OKN and lower pursuit gain.

On the basis of a retrospective re-evaluation of the evolution of the scoliosis and two years follow-up we found that the children in neurotological group A had usually lumbo-sacralis scoliosis and that these scoliosis had a slow progression while the pt in group B had usually dorsal scoliosis with a fast and continuous progression despite the treatment adopted.

DISCUSSION

The vestibular system receives information from the muscles and the joints of the spine and it modifies either the VOR or the eye movements, especially the smooth pursuit eye movements. It is known the the neck paravertebral muscles influence the vestibular nuclei of the opposite side while they are controlled by the nuclei of the same side.

We hypothize that in the pt of group A the neurotological alterations are depending on spine alteration and that the VOR directional preponderance is the expression of a vestibular inbalance provoked by the contralateral neck paravertebral muscles hyperactivity: ascending kind of scoliosis.

As far as pt in group B is concerned, we hypothize that the scoliosis is provoked by a vestibular system alteration and that the directional preponderance causes the prevalence of neck paravertebral muscles of the same side: descending scoliosis.

The strict correlation between the spine and the vestibular system is demonstrated also by the effects of superficial paravertebral electrical stimulation.

Traumatologists have in fact observed that the results of SPES are not the same in similar pt and that the results could not be explained only on the basis of muscle enforcement.

In our opinion the results of SPES are depending on the activity of the vestibular system and the effects are not a direct muscles enforcement but they are due to a reflex vestibular modification.

In conclusion we would like to underline the importance of neurotological assessment of the scoliosis in the evolutive age especially at the onset of the disease to plan the more effective treatment, treatment that will be more conservative in ascending scoliosis than in descending scoliosis.

REFERENCES

1. Yamada K, Ikatata T, Yamamoto H, Makagawa T (1974) Equilibrium function in scoliosis and active corrective plaster jacked for treatment. J. Bone J.T. Surg. 1764

2. Sahlstrand T, Petruson B (1978) Postural equilibrium in adolescent idiopathic scoliosis. Acta Orthop. Scand. 50, 275.

3. Sahlstrand T, Petruson B (1979) A study of labyrinthine funtion in patients with adolescent idiopathic scoliosis. Acta Orthop. Scand. 50, 769.

4. Sibilla P (1983) Effects of electrical stimulation in scoliosis on muscle fibre diameters and ENG. Ist European Congress on Scoliosis and Kiphosis, Dubrovnik.

ND AGING

T LEDIN, C MÖLLER, M MÖLLER, LM ÖDKVIST.

Dept of ENT, University Hospital, Linköping, and Dept of Research and Development in Primary Health Care, Mjölby, Sweden.

ABSTRACT

All persons aged 70-75 years (n=457) in a Swedish community were invited to participate in a balance study using dynamic posturography. Out of 55 interested subjects 29 were chosen at random. Dynamic posturography comprises a sensory organization test in which the platform and visual surround is either stable or referenced to the patient's sway, furthermore the eyes are open or closed. The data of this age group differed from previously obtained data in the age groups 20-59 and 60-69 years. It is concluded that balance function is deteriorated in this high age group compared to the younger groups. When testing elderly patients they must be compared to normative data from their age group. For practical purposes balance training is of value in the elderly.

INTRODUCTION

The hip fracture incidence, even corrected for the growing number of elderly, is steadily increasing, being approximately doubled during the recent decades in Sweden (Johnell et al 1984). The incidence of hip fractures is probably associated to the frequency of falling among elderly. Gryfe et al (1977) report that 6% of falls in an elderly population result in fractures and that 1% are fractures of the hip. Patients with radial bone fractures have been postulated to display impaired postural equilibrium compared to controls (Ring et al 1988). The subjective ability to keep good equilibrium is markedly reduced in elderly about 65 years and older (Gerson et al 1989, Ödkvist et al 1988). Another important factor to consider in assessing postural equilibrium is medication and social conditions (Wickham et al 1989).

Standing equilibrium requires the cerebellum and the brainstem to integrate signals from the somatosensory, visual and vestibular systems to correct for equilibrium disturbances. The body sway under stable conditions has been studied using various forms of static posturography (Diener et al 1984, Dichgans et al 1976, Kapteyn 1972, Ledin et al 1986, 1989).

The present study was designed to study a group of elderly healthy volunteers. Assessment of balance by means of dynamic posturography, with options to have the support surface or visual surround referenced to the body sway, was used as a more sophisticated testing of equilibrium performance than static posturography only, thus resembling the dynamic disturbances of balance during daily life activities.

MATERIAL AND METHODS

From the Swedish population register in the county of Vadstena (total population 7500) all persons aged 70-75 years were retrieved (n=457). All subjects not known to have handicaps or diseases (427) were given an invitation to participate, a total of 55 subjects replied. To be included, the subject should not suffer from severe vertigo, epilepsy, Parkinson's disease, stroke, rheumatoid arthritis, total hip replacement, severe heart disease, severe hypertension or abuse of alcohol. Medication with sedatives or anxiolytics were not allowed. The studied group consisted of 15 women and 14 men with mean age 73 years (SD 1.5 years).

Dynamic posturography (Equitest, Neurocom Int Inc, Clackamas, Oregon, USA) was performed as described by Nashner (1987) and Cyr et al (1988). In the dynamic posturography, the subject is standing on a dual forceplate enclosed by a visual surround. Both the forceplate and the surround can be made to move with the person's antero-posterior (AP) sway or independent of the sway, thus enabling programmed disturbances of the equilibrium. The dual forceplate records the forces between feet and ground as well as shear forces, thereby allowing estimation of the position of the swaying body as well as the pattern of sway in terms of hip or ankle strategy.

The investigation is divided into two main sections: sensory organization test (SO) and movement coordination test (MC). The present paper is only concerned with the SO part, which is divided into six separate tests, lasting 20 seconds each with test 4, 5 and 6 repeated three times. SO 1 is a quantified version of Rombergs test. The subject stands with eyes open and the surrounding as well as the ground is stable. SO 2 is equal to SO 1 except that the eyes are closed. In SO 3, performed with eyes open, the surrounding moves in response to the body sway. In test SO 4 the platform is sway referenced and the surrounding stable. In test SO 5, with eyes closed, the platform is sway referenced, and in test SO 6 both the platform and surrounding are sway referenced. Note that in SO 3 and SO 6 some orientation information from the surrounding is available as it is only moving in the AP and not in the lateral direction.

From each test an equilibrium score is computed. The score is 100 for absolutely no sway, decreasing with increasing sway amplitude, and zero in case of falling. A strategy score is computed expressing the degree of ankle or hip movements- 100 means solely ankle and no hip movements and zero means exclusively hip movements. These calculations are related to the amount of shear force exerted. Alignment data is also calculated showing the angle between body and earth vertical during the trial. Initial alignment describes the conditions before the start of the each test and dynamic alignment is the angle during the test. The movement coordination (MC) part is divided into eight separate tests: Small, medium and large backwards and forwards translation perturbations of the platform are repeated three times each to simulate falling forwards and backwards, respectively, and furthermore the platform is tilted toes-down and toes-up five times each (Strategies, alignments and, as said above, the MC part is not the subject of this paper).

The equilibrium scores were compared to the normative data for younger age groups supplied by Neurocom Int Inc. As normative data means and standard deviations of 112 subjects aged 20-59 years and 20 subjects aged 60-69 years were provided.

Student's t-test were used to compare groups. Probability levels below 5% were considered significant.

RESULTS

Significant differences between the group of 70-75 years old compared to the 60-69 years old were found when the surround was moving and support surface stable (condition SO 3, p<0.05) and when the support was moving and vision was absent (SO 5, p<0.01). When comparing to the 20-59 years old, highly significant differences (p<0.001) occurred in all conditions except Romberg's test with eyes open (SO 1) and sway-referenced platform with normal vision (SO 4).

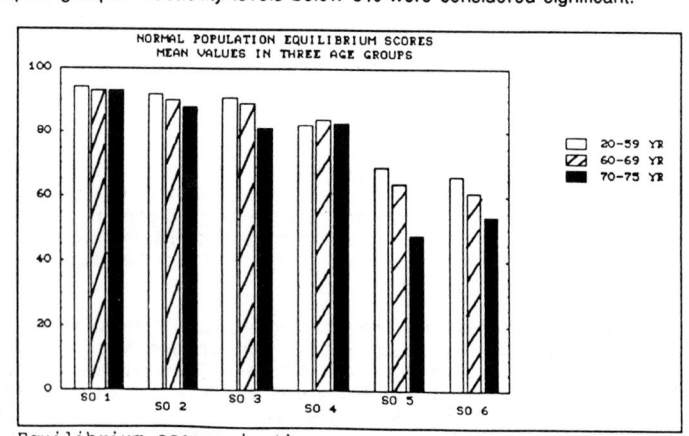

Equilibrium scores in three age groups.

DISCUSSION

With aging there is a loss of cells both in the peripheral and central part of the vestibular system (Rosenhall 1973, Bergström 1973), and in addition nerve cell loss in the somatosensory system plays a part as does diminished visual acuity. For practical and psychological reasons the elderly also have a diminished drive for activities with body movements. These two factors might significantly contribute to decreased performance in tasks that demand postural reactions. It is also well known that central compensation after vestibular disturbances is delayed and in some cases less effective in elderly people (Norre and Beckers 1988). The effect of aging on vestibular function and nerve cell loss seem to accelerate around the age of 70 years (Bergström 1973, Rosenhall 1973, Ödkvist et al 1988).

Comparing the subjects, probably active people as they volunteered for the study, with the normative data provided by Neurocom Int Inc revealed significant differences in most SO conditions when comparing the 70-75 years group with the 20-59 years group, and in a few conditions when comparing to the 60-69 years group. Albeit the normative data refer to an American population, the differences suggest that there is a decrease in balance performance around the age of 70 years, in agreement with other authors (Ödkvist et al 1988, Overstall et al 1977).

The Romberg tests with feet together and eyes open or closed resemble SO 1 and 2. These tests are really not challenging the limits of stability to any considerable degree. Albeit significant, the difference compared to the youngest group is still small, as the mean absolute value of body sway in SO 2 in the oldest group still corresponds to only 1.5 degrees of sway motion during 20 seconds, which is probably too little to classify a subject as pathological in clinical testing. Thus, healthy subjects even at high age should be able to perform perfect in Romberg tests, which are not always indicators of a perfect balance function.

Often the vestibular system is investigated in a static way and the procedure limited to the vestibulo-oculomotor reflex. Testing a system as dynamic and complex as the vestibular one is best performed when the ultimate resulting output is recorded i.e. actual balancing ability and subsequently the test method should take into consideration the input and the output movements.

Decreased balance in elderly probably relates to falls and thereby to fractures (Gryfe et al 1977), thus causing unnecessary suffering and hospitalization costs. The increased incidence of osteoporosis in elderly aggravates this relation. Lichtenstein et al (1989) used balance training to try to improve postural control in elderly, and found effects in some aspects. Physical exercises expose the vestibular, visual and somatosensory systems to new challenges and thereby enhancing central nervous system balancing mechanisms.

If physical exercises, which have been shown to both improve muscular strength (Souminen et al 1977) and prevent osteoporosis (Chow et al 1987), could be implemented among the elderly, it would most certainly improve balance, general health and decrease the high incidence of falling and subsequent fractures in the growing population of elderly.

When dealing with elderly in medical practice, it is maybe not most important to conduct all clinical investigations available for every subject, rather we should perhaps emphasize the positive effects of physical exercises. It is also important to realize, that normality in an elderly subject must be evaluated relative to control subjects of the appropriate age, and not to materials of young volunteers.

REFERENCES

Bergström B. Morphology of the vestibular nerve. II. The number of myelinated vestibular fibers in man at various ages. Acta Otolaryngol (Stockh) 1973: 76: 173-179.

Chow R, Harrison JE, Notarius C. Effect of two randomised exercise programmes on bone mass of healthy postmenopausal women. British Medical Journal 1987: 245: 1441-1444.

Cyr DG, Moore GF, Möller CG. Clinical application of computerized dynamic posturography. Ear, Nose and Throat Journal (suppl) 1988: Sep: 36-47.

Dichgans J, Mauritz KH, Allum JH, Brandt T. Postural sway in normals and atactic patients: analysis of the stabilizing and destabilizing effects of vision. Agressologie 1976: 17: 15-24.

Diener HC, Dichgans J, Bacher M, Gomph B. Quantification of postural sway in normals and patients with cerebellar disease. Electroencephalography and Clin Neurophysiology 1984: 57: 134-142.

Gerson LW, Jarjoura D, McCord G. Risk of imbalance in elderly people with impaired hearing or vision. Age and Ageing 1989: 18: 31-34.

Gryfe CI, Amies A, Ashley MJ. A longitudinal study of falls in an elderly population: I. Incidence and morbidity. Age and Ageing 1977: 6: 201-210.

Johnell O, Nilsson B, Obrant K, Sernbo I. Age and sex pattern of hip fractures- changes in 30 years. Acta Orthop Scand 1984: 55: 290-292.

Kapteyn TS. Data processing of posturographic curves. Agressologie 1972: 13 (suppl B): 29-33.

Ledin T, Tropp H, Odenrick P, Ödkvist LM: Postural sway and corrections. In: Vertigo, nausea, tinnitus and hearing loss in cardio-vascular diseases. Eds CF Claussen and MV Kirtane. Excerpta Medica International Congress Series 708, p 371-376, 1986.

Ledin T, Ödkvist LM, Möller C: Posturograpy findings in workers exposed to industrial solvents. Acta Otolaryngol (Stockh) 1989: 107 : 357-361.

Lichtenstein MJ, Shields SL, Shiavi RG, Burger MC. Exercise and balance in aged women: A pilot controlled clinical trial. Arch Phys Med Rehabil 1989: 70: 138-143.

Nashner LM. A systems approach to understanding and assessing orientation and balance disorders. Advances in diagnosis and management of balance disorders conference, Boston, MA, Oct 1987 (can be obtained from Neurocom Int Inc).

Norre ME, Beckers A. Benign paroxysmal positional vertigo in the elderly. Treatment by habituation exercises. Journal of the American Geriatrics Society 1988: 36: 425-429.

Ödkvist LM, Malmberg L, Möller C. Age-related vertigo and balance disorders according to a multiquestionnaire. In: Vertigo, nausea, tinnitus and hypoacusia in metabolic disorders. Eds: Claussen CF, Kirtane MV, Schlitter K. Elsevier Science Publishers B.V. 1988: pp 423-427.

Overstall PW, Exton-Smith AN, Imms FJ, Johnsson AL. Falls in the elderly related to postural imbalance. Br Med J 1977: 1: 261-264.

Ring C, Nayak L, Isaacs B. Balance function in elderly people who have and who have not fallen. Arch Phys Med Rehabil 1988: 69: 261-264.

Rosenhall U. Degenerative pattern in the aging human vestibular neuro-epithelia. Acta Otolaryngol (Stockh) 1973: 76: 208-220.

Suominen H, Heikinen E, Liesen H, Michel D, Hollman W. Effects of 8 weeks endurance training on skeletal muscle metabolism in 56-70-year-old sedentary men. Eur J Appl Physiol 1977: 37: 173-180.

Wickham C, Cooper C, Margetts BM, Barker DJP. Muscle strength, activity, housing, and the risk of falls in elderly people. Age and Ageing 1989: 18: 47-51.

Acknowledgements: The technical assistance in the dynamic posturography investigations by Mr Johan Deblen and Mrs Lisbeth Noaksson is gratefully acknowledged.

Correspondence to: T Ledin, Dept of ENT, University Hospital, S-581 85 Linköping, Sweden.

© 1991 Elsevier Science Publishers B.V. All rights reserved.
Vertigo, nausea, tinnitus and hypoacusia due to head and neck trauma.
C.-F. Claussen and M.V. Kirtane, editors.

SQUARE WAVE PERTURBED POSTUROGRAPHY- EFFECTS OF VISION, DIRECTION AND AMPLITUDE

T LEDIN, LM ÖDKVIST.

Dept of ENT, University Hospital, S-581 85 Linköping, Sweden.

ABSTRACT

Perturbed posturography on the EquiTest movable platform was utilized to study the force reactions to sudden antero-posterior perturbations between 13 and 127 mm in both backwards and forwards directions in ten healthy men 23-58 years old (mean 36). In addition, the effect of vision was investigated. The acquired information was processed in Matlab mathematical software package for further information extraction.

The experiment unveiled that the distance a subject moves the center of pressure (CP) as well as the latency to maximum CP deflection during a perturbation is an increasing function with perturbation amplitude. The latency to maximum CP deflection was larger for conditions with vision present, however no dependency on perturbation direction was found. Regression analysis showed that in backwards perturbations the differential increase in CP deflection amplitude was larger than in forwards perturbations. For backwards perturbations, larger differential CP displacements were allowed with vision present compared to absent.

INTRODUCTION

Sudden perturbations of the support surface in standing man activate automatic motor programs that bring the vertical projection of center of gravity (CG) back into the stable area of support. This process involves visual influences, somatosensory information from muscle spindles and joints, vestibular signals as well as central coordination. Nashner and Berthoz (1978) studied visual influence on early EMG activity and sway amplitudes when the subject was exposed to different visual conditions during platform perturbations. The vestibular organs are highly sensitive to perturbations. Nashner (1971) estimated that the semicircular canals were more sensitive than the otoliths, also in antero-posterior (AP) perturbation stimuli, with a detection threshold of about 0.05 deg/s^2 for rotatory AP acceleration.

Corrective movements are organized as modifiable preprogrammed patterns (for a general outline, see Nashner and McCollum 1985). A given peripheral stimulus, such as support surface translation, may cause different patterns of postural responses depending on e.g. initial posture and surface conditions (Diener et al 1983, Horak and Nashner 1986, Marsden et al 1981, Moore et al 1986). It has been argued that more complex postural behaviors, such as standing on a very short surface, inactivate the automatic mechanisms, forcing the subject to rely on higher level learned mechanisms (Roberts 1978). When the standing condition is altered, the response pattern is often gradually modified over several exposures to the new condition (Horak et al 1985, Horak and Nashner 1986, MacPherson et al 1986, Nashner 1976). However, a study concerning postural movements during walking (Nashner and Forssberg 1986) and an above-mentioned study on horizontal perturbations on a short surface (Horak and Nashner 1986) have shown that altered muscular strategies of movement are not associated with increased latencies to EMG onsets, i.e. the processes probably take place within the automatic control system, rather than relapsing to higher conscious level control of posture. It is therefore probable that these processes are under the influence of higher centra, albeit not in a conscious way.

Measurement of human equilibrium has for long mostly included static standing, either in the Romberg test, conducted in everyday medical practice, or in static posturography, i.e. standing on a stable force platform that measures the forces between feet and ground. Recently the study of reactions to disturbances of stance has come into interest. Dynamic posturography (EquiTest, Neurocom Int Inc) offers the user a small set of perturbations in the AP direction, and also in the form of toes-up and toes-down tiltings of the support surface.

As the perturbation possibilities of EquiTest were rather limited, a user-friendly, menu-driven, multi-purpose interface software to the hardware in EquiTest was developed (Ledin et al 1990). The concept of perturbed posturography enables the user to design his own perturbation protocol with a multitude of possibilities. Data evaluation is expected to be conducted offline in the signal processing software of choise.

The influence of stimulus duration, velocity and amplitude in backwards AP support surface translations on muscular latencies and EMG activity were investigated by Diener et al (1988). They found that for short enough stimuli (less than 75 ms), no scaling of the postural responses occured. The middle portion of EMG activity amount in postural muscles (75-150 ms post stimulus) was determined by stimulus velocity and the long term (150-500 ms post stimulus) corrective EMG activity was determined by stimulus amplitude. The measurement of torque (i.e. vertical forces on the platform) around the ankles was briefly mentioned, but not discussed further in detail.

The present study was undertaken to test a simple method to evaluate the effect of sudden AP perturbations on standing man. Both backwards and forwards directions were used. The effects of vision as well as varying amplitudes were investigated.

MATERIAL AND METHODS

Ten healthy male volunteers aged 23-58 years (mean 36, SD 11) were investigated. All subjects denied alcohol abuse or having a family history of alcoholism in first degree relatives. No subject was working with volatile solvents. No subject had any history of otological or neurological disease.

The concept of perturbed posturography (Ledin et al 1990) was employed to expose the subjects to backwards and forwards perturbations of the support surface. Perturbed posturography is a way of enhancing the perturbation possibilities of the apparatus used in dynamic posturography (EquiTest, Neurocom Int Inc, Clackamas, Oregon, USA), enabling the user to select his own stimulation pattern, by means of software written in Turbo-Pascal. Dynamic posturography (Nashner 1987, Cyr et al 1988) comprises a dual forceplate enclosed by a visual surround, where the forceplate and the visual surround can be made to move actively, or in phase with the tested subject's sway. The perturbation possibilities in EquiTest include AP translations of three amplitudes in both directions and repeated support surface tiltings (toes-up and toes-down) of one amplitude. The force responses are evaluated to find the latency from translation perturbation onset until a torque around the ankles is generated to counteract the movement, furthermore the amount of reaction is calculated along with data to compare the weight bearing of each leg. The tiltings are evaluated using an energy function to illustrate the decline in energy to correct for repetitive stimuli.

In perturbed posturography, the user is presented a menu driven interface to access the translation, rotation and visual actuators of the EquiTest platform. A number of signal types with complete possibilities to adjust describing parameters are available. Furthermore, the software can easily be extended by simple programming in the user-friendly environment of Turbo-Pascal. The force data from the EquiTest platform are collected and presented to the user in unprocessed form. The user is then expected to export data to external signal processing software for offline, preferrably interactive, analysis, thus enhancing inventiveness.

In the present study, the responses to forceplate movements in the AP direction were studied. Translation amplitudes of 13, 25, 63, 102 and 127 mm were used. The translation speed was the highest permissible, about 0.21 m/s (Ledin et al 1990). A sampling frequency of 25 Hz was used. For each amplitude six perturbations in each direction (forwards/backwards) were presented in alternating order during the 59 seconds measurement period. The time between successive perturbations was 4.5 seconds. No subject had any difficulty in regaining normal body posture between perturbations. For all five amplitudes, one test with eyes open and one with eyes closed was conducted. Sufficient time to relax between tests was given.

Measurement data were processed in the mathematical software package Matlab (The MathWorks Inc, USA) for its simplicity, extensive capabilities and interactive as well as batch oriented mode of operation.

The data processing for each subject comprised computing the location of the CP in the AP direction as a function of time. The first CP deflection after each perturbation was automatically detected, and its amplitude relative to baseline value prior to test as well as latency from initiation to maximum CP deflection computed. In cases of a gradual slow response, a defined peak could not always be found. In some cases very sharp peaks prior to proper AP CP deflection responses were identified. For these cases a minimum allowable peak duration was determined, to detect and discard artifact peaks. Finally, CP deflection parameters were statistically evaluated and graphically presented.

For each subject a regression line between perturbation amplitude and resulting CP deflection amplitude as well as latency to maximum CP deflection was constructed. The regression was based on all perturbation amplitudes, but also on the three middle amplitudes only (25, 63 and 102 mm), as there was an apparent loss of linearity at the endpoints in maximum CP deflection amplitude data. The slope of the regression line is a measure of the differential increase in CP deflection (or the corresponding latency) in response to an increase in perturbation amplitude. As the body height influences the location of CP, all parameters were also checked for depency upon body height.

Differences between conditions were evaluated using Student's t-test for paired samples. A probability level of 5% was considered significant.

RESULTS

The CP deflection trace from one experiment is presented (amplitude 127 mm, eyes open, figure 1), along with the extracted response to a particular perturbation (backwards, eyes open, figure 2). For both figures, the y-axis is in 100 mm units and the x-axis in sampling units (40 ms). The y-axis is directed ahead. Forwards perturbations cause backwards CP deflections, and vice versa. The timing of perturbation initiations are obvious in figure 1 and indicated by an arrow in figure 2.

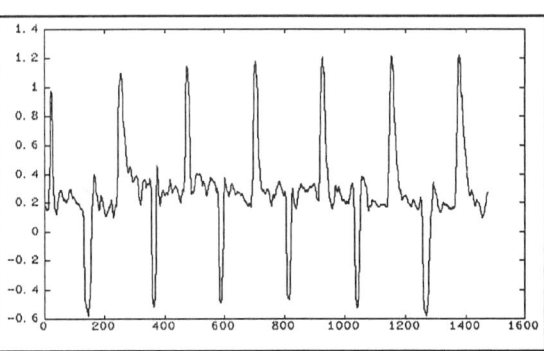

Figure 1. CP deflection trace, 60 s test.

The relationship between perturbation amplitude and CP deflection amplitude showed that the linearity was good for the three innermost amplitudes, but less evident for the extremes. Average values of CP deflection amplitudes as functions of perturbation amplitude are presented in figure 3. The four graphs are identified by observing the order at 127 mm perturbation size; from top the backwards eyes closed, backwards eyes open, forwards eyes open and forwards eyes closed functions are shown. Except for an apparent relation showing increasing amplitudes of CP deflection with increasing perturbation amplitude, no obvious differences between perturbation conditions could be found.

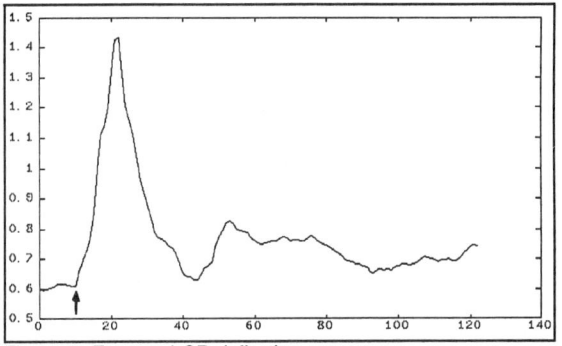

Figure 2. Extracted CP deflection response.

The latency from perturbation initiation to maximum CP deflection was found to be dependent upon stimulation amplitude and vision, but not on perturbation direction. Average latencies are shown in figure 4. Note eyes closed conditions having lower values than eyes open conditions. At 127 mm perturbation size, from top the forwards eyes open, backwards eyes open, backwards eyes closed and forwards eyes closed functions are shown.

Amplitudes (table 1) and latencies (table 2) for all conditions are displayed in tables. In addition to means and standard deviations, comparisons between neighboring conditions (eyes open (EO) vs eyes closed (EC) and forwards vs backwards) are shown (*=p<0.05, **=p<0.01, omitted=NS).

When studying different impacts of perturbation amplitude on CP deflection amplitudes and latencies to maximum CP deflections, the regression line was based on all five amplitudes 13 to 127 mm as well as the three center amplitudes alone. The relation between perturbation amplitude and CP deflection using only the three center amplitudes was by visual inspection found to be the more linear one. Means and standard deviations of the regression coefficients for each testing condition as well as statistically significant differences between conditions for both amplitudes (table 3) and latencies (table 4) are shown in tables.

From the regression coefficients based on the three center perturbation amplitudes, it is concluded that with vision present, a greater incremental displacement of CP is allowed than with vision absent. Furthermore, backwards perturbations result in larger incremental displacements of CP than forwards do. From the regression coefficients for the latencies to maximum CP deflection, a significant difference was found between forwards and backwards perturbations in the testing condition with vision absent.

No dependency on body height was found in any parameter.

Table 1. Average CP deflections (mm) for all perturbation conditions and amplitudes.

		\multicolumn{10}{c}{Perturbation amplitudes}

Condition		13 mm		25 mm		63 mm		102 mm		127 mm	
		EO	EC	EO	EC	EO	EC	EO	EC	EO	EC
		p<		p<		p<		p<		p<	
Forwards	m	27.8	28.5	35.0	36.5	65.4	65.8	83.1	79.8	88.9 *	84.4
	SD	6.2	8.5	6.1	8.0	8.0	8.9	10.3	8.7	9.0	8.7
p<						*		*		**	
Backwards	m	29.2	31.7	34.9 **	40.3	65.7 **	72.3	90.3	91.0	90.9	92.2
	SD	7.9	7.9	7.2	7.5	6.6	7.0	8.1	7.7	7.4	7.0

Table 2. Average latency to maximum CP deflections (ms) for all perturbation conditions and amplitudes.

Condition		13 mm		25 mm		63 mm		102 mm		127 mm	
		EO	EC	EO	EC	EO	EC	EO	EC	EO	EC
		p<		p<		p<		p<		p<	
Forwards	m	351	349	461	376	534 **	417	542 *	462	562 *	464
	SD	99	113	151	83	104	45	96	95	105	55
p<											
Backwards	m	433	366	487 *	399	539 *	436	512 **	445	531 *	479
	SD	156	97	129	68	137	53	90	52	102	60

Table 3. Regression coefficient between perturbation amplitude (mm) and CP deflection amplitude (mm).

		\multicolumn{4}{c}{Slope of regression line}

		All amplitudes		Reduced set of amplitudes	
Condition		EO	EC	EO	EC
			p<		p<
Backwards	m	0.592	0.564	0.727 *	0.665
	SD	0.083	0.100	0.124	0.094
p<				*	*
Forwards	m	0.559 *	0.508	0.632	0.569
	SD	0.111	0.083	0.147	0.109

Table 4. Regression coefficient between perturbation amplitude (mm) and latency to maximum CP deflection amplitude (ms).

		All amplitudes		Reduced set of amplitudes	
Condition		EO	EC	EO	EC
			p<		p<
Backwards	m	0.67	0.89	0.33	0.49
	SD	1.27	0.70	1.70	1.04
p<					*
Forwards	m	1.55	1.01	1.06	1.14
	SD	1.15	0.88	1.83	0.87

DISCUSSION

Ground force responses to increasing amplitudes of square wave perturbations were studied. A menu-driven software introducing AP perturbations to augment the EquiTest dynamic posturography method was utilized. The effects of vision, perturbation direction and amplitude on response amplitudes of and latencies to maximum CP deflections in the AP direction were investigated. The acquired information was explored in an easy-to-use mathematical software. An increasing amplitude of movement was found to cause an increasing amplitude of CP deflection, however not in strict proportion to actual deflection. At small amplitudes the CP deflection exceeded perturbation size, at larger amplitudes not. This is in contrast to a purely passive process, and consequently we agree in that active motor programs at least in part determine the corrective maneuvres.

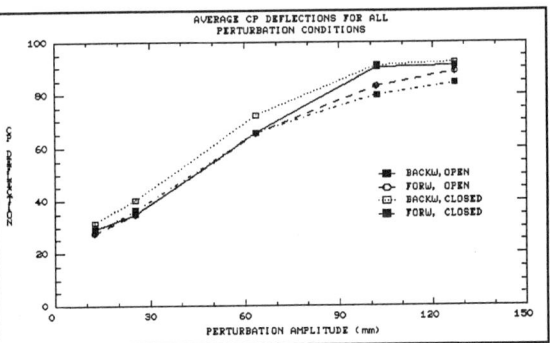

Figure 3. CP deflection amplitudes (mm) as functions of perturbation amplitudes (mm).

Apart from the observation that larger amplitudes of translation perturbations cause both larger displacements of CP as well as longer latencies to maximum CP deflections, maybe the most striking finding in this study was that the latencies were found to depend on vision, with longer latencies with vision present. Maybe the subjects felt more confident when they were allowed to have their eyes open, thereby using a less tense muscular apparatus to correct for the predictable perturbations. Hence increased latencies compared to conditions with vision excluded were allowed.

The latencies were in the order of 350-550 ms depending on conditions and amplitudes. This can be compared to the

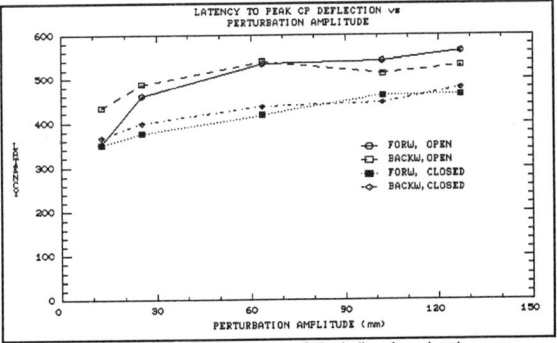

Figure 4. Latencies to maximum CP deflection (ms) as functions of perturbation amplitudes (mm).

latencies proposed for onset of EMG responses to translation perturbations, about 100 ms for gastrocnemius muscle EMG after backwards perturbations (Diener et al 1988). The difference is obviously the time required for the muscle to exert peak torque in correcting for the disturbance. The situation in forwards perturbations, with the tibialis anterior muscle being stretched instead of the gastrocnemius muscle, obviously did not change the latency conditions significantly. As said above, an increased latency was found to follow increased perturbation size, albeit the increment was not purely the effect of increased time to complete a longer perturbation distance. From the regression coefficients, it is found that 1 mm increment in perturbation amplitude causes about 1 ms longer latency to maximum CP deflection. When comparing to the fact that the platform requires about 5 ms to complete 1 mm of movement, it is obvious that the corrections are not passive processes.

Different body positions in a given perturbation situation may cause different responses from the corrective processes (Moore et al 1986). It is possible that the subjects involuntarily prepared themselves by adjusting body posture prior to the next perturbation as the series was predictable. However, instructions were given not to prepare for the next perturbation. They could also have tensed their muscles to prepare, but if a subject appeared tense, instructions to relax were given and the test repeated.

As the dynamic location of CP was studied, it should be noted that the CP is not identical to the vertical projection of CG. CP is composed of the location of CG, a static component, and the acceleration forces due to body movement, a dynamic component. Thus, only in very low frequency and amplitude movements, CP is a good estimation of CG projection (Murray et al 1967, 1975, Gurfinkel 1973, Lidström et al 1990).

It would have been interesting to study CG instead of CP. However, the suggested method in EquiTest (Neurocom 1988) to compute CG from CP data, using time-averaged CP data and antropometric relations, has not been implemented in the application in this paper. This is due to validity problems. As the frequency content of body movements increase, like in sudden perturbations, the errors in CG estimation increase. In general it can not be assumed that these CG calculations are valid in perturbed posturography. The idea of separating CG from CP by means of Fourier transformation and a filtering function derived from solid inverted pendulum mechanics (Lidström et al 1990) is critically dependent on the inverted pendulum hypothesis of body sway, which is probably not applicable to perturbed posturography. Attempts to filter data using more complicated multisegmental models of body movement quickly increase the computational work to undesired levels.

Estimating the dynamics of the human equilibrium system in response to perturbations is a difficult problem. The system displays saturation phenomena in that foot length is highly restricted, thus allowing only a limited torque to correct for a disturbance. Furthermore, the measurement situation in posturography can not easily account for corrective movements that include e.g. stepping. A subject can hardly be expected to take part in an experiment where he may lose his balance and fall, without knowing that security measures are taken to avoid any harm to his body. Therefore, any method to estimate human balancing dynamics must rely on extrapolation of data from experiments that are conducted within restricted subsets of parameter values, enhancing safety. The utilization of regression procedures is much in use, albeit not applicable outside the linearity range, as observed regarding maximum CP deflections at the two outermost amplitudes in this study.

Randomized stimuli would have been preferred instead of a predictive one, as the CNS quickly learns to predict a repetitive stimulus. But as it was also concluded that the larger amplitudes were the more reliable, in that they presented smaller coefficients of variation (defined as mean/SD), the limited length of the platform made it impossible to expose the subjects to randomized directions, at least for the larger amplitudes. The measurement time would also have been longer if randomization had been undertaken. Yet, valuable information (Diener et al 1988) may be acquired, also in the case of predictive stimuli. In a series of papers, Maki (1986a, 1986b, 1988) and Maki et al (1987) explored pseudorandom translation perturbing stimuli in identifying human balancing dynamics, and encountered difficulties in identifying subjects liable to lose their balance and experience a fall (Maki et al 1987). This is partly due to inherent problems of statistical inference (Bartlett et al 1986), but can also reflect the complexity of the equilibrium system and its interaction with environmental factors. The real world is an eternal surprise to scientists, trying to model it.

In conclusion, this paper has demonstrated how to acquire and process posturographic data from an experiment with predictable AP support surface perturbations, using a simple concept. The user is able to furnish his own protocol, giving him full control over the analysis, yet not sacrificing the possibilities of automatic analysis once his concept is fully developed. To us, this seems an attractive way to control our investigation procedures in the future, having the possibility to develope the concepts further by ourselves whenever there is a need.

REFERENCES

Bartlett SA, Maki BE, Fernie GR, Holliday PJ, Gryfe CI. On the classification of a geriatric subject as a faller or nonfaller. Med & Biol Eng & Comput 1986: 24: 219-222.

Cyr DG, Moore GF, Möller CG. Clinical application of computerized dynamic posturography. Ear, Nose and Throat Journal (suppl) 1988: Sep: 36-47.

Diener HC, Bootz F, Dichgans J, Bruzek W. Variability of postural "reflexes" in humans. Exp Brain Res 1983: 52: 423-428.

Diener HC, Horak FB, Nashner LM. Influence of stimulus parameters on human postural responses. J Neurophysiol 1988: 59: 1888-1905.

Gurfinkel EV. Physical foundations of the stabilography. Agressologie 1973: 14C: 9-14.

Horak FB, Diener HC, Nashner LM. Influence of stimulus parameters and set on human postural synergies. Soc Neurosci Abstr 1985: 11: 704.

Horak FB, Nashner LM. Central programming of postural movements: adaptation to altered support surface configurations. J Neurophysiol 1986: 55: 1369-1381.

Ledin T, Hedbrant J, Ödkvist LM. Perturbed posturography - an experimental setup and simple applications. Proceedings 17th Neurootological and Equilibriometric Society Congress Proceedings, Bad Kissingen, 1990 (this volume).

Lidström J, Friberg S, Lindström L. Refinement of postural sway measurements in scoliosis research. J Orthop Res, in press, 1990.

MacPherson JS, Rushmer DS, Dunbar DC. Postural responses in the cat to unexpected rotations of the supporting surface: evidence for a centrally generated synergic organization. Exp Brain Res 1986: 62: 152-160.

Maki BE. Interpretation of the coherence function when using pseudorandom inputs to identify nonlinear systems. IEEE Trans Biomed Eng 1986: 33: 775-779.

Maki BE. Selection of perturbation parameters for identification of the posture control system. Med & Biol Eng & Comput 1986: 24: 561-568.

Maki BE. Addendum to "Interpretation of the coherence function when using pseudorandom inputs to identify nonlinear systems". IEEE Trans Biomed Eng 1988: 35: 279-280.

Maki BE, Holliday PJ, Fernie GR. A posture control model and balance test for the prediction of relative postural stability. IEEE Trans Biomed Eng 1987: 34: 797-810.

Marsden CD, Merton PA, Morton HB. Human postural responses. Brain 1981: 104: 513-534.

Moore SP, Horak FB, Nashner LM. Influence of initial stance position on human postural responses. Soc Neurosci Abstr 1986: 12: 1301.

Murray MP, Seireg A, Scholz RC. Center of gravity, center of pressure, and supportive forces during human activities. J of Appl Physiology 1967: 23: 831-838.

Murray MP, Seireg AA, Sepic SB. Normal postural stability and steadiness: Quantitative assessment. The Journal of Bone and Joint Surgery 1975: 57-A: 510-516.

Nashner LM. Adapting reflexes controlling the human posture. Exp Brain Res 1976: 26: 59-72.

Nashner LM. A model describing vestibular detection of body sway motion. Acta Otolaryngol (Stockh) 1971: 72: 429-436.

Nashner LM. A systems approach to understanding and assessing orientation and balance disorders. Advances in diagnosis and management of balance disorders conference, Boston, MA, Oct 1987 (can be obtained from Neurocom Int Inc).

Nashner LM, Berthoz A. Visual contribution to rapid motor responses during postural control. Brain Res 1978: 150: 403-407.

Nashner LM, Forssberg H. Phase-dependent organization of postural adjustments associated with arm movements while walking. J Neurophysiol 1986: 55: 1382-1394.

Nashner LM, McCollum G. The organization of human postural movements: A formal basis and experimental synthesis. Behav Brain Sci 1985: 8: 135-172.

Neurocom Int Inc. EquiTest Technical Manual, 1988 (can be obtained from Neurocom Int Inc).

Roberts TDM. Neurophysiology of postural mechanisms (2nd ed). Butterworths, London, 1978.

Acknowledgements: Special acknowledgement to Johan Hedbrant MSc for stimulating discussions on control theory. The financial support of the County of Östergötland Research Funds, Sweden is gratefully acknowledged.

Correspondence to: T Ledin, Dept of ENT, University Hospital, S-581 85 Linköping, Sweden.

PERTURBED POSTUROGRAPHY - AN EXPERIMENTAL SETUP AND SIMPLE APPLICATIONS

T LEDIN, J HEDBRANT, LM ÖDKVIST.

Dept of ENT, University Hospital, S-581 85 Linköping, Sweden.

ABSTRACT

A menu-driven software was constructed to enable the user to select any of the three possible perturbation modes (support surface translation or tilting as well as surround inclination) in the EquiTest dynamic posturography concept. A number of waveforms with complete possibilities to adjust parameters are available. Data from four vertical force transducers are acquired, along with a shear force in the horizontal direction. Additional data inputs are available for external signal sources. The information is presented by the software in unprocessed form, and possibilities are given to export textfiles of data to external software for further information extraction. In three simple applications, the capabilities of the system have been demonstrated. Acquired data have been processed in Matlab mathematical software package, an easy-to-use, interactive as well as batch oriented way of data processing giving the user complete possibilities to extract any desired information.

INTRODUCTION

The problem of falling is a cause of substantial morbidity in advanced age (Johnell et al 1984). In a growing population of elderly attempts ought to be made in understanding the causes of falls. In many cases an impaired equilibrium plays an important part (Ring et al 1988b, Fernie et al 1982). Thus, it might be important to identify individuals at risk of falling, who could be subject to preventive measures, e.g. dietary recommendations, physical exercises or simply information programs.

The classical way of estimating falling liability is that of spontaneous sway measurements (static posturography) in standing man (Kapteyn 1972, Njiokiktjien and de Rijke 1972, Sahlstrand et al 1978), albeit early investigations using simple arrangements (Begbie 1963) produced conditions that closely resemble dynamic equilibrium testing. Increased spontaneous sway in a group of subjects is, however, not an entirely successful predictor in identifying individuals at risk of falling (Bartlett et al 1986). Clement et al (1984) studied cosmonauts after exposure to weightlessness, and suggested that postural control may be composed of two components; a stable reference system based on past knowledge, and a process that corrects for sudden disturbances. The measurement situation in static posturography does not resemble the dynamic conditions that characterize daily life. Falls are not likely to occur in stable standing, rather in situations of unexpected equilibrium disturbances, which require fast corrections of body position, demanding both muscular strength and an adequate muscular coordination. Thus, balance testing would benefit from a more dynamic measurement situation.

Dynamic posturography (Equitest, Neurocom) is a new investigation procedure that enhances measurement of spontaneous sway by exposing the subject to conditions where the surround as well as the support platform can be made to follow the sway, increasing the difficulties to correct disturbances of equilibrium. The platform can also move actively in simple translations or support surface rotations around the ankle axis. The user is given the possibility to extract data from the system using special software for further offline processing.

This paper describes a computer-controlled, user-friendly, menu-interfaced concept to enhance the perturbation possibilities of EquiTest, introducing a new dimension in equilibrium system testing. Various waveforms are available and it is possible to select several parameters that describe the perturbation signal. The system allows easy export of data for further information extraction in powerful external signal processing software.

HARDWARE DESCRIPTION

The apparatus used in dynamic posturography (EquiTest, Neurocom Int Inc, Clackamas, Oregon, USA) was used as hardware to be interfaced to the user by means of a software package developed at the department. The concept of dynamic posturography (Nashner 1987, Cyr et al 1988) comprises a dual forceplate enclosed by a visual surround. Both the forceplate and the surround can be made to move actively in the antero-posterior (AP) direction, either independent of the sway, thus enabling programmed disturbances of the equilibrium, or in phase with the tested subject's sway.

The dual forceplate records the forces between feet and ground as well as shear forces, thereby allowing estimation of the position of the swaying body as well as the pattern of sway in terms of hip or ankle strategy. Vertical force transducers are located in all four quadrants of the dual forceplate. The AP distance between each pair of transducers beneath each foot is 100 mm, the lateral distance between transducers under opposite feet is 114 mm. The shear force transducer is positioned in the middle of the dual forceplate.

Denoting the vertical forces by F_{ab}, where a is the side (left/right) and b specifies front/rear of each foot, simple mechanical equilibrium yields for the center of pressure (CP) location, assuming the x-axis to be in the AP direction and the y-axis in the lateral direction:

CP_x = (forces at front - forces at rear) / total force * 100 mm =

$$= \frac{(F_{lf} + F_{rf}) - (F_{lr} + F_{rr})}{(F_{lf} + F_{rf}) + (F_{lr} + F_{rr})} * 100 \text{ mm}$$

CP_y = (forces at right - forces at left) / total force * 114 mm =

$$= \frac{(F_{rf} + F_{rr}) - (F_{lf} + F_{lr})}{(F_{rf} + F_{rr}) + (F_{lf} + F_{lr})} * 114 \text{ mm}$$

The location of CP is dynamic, thus we are merely interested in studying the changes in the location and not the exact position, which is sensitive to feet positioning and body posture. It should be noted that the CP does not represent the vertical projection of center of gravity (CG). CP is composed of a static component, the location of CG, and a dynamic component, the acceleration forces due to body movement. Only in very low frequency and amplitude movement, CP is a good estimation of CG projection (Murray et al 1967, 1975, Gurfinkel 1973, Lidström et al 1990).

HARDWARE INTERFACING SOFTWARE

The user is presented a menu driven interface to perturbed posturography. All routines are written in Turbo-Pascal and can easily be modified in an integrated environment. The system operates on any IBM compatible personal computer. A math coprocessor is necessary to operate the EquiTest and highly advisable when measurement data shall be processed further in associated mathematical software (see below), albeit not necessary to operate the interfacing software. On a special license agreement with the manufacturer of EquiTest software access to the electronic circuitry was established. Thus translation, rotation and visual actuators were made available in order to perturb the apparatus in its three degrees of freedom. The force measured by the four vertical and the shear force transducer are read and stored for further calculations. The eight auxiliary channels prepared to receive external data in EquiTest are also ready to be used.

A spectrum of perturbation signal types are available, with complete optional possibilities to modify signal parameters. The signals determine the position of the actuators at steady state. Thus, one must take great care in not assuming the actuators to move quicker than their maximum capacity. The signal types in the present setup are pulse, step, ramp, sine wave, triangle wave, square wave, pseudo-random binary noise (PRBN) and a random sequence. The latter two are furthermore available with an option to randomize the data sequence through the use of a user-chosen seed value. The probability of state switch of the PRBN signal can be specified at any value from 0 to 100 %.

Any perturbation signal can be modified in a number of ways. The amplitude can be varied from zero up to 10 V absolute value (the actuators in EquiTest are designed to accept a maximum of 10 V input voltage). For translation 1 V output increment is equivalent to 6.4 mm of motion. For rotation about the ankle axis and visual surround inclination the corresponding value is 1 degree motion per 1 V input voltage (Neurocom 1988). The slew-rate (rate of increase/decrease per time unit) of the signal can be maximized. The period time of repetitive signals can be specified. The measurement time can be chosen to any of 15, 30, 45 or 59 seconds, the sampling frequency can be chosen from 25 Hz and below. A delay time before perturbation starts can be specified. For randomized signals (PRBN and random) an optional user specified seed can be used to produce a unique random sequence for each seed specified. A smoothing parameter between zero and one can be specified. Each signal sample value is then reduced by that fraction of the prior sample.

Possibilities are given to enter patient data and to save and read stimulation signals and measurement data to and from disk. Measurement data can be stored in either a compact internal format for the program itself, or as text files for export of all data or fractions thereof to subsequent offline analysis in other mathematical or signal processing software.

MEASUREMENT DATA PROCESSING

Acquired data from force transducers (and optionally data from EquiTest auxiliary channels) along with the perturbation signal are supposed to be subject to offline analysis, and efforts have been spent on different ways to export data. The available graphical presentation possibilities of the interfacing software are by no means complete (figure 1), neither intended to be. Rather, the user is expected to continue exploring the data by himself. Thus, ingenuity is enhanced.

We have chosen to process measurement data in the mathematical software package Matlab (The MathWorks Inc, USA) for its extensive capabilities and interactive mode of operation. Instructions can be entered from the keyboard as well as from external textfiles with sequences of instructions prepared. Any instruction file can without

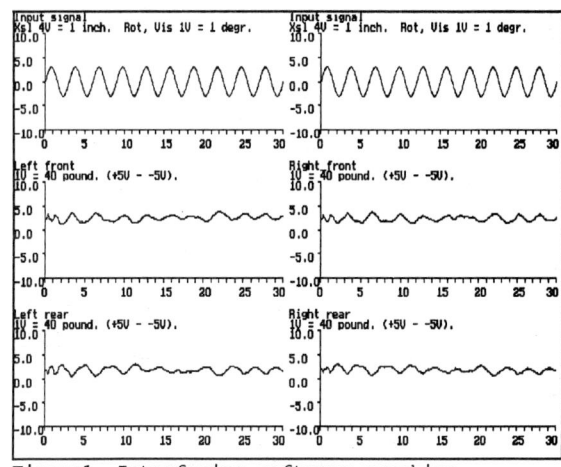

Figure 1. Interfacing software graphics.

restrictions refer to another file. Thus the programming in Matlab furnishes the hierarchy of top-down programming. A number of useful instruction files are provided with the system, as well as an advanced set of internal commands. Optionally, prepared files with Matlab instructions are available in a variety of subjects. Within hours, the beginner is well off on his Matlab crusade.

APPLICATION 1: EVALUATING THE MAXIMUM TRANSLATION SPEED OF THE MOVABLE PLATFORM

In order to estimate the maximum possible translation speed of EquiTest movable platform Newton's second law was used. Non-deformable bodies weighing approximately 25 and 50 kg were placed on the platform and the shear force measured as the objects were translated at maximum speed for three different distances with a maximum of 127 mm. A sampling frequency of 25 Hz was used.

The appearance of shear force at start of movement as well as its disappearance at end was noted and the time difference was computed. Dividing manually checked perturbation amplitudes by elapsed times yielded a maximum speed of about 21 cm/s for translation, independent of the weight attached to the platform and the perturbation amplitude. Integration of shear force with respect to time (estimates the velocity profile) supported the results above. Integrating again with respect to time was not successful in trying to find the position of the platform, due to velocity offset problems. Figure 2 shows, from the bottom, the ideal perturbation signal, measured shear force, estimated velocity and estimated position of the forceplate. The X-axis is in sampling units (40 ms), the y-axis is in arbitrary units for each curve.

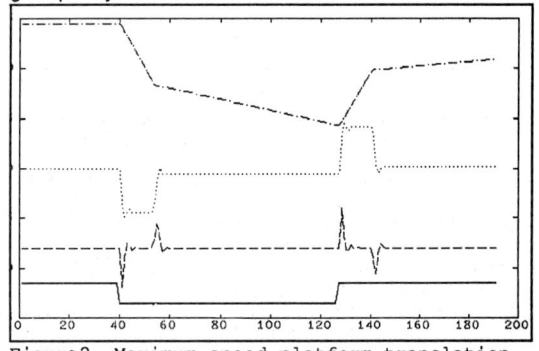

Figure 2. Maximum speed platform translation.

APPLICATION 2: STATIC POSTUROGRAPHY

Static posturography is a well known method and is conducted on a stable platform with or without superimposed rubber foam. The effects of absent or distorted vision (Ring et al 1988a) may be tested, and disturbed muscle proprioception may be provided using mechanical vibrators attached to the calves (Pyykkö et al 1986a, 1986b, Johansson et al 1989). We may define static posturography to be conducted on a non-movable force platform, albeit this does not cover all experimental setups (e.g. Overstall et al 1977).

Previously conducted static posturography according to Sahlstrand et al (1978) has proven useful in assessment of effects of solvents on CNS equilibrium functions (Ledin et al 1986, 1989). The procedure is to measure the position of CP in AP as well as lateral direction during one minute of quiet, upright, double-leg standing in a darkened room, with arms hanging and feet in approximately military position. The CP positions are treated as sampled from a bivariate normal distribution, and a confidence ellipse at level $e^{-1/2}$ is computed. The area of the confidence ellipse is an estimation of body sway. The test is often conducted three times with eyes open and three times with eyes closed, the averages for eyes open and closed, respectively, are the ultimate outcome of the investigation procedure (Ledin et al 1986, 1989).

The hardware interface program was in this case used a bit out of its normal scope, as no perturbation signal was used (in practice, amplitude zero was selected). Measurement time was 59 seconds. A sampling frequency of 25 Hz was used.

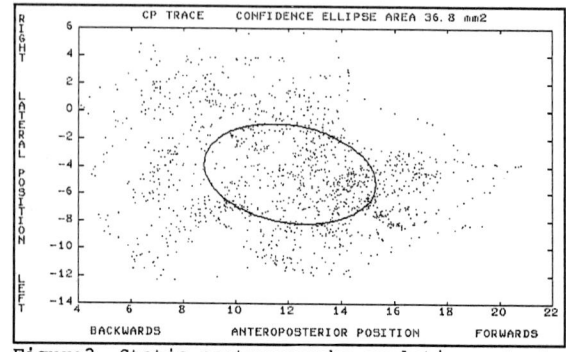

Figure 3. Static posturography emulation output.

Denoting x = CP position in AP direction
y = CP position in lateral direction
m_i = mean of variable i
s_i = standard deviation of variable i
r_{ij} = cross correlation coefficient between variables i and j,

and for brevity $X = (x-m_x)/s_x$ "normalized" x variable
$Y = (x-m_y)/s_y$ "normalized" y variable,

the bivariate normal distribution density function assumes the simple form

$f(x,y) = A\ e^{-c(x,y)}$

where

$A = (2\ pi\ s_x\ s_y)^{-1}\ (1-r_{xy}^2)^{-1/2}$

$c(x,y) = 1/2\ (1-r_{xy}^2)^{-1}\ (X^2+Y^2-2r_{xy}XY)$

Thus, the confidence ellipse at level $e^{-1/2}$ is found when $c(x,y)=1/2$ is solved for pairs (x,y).

The Matlab script, a few simple instructions, computes the basic statistics above, the ellipse area, and presents a scatterplot of all measured CP positions (x,y) with the confidence ellipse superimposed (fig 3).

APPLICATION 3: VISUAL INFLUENCE ON EQUILIBRIUM

Using a sine wave (period 5 seconds, amplitude 6 degrees top-to-top) the visual surround was perturbed in the AP direction. A healthy subject with adequate vision was tested. Sampling frequency was 25 Hz. The relation between the visual stimulation signal (in degrees, positive values mean surround moving away from subject) and the resulting AP sway (CP deflection in mm in AP direction, positive values mean leaning forwards) is shown in figure 4. Obviously there is a relation between visual surround inclination and the angle of the subject with a gain of approximately 0.3 at 0.2 Hz. CP is assumed to be at 55% of body height and the body is modelled as an inverted pendulum.

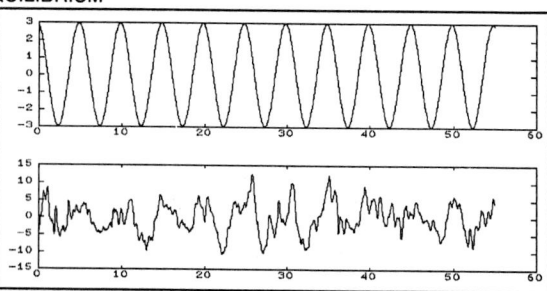

Figure 4. Visual influence on equilibrium.

DISCUSSION

This paper has presented a menu-driven software enabling the user to introduce perturbations to augment and extend the EquiTest dynamic posturography concept. The acquired information is presented by the software in unprocessed form, suggesting the user to explore it in external software for further information extraction. In three simple applications, the capabilities of the system have been demonstrated. The simplicity and feasibility of processing data in Matlab mathematical software have been indicated.

In the first experiment, Newton's second law of inertia was used to estimate the maximum speed of EquiTest support surface translation. The mere occurrence of acceleration and deceleration forces was measured, rather than pure integration with respect to time of the shear force. Despite apparently successful results, such an integration is sensitive to signal offset, and furthermore the weight of the platform itself affecting the shear forces is unknown. The attempt to integrate the velocity in order to compute platform position unveiled the problems of signal integration when systematic errors have been introduced. The velocity was apparently independent of translation amplitude and platform load. This is what would be expected, since the step motors used in the equipment makes it insensitive to actual load within the range of operation. However, with decreasing amplitude, the number of sampling intervals required to move the distance decrease and rounding errors become more important. Thus, calibration experiments are better conducted using as large an amplitude as possible, together with the maximum available sampling frequency, in order to increase resolution.

In a second experiment, the static posturography method of Sahlstrand et al (1978) was implemented on the EquiTest using a few lines of Matlab programming code. Obviously the owner of an EquiTest equipment can easily conduct the well known static posturography procedures. It is a minor task to implement any kind of static posturography (Sahlstrand et al 1978, Diener et al 1984, Taguchi et al 1978, Lidström et al 1990) using our concept of perturbed posturography software and an easy-to-use signal processing software. Thus, modern computer technology provides the possibilities to compare different approaches to static posturography, using inexpensive equipment and software.

Third, visual influence on static stance, in agreement with Ring et al (1988b), was demonstrated by letting the visual surround move in a sinusoidal fashion, causing the subject to follow the oscillating movement.

In vestibular and oculomotor testing, randomized stimuli have proved to be helpful in unveiling CNS disturbances that sinusoidal tests fail to diagnose, as the CNS quickly learns to predict a repetitive stimulus. Even in dynamic posturography, with its enhanced possibilities to detect balance disorders in a dynamic environ-ment, randomized stimuli should be of value in approaching balance disorders in their full context. The present study indicates a possible way to encounter the problem, enabling the scientist to design his perturbation concept in an easy way, and providing him the simple, yet powerful, tools to evaluate it. Thus, the incentives of an open minded research environment are enhanced, albeit not created.

REFERENCES

Bartlett SA, Maki BE, Fernie GR, Holliday PJ, Gryfe CI. On the classification of a geriatric subject as a faller or nonfaller. Med & Biol Eng & Comp 1986: 24: 219-222.

Begbie GH. The effects of alcohol and of varying amounts of visual information on a balancing test. Ergonomics 1966: 9: 325-333.

Clement G, Gurfinkel VS, Lestienne F, Lipshits MI, Popov KE. Adaptation of postural control to weightlessness. Exp Brain Res 1984: 45: 126-132.

Cyr DG, Moore GF, Möller CG. Clinical application of computerized dynamic posturography. Ear, Nose and Throat Journal (suppl) 1988: Sep: 36-47.

Diener HC, Dichgans J, Bacher M, Gompf B. Quantification of postural sway in normals and patients with cerebellar diseases. Electroencephalography and clinical neurophysiology 1984: 57: 134-142.

Fernie GR, Gryfe CI, Holliday PJ, Llewellyn A. The relationship of postural sway in standing to the incidence of falls in geriatric subjects. Age & Ageing 1982: 11: 11-16.

Gurfinkel EV. Physical foundations of the stabilography. Agressologie 1973: 14C: 9-14.

Johansson R, Magnusson M, Åkesson M. Identification of human postural dynamics. IEEE Transactions on Biomedical Engineering 1988: 35: 858-869.

Johnell O, Nilsson B, Obrant K, Sernbo I. Age and sex patterns of hip fracture - changes in 30 years. Acta Orthop Scand 1984: 55: 290-292.

Kapteyn TS. Data Processing of Posturographic Curves. Agressologie 1972: 13B: 29-34.

Ledin T, Tropp H, Odenrick P, Ödkvist LM: Postural sway and corrections. In: Vertigo, nausea, tinnitus and hearing loss in cardio-vascular diseases. Eds CF Claussen and MV Kirtane. Excerpta Medica International Congress Series 708, p 371-376, 1986.

Ledin T, Ödkvist LM, Möller C. Posturography findings in workers exposed to industrial solvents. Acta Otolaryngologica 1989: 107: 357-361.

Lidström J, Friberg S, Lindström L. Refinement of postural sway measurements in scoliosis research. J Ortoph Res, in press, 1990.

Murray MP, Seireg A, Scholz RC. Center of gravity, center of pressure, and supportive forces during human activities. J of Appl Physiology 1967: 23: 831-838.

Murray MP, Seireg AA, Sepic SB. Normal postural stability and steadiness: Quantitative assessment. The Journal of Bone and Joint Surgery 1975:57-A: 510-516.

Nashner LM. A systems approach to understanding and assessing orientation and balance disorders. Advances in diagnosis and management of balance disorders conference, Boston, MA, Oct 1987 (can be obtained from Neurocom Int Inc).

Neurocom Int Inc. EquiTest Technical Manual, 1988.

Njiokiktjien C, de Rijke W. The recording of Romberg test and its application in neurology. Agressologie 1972: 13C: 1-7.

Overstall PW, Exton-Smith AN, Imms FJ, Johnsson AL. Falls in the elderly related to postural imbalance. Br Med J 1977: 1: 261-264.

Pyykkö I, Starck J, Scholtz HJ, Meyer E, Aalto H, Enbom H. Evaluation of vestibular deficiency using posturography. In: Vertigo, nausea, tinnitus and hearing loss in cardio-vascular diseases. Eds CF Claussen and MV Kirtane. Excerpta Medica International Congress Series 708, p 363-370, 1986.

Pyykkö I, Toppila E, Starck J, Aalto H, Enbom H, Seidel H. Computerized posturography: Development of stimulation and analysis methods. In: Vertigo, nausea, tinnitus and hearing loss in cardio-vascular diseases. Eds CF Claussen and MV Kirtane. Excerpta Medica International Congress Series 708, p 353-362, 1986.

Ring C, Matthews R, Nayak L, Isaacs B. Visual push - a sensitive measure of dynamic balance in man. Arch Phys Med Rehabil 1988: 69: 256-260.

Ring C, Nayak L, Isaacs B. Balance function in elderly people who have and who have not fallen. Arch Phys Med Rehabil 1988: 69: 261-264.

Sahlstrand T, Örtengren R, Nachemsson A. Postural equilibrium in adolescent idiopathic scoliosis. Acta Ortop Scand 1978: 49: 354-365.

Taguchi K, Iijima M, Suzuki T. Computer calculation of movement of body's center of gravity. Acta Otolaryngol (Stockh) 1978: 85: 420-425.

Acknowledgements: The financial support of the County of Östergötland Research Funds, Sweden and the helpful attitude of Neurocom, USA in sharing details of EquiTest are gratefully acknowledged.

Correspondence to: T Ledin, Dept of ENT, University Hospital, S-581 85 Linköping, Sweden.

LESIONS IN THE VESTIBULAR-SPINAL SYSTEM IN CHILDREN AND THEIR DETERMINATION BY CRANIO-CORPO-GRAPHY AND POSTUROGRAPHY

GOTTFRIED AUST

Beratungsstelle für Hörbehinderte

Paster-Behrens-Straße 81, D 1000 Berlin 47 (West Germany)

In cases of vertigo in children, especially small children, the examiner must rely on the observations and details of the children's parents or relatives. Later on, with school-age children, one can rely on their own information. However, to clarify the child's vertigo, a detailed neurotologic examination is necessary.

Diagnostic measurements in small children are more difficult, because it takes more time to get a child used to the examination situation. Further problems arise when during extensive diagnostic procedures batteries of single stressing tests are necessary. Since children normally are more sensitive and restless than adults, they sometimes react more anxiously due to previous experience with medical doctors. Very often the child does not realize the examiner's questions and intention. As a consequence, its development, and its ability to cooperate must be considered in neurotologic examinations. Additional difficulties arise from sensory, intellectual and physical impairment, which reduces the child's cooperation (1,4,5,6,8).

Besides the rotatory tests, vestibular spinal examinations are suitable measurements in children. They need only a short time, and their results are reliable, especially as screening tests.

ROMBERG-TEST

The examination of the standing reactions is feasible, as soon as the child is able to stand firmly. The standing reactions can be observed during Romberg-position. The recording techniques Posturography and Cranio-Corpo-Graphy (CCG), however, provide us with more detailed information. The test results are recorded in a document, which can be evaluated. This is of importance in follow-up studies.

The photo of the Romberg test, recorded by the Cranio-Corpo-Gram, shows four white spots representing the sway of the patients' head and shoulders. The square measure of the spots can be determined by planimetry. For this study, the Romberg test was performed over a period of 30 seconds in total darkness and recorded by the CCG-device from Hortmann/Germany in combination with a wide-angle lens and camera from Mamiya/Japan. The CCG was evaluated by measuring the lateral and the anterior-posterior deviation in millimeters (2,3).

In the posturogram the patients' body-sway is recorded by tracing it over a defined time, in our examination over 30 seconds. We used the so-called "Luzerner Messplatte" from Happersberger-Otopront/Germany in combination with a plotter for printing the deviations of the body's center of gravity (7,9,10). The broader the patients' sway, the larger the dislocation of the center of gravity of the body and also the surface area in the plot. In our study we measured the sway-amplitudes in millimeters in the lateral and the anterior-posterior extension during 30 seconds under the following test-conditions first, standing on the platform with a fixation on a target, and second, standing with closed (blindfolded) eyes.

UNTERBERGER/FUKUDA STEPPING TEST

The dynamic Fukuda-Unterberger stepping test is one of the best examinations for measuring the vestibular-spinal system when the child is able to walk firmly. The test can be performed by observing the child's movement pattern. More detailed information can be received, when the test result is recorded by Cranio-Corpo-Graphy. The photographic test result consists of four light traces from the two head- and the two shoulder-lamps, which are evaluated for the following parameters: total length, lateral sway, lateral deviation, and spin. Additional information comes from the qualitative evaluation, e.g. knotted pattern (3).

We have compared the vestibular-spinal test results from 15 hearing disabled children of pre-school age and from 15 children with normal hearing in the same age group. We found that hearing disabled children showed no significant differences in their body equilibrium performance, expressed by the Romberg and the stepping test, compared with the normal hearing group. This indicates, that peripheral vestibular disorders as expected in hearing disabled children, cannot be identified by the vestibular spinal routine tests. To recognize peripheral vestibular lesions we must perform caloric and rotatory tests. We could, however, identify three hearing disabled children with pathologic vestibular test results. In these three children, with the help of our vestibular spinal test, we could confirm additional disturbances of the body equilibrium, caused by minimal cerebral dysfunction. Neurotologic tests are also possible in children, as we could show in more recent publications (1,2,3,5). In these patients it is important, to pay attention to special child-oriented tests and child-oriented test situation. Under these conditions and in such an environment it is possible in most cases, perhaps with test repetition, to receive valuable test responses even in small children. Vestibular spinal tests using posturography and Cranio-Corpo-Graphy are of importance in this relation.

When both recording techniques, Posturography and Cranio-Corpo-Graphy, are compared in terms of application to children, it can be stated that Posturography is appropriate for the static measurement (Romberg test). Small patients quickly learn the test performance. This is important in hearing disabled children, because they understand speech less than normal hearing children. The resolution of changes of the center of gravity in respect to the time is satisfactory. The graph gives further information about qualitative changes of the movement pattern, e.g. frequency of the body movement, repetitive deviations and falling tendency in one direction. The examination is possible with eyes open and fixated, and with eyes closed. Further test variations are practicable without difficulties, e.g. standing on a rubber foam plate to reduce the foot contact to the floor. One of the disadvantages of our "Luzerner Messplatte" is the decrease of information by less body weight. When comparing patients with varying body weight, one must use a correcting factor. Another disadvantage is the software. The evaluating computer program of the platform should be extended by the calculation of the total length, by the analysis of the frequency of the body-sway, and by the automatic correction of the body weight.

The Romberg test with registration in the CCG is easy to perform on children. Difficulties arise for children by testing them in total darkness and by using the big and heavy helmet. We constructed a variable-sized band for children made from synthetic material, which carries the light diodes, the battery and the switch. However, the resolution of the Romberg test in the CCG, expressed by the white spots in the photo is not as high as in posturography.

The recording of the stepping test by a polaroid camera in combination with the variable head band is an excellent examination procedure of the vestibular-spinal system in older children. The test result is ready for manual evaluation only a few seconds after the end of stepping. Higher test comfort will be achieved in the future by using video technology combined with evaluation and calculation by computers.

REFERENCES

1. Aust G (1976) Verhdlg.GNA Bd.V, 15
2. Aust G (1976) Laryng.Rhinol. 55:855
3. Aust G (1978) Verhdlg.GNA Bd.VI,1:191
4. Aust G (1985) Das sensorische Rezeptorverhalten in Zeit und Raum. Habilitationsschrift Freie Universität Berlin
5. Claussen CF (1981) Schwindel. Symptomatik, Diagnostik und Therapie. Ein Leitfaden für Klinik und Praxis. edition m+p dr.werner rudat, Hamburg und Neu-Isenburg
6. Claussen CF, Aust G, Schäfer WD, v.Schlachta I (1986) Atlas der Elektronystagmographie. Atlas der neurootologischen Untersuchungstechnik - Registrierkurven, Befundauswertung, Schwindeldiagnostik. edition m+p dr.werner rudat & co nachf. Hamburg
7. Fried R, Arnold W (1987) Laryng.Rhinol.Otol. 66, 433
8. Goebel P, Aust G (1978) Arch.Oto-Rhino-Laryng. 220:265
9. Hamann K-F (1987) Training gegen Schwindel. Mechanismen der vestibulären Kompensation und ihre therapeutische Anwendung Berlin, Heidelberg, Springer Verlag
10. Norre ME, Forrez G, Beckers A (1987) Clin.Otolaryngol. 12: 215-220

DYNAMIC POSTUROGRAPHY

Wallace Rubin, M.D.

Otorhinolaryngology and Biocommunication, Louisiana State University School of Medicine, New Orleans, Louisiana, U.S.A.

Posturography became clinically relevant because objective tests of vestibular function in use only assessed responses of the horizontal semicircular canals (rotary and caloric tests). Vestibulospinal tests such as dynamic posturography are tests of the vertical canal systems and probably the otolith organs as well.

Posturography, however, is not a screening device. The test cannot stand alone as a vestibular testing modality. It does correlate well with caloric tests in acute vestibular conditions. It does correlate well with rotation tests and adds information otherwise not available in terms of monitor follow-up. Furthermore it is the only objective technique available that measures the proprioceptive and ocular imputs concurrently with the vestibular input. This advantage allows dynamic posturography to elicit and confirm abnormalities in a small number of cases in which other ENG techniques do not reveal abnormalities.

There are also reports in the literature that state that posturography testing:
1. Detects abnormality in sixty-four percent of patients with unilateral peripheral vestibular disease and nearly one-hundred percent in those with central nervous system disease.
2. Distinguishes patients with peripheral and central vestibular pathologies from those with other CNS disease in eighty percent of the cases.

3. Correctly distinguishes between sensory losses and "distortions" due to trauma, fistula, and positional vertigo in eighty to eighty-five percent of cases.

Posturography testing is divided into two parts. Sensory organization testing provides information with regard to the functional impact, the site of pathology and the implications for treatment. The movement coordination portion of the testing provides further information with regard to the functional impact and the type and site of the pathology. The information from both of these portions of the posturography testing are helpful in designing and predicting the prognosis with regard to the rehabilitation aspects of vestibular system therapy.

Vestibular rehabilitation fits into the logical scheme of specific etiologic medical management. Only those medications that are specific for treating causative mechanisms are used. Vestibular suppressive medications are counter productive and are used only when acute symptoms occur and at that time they are only used on an acute basis. Vestibular rehabilitative techniques are specific forms of therapy designed specifically. Posturography results from both the sensory organization and movement coordination portions of the test are utilized to design the vestibular rehabilitation program.

POSTTRAUMATIC NEUROOTOLOGICAL DISTURBANCES DUE TO CERVICAL LESIONS

VERTIGO DUE TO WHIPLASH INJURY

SAGNELLI M.   POLLASTRINI L.   BARETTI F.   PATRIZI M.

1st E.N.T. Department - "La Sapienza" University of Rome

INTRODUCTION

Whiplash injury is the most common traumatic lesion of the cervix, caused in almost all cases by car accidents. The vertebral column, all one with the car, is thrust forwards whilst the head, due to inertia, is thrown backwards. Hence, an over-extension of the head ensues reaching 140 degrees (under normal conditions it reaches 45 degrees). In the absence of other lesions, a whiplash injury can involve the vestibular system resulting in vertigo associated or not with cochlear and/or neurological symptoms.

The aim of the present study is to define the characteristics of vertigo due to whiplash injuries and the etiopathogenetic mechanisms from which they derive.

MATERIAL AND METHODS

An otoneurological examination was carried out on a group of 75 subjects who came to our Centre complaining of vertigo, headache, cervical stiffness and neck pain, associated or not with hearing loss and neurological disorders, arising after car accidents and referable to whiplash injury.

The cause/effect relationship between the accident and the onset of symptoms was established. All patients then underwent: 1) a general medical examination with target clinical history relative to possible episodes of otolabyrinthitis; 2) a neurological examination; 3) a complete ENT visit in order to exclude existing aural pathology; 4) pure tone threshold audiometry.

Subsequently, the patients all underwent vestibular testing including spontaneous balance procedures (tonic-segmentary deviations) and instrumental (caloric and ENG) tests for the study of spontaneous and optokinetic nystagmus.

63 of the 75 patients showed pathological findings and were subdivided into two groups, selected according to the type of vertigo: group A, included 45 subjects with non-rotatory vertigo; group B, consisted of 18 subjects with rotatory vertigo.

RESULTS

The 45 subjects in group A complained of instability and various, badly defined, sub-continuous neurovegetative phenomena, including headache and neck pain. In 36 cases spontaneous nystagmus of central origin was found (one degree horizontal or pure rotatory, in some cases pure vertical). After caloric and rotatory stimulation, 34 subjects presented bilateral vestibular hyperreflexia (disinhibited response) and 11 an asymmetric or non-asymmetric bilateral hyporeflexia. In 60% of cases with spontaneous nystagmus there were noticeable signs of bilateral symmetric hyperreflexia. The ENG traces are abnormal for amplitude, form and rythmn of nystagmus. Spontaneous vestibular tests gave contrasting results with vestibular syndromes which were both harmonic (probably due to the irritation of the lower brainstem) and disharmonic (due to prevalently cranial sites of lesion). The optokinetic nystagmus was modified (either hyper or hypo, mainly on the horizontal plane) in 29 cases, which would seem to suggest – in agreement with other Authors (1) – the existence of a vestibular disorder of central origin due to a widespread lesion of the brainstem. The vertigo was not associated to hearing loss and this finding distinguished it from rotatory vertigo of peripheral origin which tends to be accompanied by a neurosensorial hearing loss with recruitment.

It is interesting to note how of the 22 patients in whom neck pain was reduced during the period of observation, 16 also showed a reduction in the subjective intensity of the vertigo, whereas 13 patients who experienced worse neck pain showed a parallel increase in vertigo.

These results confirm the hypothesis suggested by Hinoki (2) whereby lesions of the soft cervical tissues (muscles, articulations, capsules, sensory nerves) are an important determining factor in vertigo due to cranial and cervical trauma. In order to verify this teory, 45 subjects underwent galvanic stimulation (25 Hz, 0.7 mA, 5 volts) with the anode placed on the nape of the neck and modifications of both nystagmus and tonic-segmentary deviations were recorded. The choice of such a method, as suggested by Hinoki in a recent study (2), is justified by the fact that the application of an anodic stimulation induces an increase in the excitability of the muscles and of the nerve endings near the electrode (3), thus enabling us to verify whether, in fact, the appearance of intensification of vestibular symptoms can be related to the hypertonia of the soft cervical tissues.

After turning off the circuit, 71.1% of the patients showed an increase of vertigo and modification of the tonic-segmentary tests. Hence, anodic stimulation would seem to favour the formation of abnormal centripetal impulses deriving from the irritated cervical areas, thus confirming the importance of role played by an over-excitation of the cervical proprioceptors in the triggering of vertigo due to whiplash injury. Hinoki (2) proposed an experimental trigger/target model in which the over-excited cervical proprioceptors act as triggers and the vestibular pathways and/or centers as targets.

Abnormal centripetal impulses deriving from the damaged soft tissues can make their way up the pathways to the brainstem, interfering with its functions. Such a dysfunction can even reach the eye, body and limb muscles causing dysfunctions and modifications of tonic-segmentary findings. The existence of neurovegetative symptoms suggests the involvment of the hypothalamus. Lastly, the cerebellum, due to its connections with the cervical proprioceptors and the brainstem, would seem to be involved in the genesis of whiplash injury; in fact, other Authors have shown cerebral ataxia to be present in almost half the subjects who had undergone whiplash injuries.

The 18 patients in group B referred rotatory vertigo, which was often intense and associated with neurovegetative phenomena of various types, including headache and neck pain. Spontaneous nystagmus was present in all patients and it was mainly horizontal-rotatory, and occasionally pure horizontal nystagmus. The optokinetic nystagmus was modified in the presence of spontaneous nystagmus. In all cases both spontaneous and instrumental vestibular tests showed a syndrome of a harmonic-deficitary nature: in 12 cases hyporeflexia was bilateral and symmetric and in 6 it was asymmetric, associated with various degrees os sensorineural hearing loss with signs of recruitment.

These findings suggest that whiplash injury can provoke labyrinthine disorders (even though in a considerably lower percentage) with objective vertigo and cochlear symptoms. As in group A, the 18 subjects in group B underwent anodic galvanic stimulation and in all patients there was an increase in subjective vertigo along with modifications of the tonic-segmentary tests. The model exemplifying the trigger/target correlation between irritated cervical and vestibular structures can, in this context, explain the etiopathogenetic relationship between vertigo and whiplash injury. In this case the trigger is represented by the proprioceptors and the sympathetic cervical endings, whilst the target is the peripheral vestibular system. Hinoki (2) has explained the high incidence in whiplash injuries of central vestibular lesions over peripheral lesions, suggesting that peripheral labyrinthine dysfunction can only manifest in cases where patients, with a pre-existing aural lesion or latent labyrinthine dysfunction, are placed under conditions of stress, even minimal, represented by whiplash injury which could show up such a dysfunction.

Cervical nystagmus was studied in all 63 patients. This is a peculiar form of nystagmus induced by stimulation of the muscular-tendineous proprioceptors of the neck and the nape of the neck, which can be seen in cases of lesions of the cervical structures (whiplash injury) so as to create an irritation of the proprioceptors. The patients, with his eyes closed, are placed on a rotating chair, and their head is held firmly by an assistant; the chair is turned manually to the right and to the left with 30 degrees oscillations in relation to the position at rest; the chair takes 10" for repositioning and stays in the extreme lateral position for a further 10". By means of ENG recordings, cervical nystagmus was found in all patients, manifesting as one or more series of well defined, regular nystagmus. Such results are further evidence of the role played by abnormal ascending impulses, deriving from the cervical proprioceptors in a state of hypertonia, in the triggering of vertigo due to whiplash injury.

In the past, Authors (4) have shown that cervical vertigo due to whiplash injury is due essentially to neurovascular disorders at a level with the vertebral or inner auditory arteries, subsequent to irritation of the cervical sympathetic nerve. Such theories, are based on electromiographic and electronystagmographic findings after administration of adrenergic substances capable of inducing an over-excitation of the posterior cervical sympathetic nerve endings which results in the over-excitation of the cervical proprioceptors and hypertonia of the deep neck muscles.

REFERENCES

1. Ushio N, Ishida I (1971) Pract Otol (Kyoto) 64:493

2. Hinoki M (1985) Acta Otolaryngol (Stockh) Suppl 419:9

3. Suzuki M (1955) J Physiol Soc Jap 17:223

4. Ushio N, Hinoki M (1975) Pract Otol (Kyoto) 68 Suppl 6:1059

CERVICAL SYNDROME DUE TO TRAUMA

REGINA BECKER, ERHARD D. MEYER

HNO-Klinik und Poliklinik (Dir.: Prof.Dr.sc.med. H.J. Gerhardt),
Bereich Medizin (Charité) der Humboldt-Universität zu Berlin,
Schumannstr. 20/21, 1040 Berlin, GDR

INTRODUKTION

The complaints and findings of patients with neck trauma were examined in a retrospective study. The question was, if there were specific symptoms or if the symptom combinations were similar to the so-called encephalic cervical syndrome of Decher (1). Both diseases practically concern the same anatomical region.

MATERIAL AND METHODS

40 patients (22 men and 18 women) after neck trauma were chosen from our patients file. The later symptoms and findings could only be recorded in this study. According to the mechanism of the accident two groups of patients were assembled:
1. Patients with whiplash injury, n = 17, avarage age: 41 years
2. Patients with head neck trauma, n = 23, avarage age: 35 years.
Group 2 consisted of 6 patients with direct neck injury and 17 patients with simultaneous cranial injury of slight degree, i.e. without symptoms as e.g. a longer loss of consciousness and amnesia. Only the 8 most frequent factors were included in this analysis. The results were demonstrated in form of histograms for each group separately.

RESULTS

The results of the anamnestic details about the complaints are shown in figure 1 and 2. The most frequent complaints in both groups were vertigo and pain (≥ 60 %). The term vertigo means in this context as well long-lasting dizziness as vertigo attacks due to head movements.
Pain means as well neck pain as occipital or frontal headache.

The results of the analysis of neurootological findings are shown in figure 3 and 4. Most frequent findings were 1. cervical nystagmus and 2. positional and positioning nystagmus in both groups.

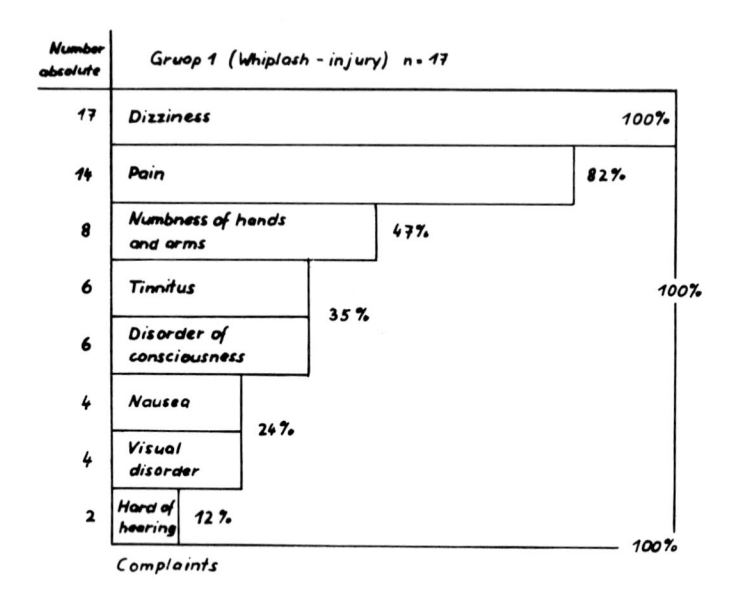

Fig. 1. Complaints, Group 1

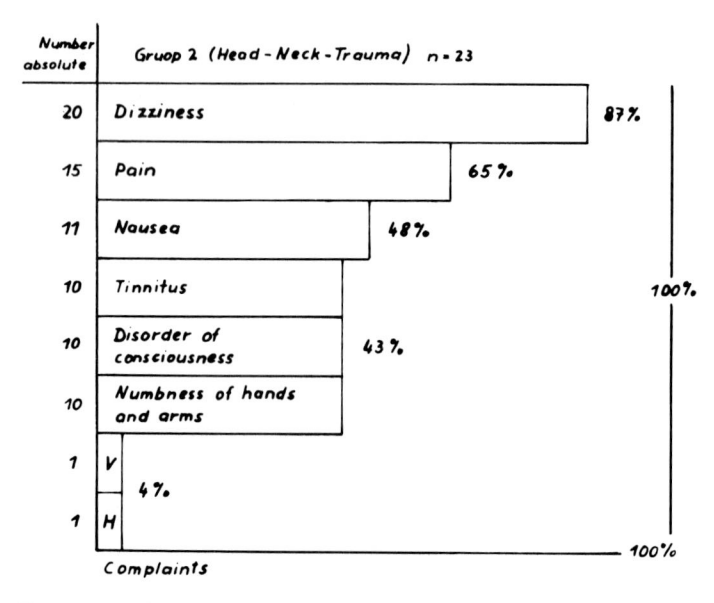

Fig. 2 Complaints, Group 2, V = Visual disorder, H = Hard of hearing

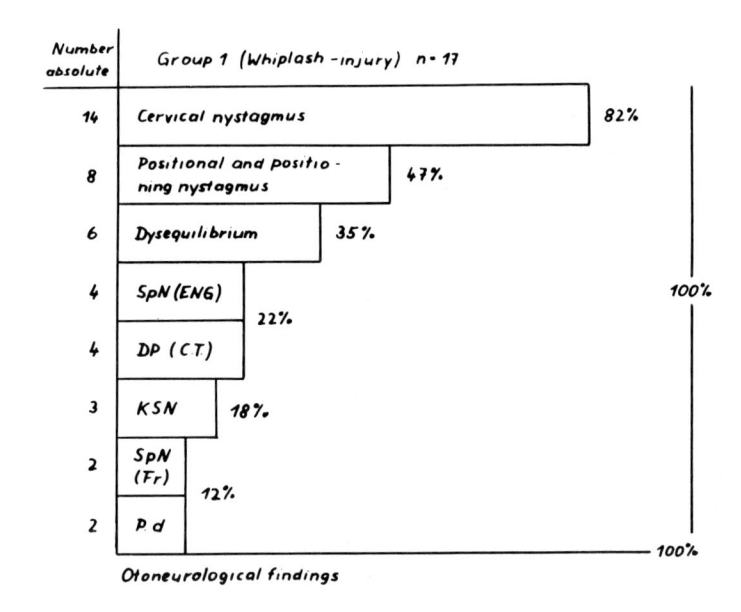

Fig. 3. Otoneurological findings, Group 1, SpN = Sponaneous nystagmus, DP (C.T.) = Directional preponderance (Caloric test), KSN = Head shaking nystagmus, P.d. = Perceptive deafness

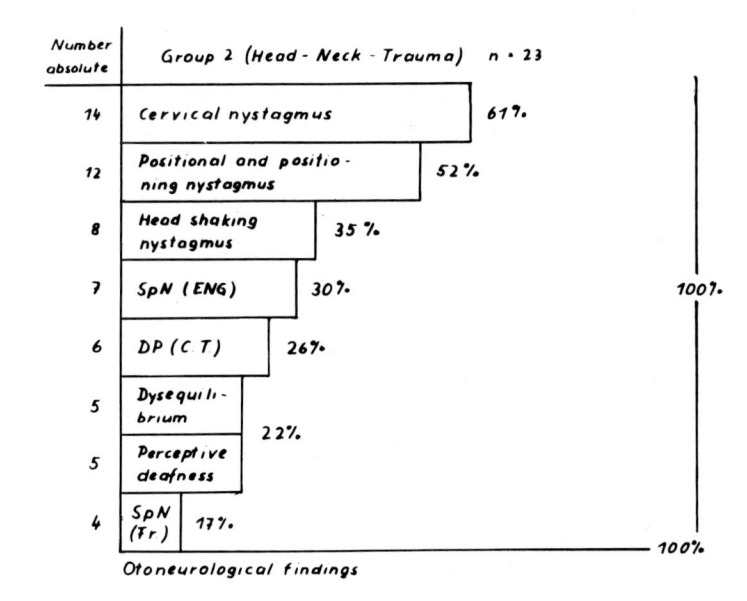

Fig. 4 Otoneurological findings, Group 2

DISCUSSION
Clinical symptoms

Decher (1) described the encephalic cervical syndrome as arrangement of symptoms, which are head and neck pain, hearing loss, tinnitus and vertigo. This definition is still valid. These symptoms can be of different character, and there are often associations to the cervical brachial syndrome. The changing symptom combination of vertigo and headache with further symptoms, e.g. tinnitus and numbness in hand and arms were also found in both groups of the present study. Specific symptoms in patients with neck trauma were not observed by us.

Other investigators (2,3) found similar results in cases of whiplash injury. Mean symptoms were also vertigo, pain and numbness at their patients. The relatively frequent appearance of numbness in arms and hands in cases of whiplash injury can be interpreted as a simultaneous damage of the lower cervical spine. The remaining provable symptoms ca be related to an affect of the brain stem, although there were no cases with clinical indications of a cerebral commotion.

Otoneurological findings

The most frequent experimental finding was the cervical nystagmus in both groups, in patients with whiplash injury more frequently compared to the head neck trauma. Decher (1) found this provoked nystagmus in 75 % in his patients with cervical syndrome. We found in more than 90 % of patients a cervical nystagmus in a former study in patients with cervical syndrome and pathological manual medical findings. The cervical nystagmus is obviously not a specific finding in patients with neck trauma, But the pathogenetic importance of this provoked nystagmus is not clear up to now.

We also found the remaining symptoms of cervical syndrome which were named by Decher by our patients, e.g. positional and positioning nystagmus: 47 % in group 1, 52 % in group 2 as well as the occurrence of all kinds of vestibular disorders (central, peripheral and combined).

A differentiation between cervical syndrome and neck trauma by otoneurological investigations was not possible corresponding to our results.

The present results are agreement with the statement of Gutmann (2), that the posttraumatic clinical symptoms don't in principle differ from the nontraumatic cervical symptom combination.

Some observations to the pathogenesis

The large degree of correspondence of the symptoms and neurootological findings is obviously caused, as mentioned above, by the common pathological - anatomical substraum.

It is widely believed, that this symptoms with cervical syndrome are caused by functional disturbances of the upper cervical spine, i.e. of the segments C0/C1 to C2/C3.

Detailed studies about neck trauma were available of Gutman (2) and Zenner (3). Zenner found in his study about whiplash injury, that the head neck joints are especially susceptiple to functional disturbances. The cause is the anatomy of the head neck joints, which differ fundamentally from the remaining cervical spine. From this approach the named clinical symptoms with neck trauma as well as with cervical syndrome are refered to the head neck joints. In this context it is thinkable that the cervical nystagmus ca be the expression of functional disorders of the head neck joints and the irritation or over - excitation of the cervical proprioceptors.

The proof of the cervical nystagmus could be a possibility for objective proof of the posttraumatic complaints, especially with younger patients. The evidence for the hypothesis is still due.

REFERENCES

1. Decher H (1969) Halswirbelsäule und Vestibulargan. Archiv für Ohren - Nasen- und Kehlkopfheilkunde 194: 188

2. Gutmann G (1988) Klinik von posttraumatischen Funktionsstörungen der oberen HWS: Symptomkombination und Symptomdauer, Frage der Latenz. In: Wolff HD (eds): Die Sonderstellung des Kopfgelenkbereichs. Vortragsband, Springer Verlag (Manuelle Medizin)

3. Zenner P (1987) Die Schleuderverletzung der HWS und ihre Begutachtung. Monographie, Dissertation

DYNAMIC POSTUROGRAPHY IN CERVICAL VERTIGO

M ÅLUND, T LEDIN, LM ÖDKVIST, C MÖLLER, S-E LARSSON.

Depts of ENT and Orthopaedic Surgery, University Hospital, S-581 85 Linköping, Sweden.

ABSTRACT

Cervical vertigo, the entity of neck disorder and associated vestibular symptoms, was investigated in 15 suspected subjects and results were compared to 15 age-matched controls. A modified dynamic posturography investigation with different head positions was used. Head position was monitored with electrogoniometry in three dimensions. Differences on a sway-referenced platform were found.

INTRODUCTION

Since Ryan and Cope (1955) introduced the term "cervical vertigo" various authors have called attention to this syndrome. Recognition of cervical vertigo is important as the patient can be spared some unnecessary and uncomfortable diagnostic procedures. Furthermore the treatment is more effective the earlier the diagnosis. Dynamic posturography is introduced in an attempt to objectify neck influence upon balance in cases of suspected cervical vertigo.

MATERIAL AND METHODS

Fifteen patients aged 32-64 years (mean 48 years) with suspected cervical vertigo were investigated. ENG and routine examination had excluded abnormality of the peripheral as well as central vestibular systems. All patients had transient equilibrium disturbances, most of them since more than one year, and all had neck pain and/or stiffness since at least one year. Four cases had tinnitus and three a feeling of fullness in the ear. Two patients had a history of whiplash trauma. Comparisons with 15 age-matched healthy controls were made. Their sex, body weight and length did not differ from the patients.

Parts of the dynamic posturography concept (Equitest, Neurocom Int Inc, Clackamas, Oregon, USA) as described by Nashner (1987) and Cyr et al (1988) were performed. In the dynamic posturography, the subject is standing on a dual forceplate enclosed by a visual surround. Both the forceplate and the surround can be made to move with the person's antero-posterior (AP) sway or independent of the sway, thus enabling programmed disturbances of the equilibrium.

The investigation is divided into two main sections: sensory organization test (SO) and movement coordination test (MC). The SO part is divided into six separate tests (see Ledin et al 1990 for figure), lasting 20 seconds each with test 4, 5 and 6 repeated three times. SO 1 is a quantified version of Rombergs test. The subject stands with eyes open and the surrounding as well as the ground is stable. SO 2 is equal to SO 1 except that the eyes are closed. In SO 3, performed with eyes open, the surrounding moves in response to the body sway. In test SO 4 the platform is sway referenced and the surrounding stable. In test SO 5, with eyes closed, the platform is sway referenced, and in test SO 6 both the platform and surrounding are sway referenced. Note that in SO 3 and SO 6 the tested subject might have some orientation information from the surrounding as it is only moving in the AP direction and not in the lateral direction. From each test an equilibrium score is computed. The score is 100 for absolutely no sway, decreasing with increasing sway amplitude, and zero in case of falling.

The movement coordination (MC) part is divided into eight separate tests: Small, medium and large backwards and forwards translation perturbations of the platform are repeated three times each to simulate falling forwards and backwards, respectively, and furthermore the platform is tilted toes-down and toes-up five times each. Results from the movement coordination (MC) part were inconclusive and are not reported.

From the SO part test conditions with absent vision were selected, furthermore the equilibrium scores with the head in several positions for both stable and sway-referenced support surface were measured: neutral upright position, in flexion and extension, in right and left rotation, in right and left lateral flexion and (for the patients) in the position most prone to elicit a feeling of vertigo or unsteadiness ("worst position"). In 11 cases measurements were also undertaken when the patient changed from neutral to the "worst" position and vice versa. The head position in three dimensions (Ålund and Larsson 1990) was monitored with a goniometer.

Groups were compared using Student's t-test, paired data using Student's paired t-test. A probability level of 5% was considered significant.

RESULTS

Equilibrium scores examined on the stable platform showed no difference between patients and controls in any head position. Scores obtained during head movements in the patients did not show any significant differences compared to the neutral position, neither on stable nor on sway-referenced platform. On the sway-referenced platform scores were significantly lower in the patients than in the controls for the neutral position, left rotation and right lateral flexion. In the patients, a significant score reduction was noted for the "worst" position as compared to the neutral position, when measured on the sway-referenced platform.

DISCUSSION

Our findings as to posturography on a stable platform are in accordance with previous reports (Holtmann and Reiman 1989) and we agree with Norre et al (1987) that static posturography is of no certain diagnostic value in suspected cervical vertigo. When proprioceptive afferents from the legs were reduced, as is the case on a sway-referenced platform, measurements were found to distinguish between patients and controls. Furthermore, these measurements showed a significant reduction of the equilibrium score in the "worst" head position as compared to neutral position. These findings give support to the assumption that common neck disorders may give rise to aberrant neck afferents and that these are normally concealed by proprioceptive influx, making dynamic posturography a valuable tool when evaluating patients with suspected cervical vertigo.

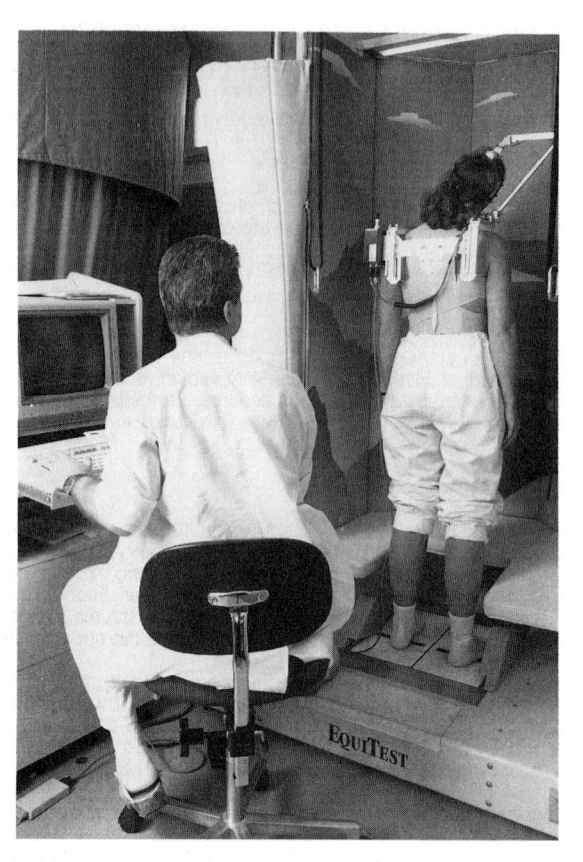

REFERENCES

Ålund M, Larsson S-E. Three-dimensional analysis of neck motion. Spine, in press, 1990.

Cyr DG, Moore GF, Möller CG. Clinical application of computerized dynamic posturography. Ear, Nose and Throat Journal (suppl) 1988: Sep: 36-47.

Holtmann S, Reiman V. Zervicale Afferenzen und ihre Einbindung in die Gleichgewichtsregulation. Laryngo-Rhino-Otol 1989: 68: 72-77.

Ledin T, Möller C, Möller M, Ödkvist LM. Dynamic posturography and aging. Proceedings Neurootological and Equilibriometric Society 17th Congress, Bad Kissingen, 1990 (this volume).

Nashner LM. A systems approach to understanding and assessing orientation and balance disorders. Advances in diagnosis and management of balance disorders conference, Boston, MA, Oct 1987 (can be obtained from Neurocom Int Inc).

Norre ME, Forrez G, Stevens A, Beckers A. Cervical vertigo diagnosed by posturography? Preliminary report. Acta Oto-Rhino-Laryng Belg 1987: 41: 574-581.

Ryan GMS, Cope S. Cervical vertigo. Lancet 1955: 2: 1355-1358.

Correspondence to: M Ålund, Dept of Orthopaedic Surgery, University Hospital, Linköping, Sweden.

**AUDIOVESTIBULAR DISTURBANCES
DUE TO HEAD TRAUMA**

CAUSES OF SENSORINEURAL HEARING LOSS IN BULGARIA

D. DIMOV, I. SPIRIDONOVA

Medical Academy, ORL-Institute, Sofia - Bulgaria

SUMMARY

Epidemiological and clinical study of the causes for deafness in 1466 infants were made for a period of 10 years (1979 - 1989). A classification of the causes and their frequency is given. Interpreting the obtained data we determined that the most frequent causes leading to sensorineural hearing loss in our country are those acting during the perinatal and postnatal periods. The virus intoxications and ototoxic aminoglycoside antibiotics have the greatest percentage of those causes. This requires for special attention to be paid in clinical practice in order to avoid those factors.

MATERIAL AND METHODS

Individuals with reduced hearing and deafness provoke medical, social and legal problems in civilized society. The abscense of hearing especially since early childhood deprives those people of socializing with others and they become disabled.

In recent years, with the use of modern functional methods of examination we succeeded in better determination of the degree of hearing loss. Particularly, the use of electrophysiological methods (ERA, BERA) makes possible the precise evaluation of the affection level from the peripheral regions up to the cortical zones. This enables a more definite classification of hearing impairments to be made. Eight thousand cases with hearing defficit and deafness are registrated in our country and gathered in the "Union of Deaf People in Bulgaria", which provides the education, rehabilitation and suitable occupation with all social acquisitions for them. The people with reduced hearing became considerably fewer recently, due to the precised diagnosis and early, adequate treatment, while the number of deafness caused by ototoxic drugs increased. This evokes justifide anxiety for the physicians, based on their therapeutical means. In order to ascertain the causes which lead to hearing impairment and deafness we made an epidemiological and clinical study of the registered cases, paying special attention to the early childhood. Examination by reflexometry was performed still at the obstetrical department and later ERA-method was used. We interpreted the data obtained from the examination of 1466 infants for a period of 10 years (1979 - 1989) and determined the most frequent causes of severe hearing affection and deafness. For better clarity the following classification of the ascertained cause for deafness is given:

I. Congenital (genetic) deafness 234 infants
II. Acquired (non-genetic) deafness 900, out of them
    1. prenatal causes   — 204 infants
    2. perinatal causes — 384 infants
    3. postnatal causes — 312 infants
III. Unknown (undefined) causes 332 infants

I. The hearidatory deafness is caused by transmission of genetic chromosomal anomalies (chromosomal aberation) by dominant and recessive way of inheritance. Autosomal-dominant deafness was proved in 152 infants, mainly in families in whome generations other deaf individuals were observed. Wardenburg's syndrome was observed in 11 infants from this group and other three had leucodystrophy. In fact this type of deafness is revealed in homozygotes. The recessive form of congenital deafness was observed when blood relationship between parents existed. It was proved in 68 infants. This type of deafness is manifested only in recessive homozygotes. The causes for these anomalies still remain unclarified as they cannot be ascertained by up – to – data examination methods.

II. Aquired (non-genetic) deafness was presented four time more as compared with the congenital one. In this case different factors and causes affect the development of the hearing organs in different phases of foetus and infant growth. Therefore they will be viewed consecutively:

1. Prenatal causes: the greatest percentage of them has the pathological pregnancy – 121 cases. Frequent virus infections of the mother during the first months of pregnancy are recorded in the anamnesis as follows: rubella – 12 cases; toxoplasmosis – 6; grippe and other virus intoxications – 27; diabetes – 2; Rh-incompatibility – 38; malformations – 24, which were observed after the Chernobil accident, x-ray treatment and others.

2. Perinatal causes: prematurity of the faetus was the most frequently observed one – 147 cases (the data shows that 16% of the small infants have reduced hearing bilaterally), natal trauma – 105; asphyxia – 97; twins – 18; infants cerebral palsy (Morbus Little) – 17. Generally speaking the oxygen insuficiancy is the one considered to be the main cause for this type of affection, as the organ of Corti of the infants is specially sensitive to it.

3. Postnatal causes: the aminoglycoside ototoxicity is the most frequent cause in this group, due to the fact that they are most often prescribed to children with different inflamatory diseases. Kanamycin, Amikacin and Gentamycin are among the most often used aminoglycosides, but possesing clinically proven cochlear toxicity. Reduced hearing and deafness were ascertained in 240 infants treated with Amikacin and Gentamycin. In this group the intoxication of organ of Corti is combined — on one hand are the aminoglycosides and on the other — the virus infections treated with antibiotics. Therefor we are not able to detrmine pure toxicity of aminoglycosides in the clinic. In this group, as a result of meningitis purulenta — 42 cases, meningoencephalitis (result of antidiphteria vaccination), parotitis and polyomyelitis in 30 cases.

III. Unknown causes: the exact cause for reduced hearing was not found in 332 infants. Latent virus infections, different preparation's intoxication and others are supposed to be the cause for it.

From the data exposed it is evident that the most frequent causes for sensorineural hearing loss in our country are those acting during the perinatal and postnatal periods, thereby the virus intoxication and ototoxic aminoglycosides having the greatest percentage. That's why the profilaxy of deafness should be directed in the first place to avoid those factors in clinical practice.

VERTIGO, NAUSEA, TINNITUS AND HYPOACUSIA AFTER IATROGENIC TRAUMATA

OTTO RIBÁRI, BÉLA BÜKI

Clinic of Otorhinolaryngology, Semmelweis University
Szigony u. 36. 1083 Budapest, Hungary

INTRODUCTION

Otological operations have a certain rate of complications which can manifest itself either during or after the operation. These complications cause symptoms such as hypoacusis, tinnitus, vertigo. The effort to diminish the rate of complications is an important task during surgery. Therefore it is important to standardize the methods of the different operations. It is also important, that residents should operate only under the strictest supervision since it is an old experience, that the rate of complications is higher when unexperienced collegues operate, than in the case of an experienced surgeon.
Intra- and postoperative bleeding and infection are frequently the result of unsufficient surgical technique. Vertigo is a frequent fenomenon during and after different otological manipulations such as the operation for chronic otitis, M. Meniere or otosclerosis. The postoperative tinnitus is luckily rare but a very unpleasant complication (3).

PATIENTS AND RESULTS

In order to establish the frequency of the postoperative hypoacusis which is also a frequently encountered complication after otological surgery we surveyed the 1572 operations for chronic otitis and 812 stapedectomies done at our ENT-Clinic at the Semmelweis University, Budapest in the past 5 years. Most of the considered operations were done at our Clinic as first operation. In this group the rate of complications was lower. In the group of the revisions (second, third operations carried out on patients who had been operated at an other Clinic before, n=279/ the rate of complications was higher (13).

Hypoacusis, vertigo and tinnitus can be caused by postoperative infection (5). Luckily the acut infections are rare as postoperative infections. Their occurence can be facilitated by the low

immunity of the patient, for instance immunodeficient states, diabetes mellitus, age. The possible causes of iatrogenic infections are bad surgical technique, long operation time. An additional factor can be the presence of virulent bacteria. The postoperative complications are: acute otitis media, labyrinthitis, meningitis, mastoiditis, cerebral abscess, sinus thrombosis. The clue to the therapy of these complications is early diagnosis with bacterial culture and antibiogramm oriented antimicrobial therapy /1,9/. In otological infections it is important to consider the possibility of an anaerobic infection. Of course surgical technique can help to diminish the possibility of infection such as elimination of all pathological tissues and adequate antibiotic therapy /6/. Hypoacusis can be caused by involuntary opening the osseous labyrinth or intraoperative acoustic trauma such as the noise of the frazer especially when in contact with the ossicles. Touching the incus with the rotating frazer can cause a severe high tone hearing loss. The luxation or breaking of the stapes or any other kind of fistula in the oval window or in the semicircular canals cause not only cochlear hearing loss but also severe rotating vertigo. This kind of lesion is not frequent recently, but it is very important to think of it, if the patient is complaining of postoperative tinnitus, permanent rotating vertigo and horizonto-rotatory nystagmus to the healthy side, both changing severity with head-positioning. These symptoms are characteristic of progressive serous, non-infectious labyrinthitis. In these cases the revision of the tympanic cavity is indicated, with the replacement of the incus or stapedectomy with closure of the oval window with connective tissue.
According to Pfalz (lo,ll) the horizontal canal is most frequently traumatized. Since it is in a prominent position we may easily break the bony wall without opening the membranous canal. If the latter is opened with a needle or the suction tube an immediate severe hearing loss and vestibular function loss is encountered. This causes severe rotating vertigo, nausea, vomiting, tinnitus and not unfrequently total deafness. There is a spontaneous horizonto-rotatory nystagmus to the healthy side with ataxy. Slight lesion causes tinnitus, positional nystagmus and high tone hearing loss. Less frequent is the lesion of the superior semicircular canal, this occurs at the removal of large

cholesteatomas. The postoperative symptoms are less characteristic, than they are in the case of the horizontal canal lesions. There is usually mild head positioning vertigo, rarely with tinnitus and hypoacusis. The diagnosis is helped by the positive fistula-sign. The existence of the above symptoms indicates an immediate surgical revision especially in case of a functioning labyrinth. The closure of the fistula is advisable by temporal fascia, perichondrium, or by bone paste and fibrin glue (4). Beside the acoustic trauma caused by drilling the thermal trauma can be mentioned. It occurs when the cooling is unsufficient. It can cause transient cochlear and vestibular symptoms. The operation for closure of labyrinthine fistula can also cause vertiginous symptoms. These kind of operation is indicated when cholesteatoma has removed the lateral wall of the horizontal semicircular canal. The fistula is either complete or partial. In these cases are also vertigo, spontaneous nystagmus and positive fistula-sign the leading symptoms. The closure needs very refined surgical solutions. The squamous epithelium is frequently interwoven with the perilympathic tissues. Therefore some surgeons leave the fistula open at the primary operation and the closure follows as a second step this is especially indicated when signs of infection can be detected at the fistula. During the second operation is the removal of the matrix more simple.

Table. Main symptoms after stapes dislocation
- Tinnitus
- Positional vertigo
- combined conductive and perceptional hearing loss
- spontaneous nystagmus towards the normal ear

The next relatively frequent kind of complication is noticed at the stapedectomies. The practiced surgeon has usually a 98 percent complete recovery, in spite of this at great numbers complications are unavoidable. The complete hearing loss occurs in 0,6-0,2 % of the cases, major statistics (8,12) found hearing loss in 1,4 per cent, conductive hearing loss is encountered in 5 % even after successful operation. When the sensorineural hearing loss is an immediate complication the pathogenetic role of a false operative technique can be postulated, for instance the direct trauma of the membranous labyrinth, the too long prothesis, the too vigorous suction, or the removal of fragments of the labyrinth. The aggressive mobilization of the stapes is also not recommended. These failures can be avoided if placing a perforation on the stapes-plate before mobilizating it. Then must not be done any effort to recover the lost stapes-plate if it is swimming in the labyrinth.

A second kind of post-stapedectomy complications follow the surgery after a few weeks. This is usually progressive hearing loss, severe tinnitus, vertigo. Untreated it progrediates to total deafness. These kind of complications can be caused by granulations, in the past for instance because of the metal-polyethylene prothesis, or talcum-powder. Sometimes a perilymph fistula can be detected as a cause. This can manifest itself sooner or later in the postoperative phase. They were rather frequent in the era of vena-wall or plastic prothesis. The use of wire prothesis has diminished the number of this kind of complication almost completely. The fistula can be treated best by an immediate surgical revision. Often it is caused by barotrauma. Since the application of the small-fenestra technique the perilymph fistulae are rather rare.

REFERENCES

1. Brook, I., Feingold, S.M.: Bacteriology of chronic otitis media. JAMA 241, 487-488, 1979.
2. Causse, J., Causse, J.B.: Eighteen years report on stapedectomy. Problems of stapedial fixation. Clin.Otol. 5, 49, 1980.
3. Fisch, U.: Postoperative complications. Proceedings of the International Conference on the Postoperative Evaluation in Middle Ear Surgery held in Antwerp on June 14-16, 1984. Ed: J.F.E. Marquet, pp. 183-185
4. Helms, J.:Labyrinthine fistulas in cholesteatoma. Results with different surgical techniques. Cholesteatoma and Mastoid Surgery, pp. 1o48-1o48, (Ed: M. Tos, J. Thomsem and E.Peitersen), 1989 Kugler and Ghedini Publications, Amsterdam, Berkeley, Milano.
5. Maniglia, A.J.:Postoperative infections secondary to ear surgery - Antimicrobial therapy. Proceedings of the International Conference on the Postoperative Evaluation in Middle Ear Surgery held in Antwerp on June 14-16, 1984. Ed: J.F.E. Marquet, pp. 186-193.
6. Marquet, J., Graff, A.: Postoperative evaluation of middle ear surgery. Audiology 21, 2o-32, 1982.

7. Marquet, J., Creton, W.L., van Camp. K.J.: Considerations about the surgical approach in stapedectomy. Acta Otol. 74, 4o6-41o, 1983.

8. Morrison, A.W. Scott Brown'n diseases of the ear, nose and throat. 4 th Edition. Ed. J. Ballantyne and J. Groves, London, Butterworths, 1979.

9. Parkin, J.L.: Antimicrobial treatment of otitis media: Penicillins, cephalosporin, sulfonamides. Otolaryngol. Head Neck. Surg. 89, 376-38o, 1981.

1o. Pfaltz, C.R.: Vestibular complications following middle ear surgery. Proceedings of the International Conference on the Postoperative Evaluation in Middle Ear Surgery held in Antwerp on June 14-16, 1984. Ed: J.F.E. Marquet, pp. 197-2o1.

11. Pfaltz, C.R.: Vertigo, edited in disorders of the neck. In: Vertigo, edited by M.R. Dix and J.D. Hood, J.Wiley, Chichester, 179-197, 1984.

12. Ribári, O., Sziklai I., Kiss, J.G.:Pathohistology of otosclerosis. Proceedings of the International Conference on the Postoperative Evaluation in Middle Ear Surgery held in Antwerp on June 14-16, 1984. Ed: J.F.E. Marquet, pp. 222-228.

IMPEDANCE AUDIOMETRIC FINDINGS IN PATIENTS WITH HEAD TRAUMA

DIETER SCHEIDHAUER, OLAF SCHWETSCHKE
Military-Medical Academy Bad Saarow, ENT-Clinic

INTRODUCTION

Preconditions of complex behaviour patterns are created in the brain stem on the basis of variable integrations of a large number of information.

Regulation of consciousness is one of the most important functions.

Therefore, among other things brain stem reflexes are used for evaluating head traumas and observing their course.

Gradual classifications of reactions controlled by brain stem as pupillary reflexes and state of consciousness are used as parameters in the GLASGOW COMA SCALE (1) to assess the severity of trauma.

The acoustically evoked potentials (AEP), especially brain stem potentials, were also introduced in the diagnostics of head traumas (3).

Some authors, ULLRICH (5) for instance, even considered it possible to make a prognosis on the basis of AEP.

The acoustic reflex (AR) is one of the brain stem reflexes. Its neuro-anatomic relay stations are located in the ventral cochlear nucleus, the superior oliva and the perifacial motor neurons of the stapedius muscle (4).

This is the basis of using impedance audiometry in retrocochlear diagnostics.

A great number of research results proved that the stapedius reflex is altered in the case of infratentorial diseases, tumours and intoxikations (2).

No evidence on the behaviour of the acoustic reflex after trauma was found in the literature.

Therefore, the question arose, whether the acoustic reflex is of diagnostic importance in head traumas.

MATERIAL AND METHODS

Two groups of 15 patients each with slight and severe head trauma were examined.

Head traumas were determined by the GLASGOW COMA SCALE as well as clinical, anamnestic, computertomographic and electroencephalographic findings.

Otoscopy was performed befor each measurement. Examinations were carried out with the impedance audiometer made by Praecitronic Dresden.

A three-channel electrocardiograph was used for registration. Resolution was 50 mm/sec. Static impedance values and the tympanogram were used to ensure equal examination conditions.

The following parameters were evaluated:
-latency
-rise time
-amplitude of the reflex

Results

No differences in acoustic reflex thresholds between the first measurement within 24 hours after trauma and the second one after 72 hours were found in patients with slight head injuries.
There were threshold values between 84 - 89 dB SPL.

A reflex loss was seen in 23 per cent of the cases at the first measurement only at a frequency of 4 KHz.

There was a mean latency of 87 - 200 msec.

No significant differences occurred in this group of patients and in comparison with a group of healthy probands.
The amplitude of the reflex represents an essential characteristic feature of dynamic impedance.

Evident qualitative changes in this parameter occurred between both measuring points.

A sharper increase in amplitude as a function of the tone stimulus was clearly seen 72 hours after the trauma.

The difference between the curves increased with rising intensity of the stimulus and was 20 - 30 acoustic Ohms (fig.1).

A check-up of impedance audiometric findings was performed in 6 patients after 3 - 4 weeks. Values obtained at 72 hours could be confirmed (+/- 9%).
Method-related restrictions had adverse effects on the measurements in patients with severe head injuries, so that patients with ear injuries or muscle relaxation could not be included in the examinations.

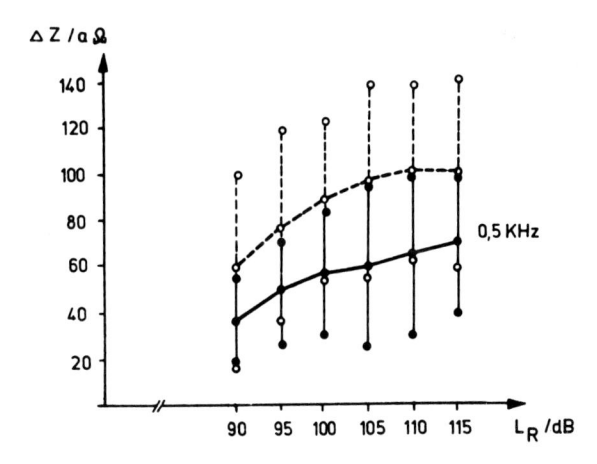

Figure 1:   Mean value and scattering of amplitude of
dynamic impedance (f_M = 220 Hz, L_M = 1.12 Pa)
Parameter: 0.5 kHz
——— measurement about 24 hours after trauma
- - - measurement about 72 hours after trauma

The evaluation revealed two trends:
- Changes in acoustic impedance were detected 24 hours after the trauma only at few frequency and intensity values. A marked decrease in amplitude and a prolongation of latency were recorded. White noise caused most changes in acoustic impedance.
The improvement of patient's general state was attended by a return to normal values of dynamic impedance.
This was seen in 11 casualties, who survived.

- Isolated changes in acoustic impedance were initially observed in 4 patients after acoustic stimulation.
Later there was a complete absence of the reflex. The clinical picture became worse.
Three patients in whom the acoustic reflex could not be elicited died.

DISCUSSION
It can be assumed that the function of the control circuit-cochlea - brain stem - stapedius muscle - is impaired even in cases of slight head traumas.
The decrease in amplitude is the impedance audiometric correlate.

Morphological lesions in severe head injuries probably lead to brain stem dysfunction and cause changes in the reflex behaviour. Results show that brain stem dysfunction due to traumas is also reflected in the behaviour of the acoustic reflex.

In addition to a qualitative assessment of reflex producibility, quantitative parameters can be included in the evaluation.

REFERENCES

1. Jennett B, Bond M (1975) Lancet 1:480-484

2. Jerger S (1980) In: Jerger J, Northern JL (eds) Clinical Impedance Audiometry. Thieme, Stuttgart, pp 128-140

3. Maurer K (1985) Z. EEG-ENG 16:148-154

4. Strutz J (1987) Laryng.Rhinol.Otol. 66:124-126

5. Ullrich A, Graser B, Rieffel M, Stöhr M (1986) Z.EEG-EMG 17:162

BILATERAL HEARING LOSS AND VESTIBULAR LOSS DUE TO A TRIFFLING TRAUMA OF THE HEAD - A CASE DEMONSTRATION

KARIN HAMANN
HNO-Ambulanz, Schillerstraße 28, Schönebeck/Elbe DDR 3300

Traumas may cause different in the inner ear. Certain lesions are accompained by the demage of the vessels of the inner ear. Bleedings may accur in and araound the membranous labyrinth leading to early and later cochlear and vestibular alterations.

I would lake to present two cases of bilateral haering loss and the bilateral failure of the vestibularcochlear organ.

Patient 1

The patient is a man at the age of 50 living in Magdeburg, who had a triffling accident 19 years ago. The accident happened in the following way: He entered his house after jogging wet sportsshoes and slipped there. He felt down without an open head injury. He lost his conscionsness for five minutes. With hearing loss, a strong vertigo, vomiting and nausea he was sent to the ORL-clinic of the Medical Academy Magdeburg.
The first examinations revealed:
- A hearing loss on both sides, in the pure tone audiometry only a feeling curve; a strong vertigo; vomiting and nausea.
- the nystagmus test showed an indicated spontaneous eye movement to the left side.
- The provocation tests with water of $44°C$, $30°C$ and icewater did not influence the nystagmus and did not reserve it. That signified a minimum of restmovement of the labyrinth on the right side.
- the EEG-examinations exhibited no pathological findings.
- by X-raying there was no longitudinal or transverse fracture of the pyramide.

The first therapy was done by giving him antibiotics. At the same time a ganglionblock of the "ganglium stellatum" was carried out 6 times on either side. After this followed a series of 12 slow intravenous injections with "Magnesium compostitum" and glucose of a high percentage. At last wi gave him 1-percentage "Procain" intravensously. Besides vasodilators, multivitamins and nicotinate preparations were adminstered. The whole treatment was without any success.

At the beginning of the 70-ties it was usual practice to inject ATP into the carotice and one year later we tried it - and again without any result.

Finally after all this unsuccessful traetment a testtympanotomy was done. "Intra operationem" we found normal conditions.

This was the last treatment and since than he had never been under treatment. Meanwhile in 1972 the 32 years old teacher had become a pensioner.

Patient 2

Now to the other case. This patient lives in Leipzig, and the accidnet happend in June 1989. The 47 years old man fell in his flat. We think, that this accident happend under the influence of alcohol. 4 days after the accidnet the patient came to the doctor for the first time. The doctor stated a wound at the back of his head, an occipital headache, a bilateral hearing loss vomiting and vertigo, when he moved his head. He was taken to the ORL-clinik of the Karl-Marx-University. On that day they found an "otitis media purulenta" on the right. The further status was regular.

After the statments of the patient and his relatives he has been hard of hearing since 1965 on the right side. The inflammation of the middle ear was cured by antibiotica.

Before the special treatment the following symptoms were found:
- hearing loss on both sides (feeling curve)
- strong vertigo: there was a nystagmus to the right side in the provocationtests. Also with cold water these nystagmus could not be reversed, perhaps a sign of a restmovement of the labyrinth.
- the CT und EEG were without any findings.
- the X-rays didn't show any fracture of the pyramide.

For the special treatment we used vasodilators and multivitamins. In recent years an oxygen inhalation is used to increase the oxygen tension. Our patient was also treated with this method. But we were not successful.

In literature is said that recovery is possible in a period of 3 - 18 months. May be, that our patient has a chance to be cured.

In January this year we repeated the examinations of both patients. Of patient one after 19 years, of patient two after half a year.
There was a coincidance of both examinations:
- the auditory analyses only represens the feeling curve of both cases,
- the vestibular tests didn't show any restmovement of the labyrinths, but without vertigo and nausea.
  The facts showed a certain state of compensation. Only in the darkessour patients feel helpless. The static tests proved that,
- the CT and EEG were without any findings,
- the FAEP couldn't be proved (hearing loss),
- the cochlear mikrophonics didn't show any important findings or results after such a long time.

Let me sum up:
1. It is possible after a trffling trauma without fracture of the skull or intracranial bleedings to suffer from a total hearing- and vestibular loss.
2. The therapy proved to be useless or without any success.
   In literature by several autors is said, that damage of the vessels running to the inner ear, may cause intracapsular or extracapsular haemorrhages of the labyrinth. Lesions may touch either the arteries or the veins and may be affected resulting in microscopic tissue damage. Corticoid administration under antibiotic pretection can decreaus hair cell demage and promote recovery of the inner ear function. But these method of treatment are not yet used in our clinics.

3. Rehabilitation is not granted by the clinics.
   The interactions between the vestibular and the visual and proprioceptive system can support vestibular compensation. But in our clinic were and are not divised physical training programmes. Our patient one carried out such physical training without supervision, and the result is very impressive.
   A hearing aid would be useless for both our patients.

Learning reading off the mouth for people with hearing loss are only offered at evening schools, but not in an short, intensiv course. Patient one, with an IO of 120 had learnt it by himself.
Because of the discribed helplessness in the dark it is very difficult for such persons to find a job. Our patient two as an alcoholic has no chance under such conditions.

4. From time to time doctors have to take a position to such cases, the diagnoses of wich is called: "comotio labyrinthi". We think that such patients should become invalids in a generous way!

DIFFERENTIAL DIAGNOSTICS IN PATIENTS SUFFERING FROM SUDDEN SENSORINEURAL HEARING LOSS

IVAN ŠEJNA

Postgraduate Medical Institute, Prague, Czechoslovakia

SUMMARY

The contribution of the objective testing of hearing for differential diagnostics is very usefull. In sudden hearing loss is evident in high percentage discovery of retrocochlear lesions. This diagnostics can also be used in the beginning phases of illness when accompenied by serious hearing loss. This one was imposseble using a conventional audiometry. No change of cochlear pathology into retrocochlear was established. The important part of this methods in diagnostics of neurinoma was proved. This method can be very usefull into diagnostics hearing losses by different origin.

INTRODUCTION

A sudden sensorineural hearing loss is still, event in the present time, an imprecisely defined nosological-etiological unit. There is still no one single opinion on its cause. Often there is a whole series of internal and external causes. Among these are influences of an infections nature, circulation, metabolic, autoimunity diseases or various influences of the external environment.

Sometimes the cause is not found after a detailed general examination. Where one is not certain of the etiology of the disease it is very difficult to cure it causally.

The determination of the degree of hearing loss can usually be carried out easil by the usual conventional pure ton audiometry or speech audiometry. The situation is different in determining the site of the lesion which caused this hearing diserder. Clarification of this point can also contribute to uncovering the etiology of the disease. Subjective Super-threshold audiometric test are not in cases of haevy hearing loss very useful. I hove tried through the introduction of objective testing methods-Impedance audiometry and Brainstem eletric response audiometry (BERA) into the routine diagnostics process, to the clarification of the following facts :

1. To ascertain the localization of the complaint in the sense of cochlear, retrocochlear or mixed lesions.
2. To compare the results acquired by the method of impedance audiometry with the recording the Brainstem potentials, acoustically evoked.
3. To determinate prognosis according to a certain typ of recording Brainstem

potentials and registrations Stapedials reflexes as one method of impedance audiometry.
4. To study dynamics of hearing changes from the curves of Brainstem responses and the permanency of BERA findings of retrocochlear lesions in connection with the result of treatment.
5. To confirm the usefulness of this objective methods in the diagnostics of acoustic neurinomas, which can also appear in the form of the sudden hearing-loss.

The threshold ton and speech audiometry was carried out on the Pracitronic MA 31 audiometer, impedance audiometry-threshold and decay of stapedial reflex, on the instruments Danplex and Madsen, evoked potentials with BERA SH 221 Hortmann.

MATERIAL AND METHODS

A set of 65 patients with sudden sensorineural unilateral hearing loss was analysed. They examined and treated et the ENT Clinic of the Postgraduate Medical Institute, Teaching Hospital Bulovka Prague, in the years 1985-1988. The set consists of 35 women and 30 men with average age of 48,13 years.

Within the framework of conventional threshold audiometry I evaluated the possible connection between the initial state of hearing after occurance, the type of hearing defect and the result of treatment. This one was the same : Vasoactive drugs and corticoids in infusions. The majority (40) are patients where all frequencies are affected. The extentof the affliction is not, however, signifficant for prognosis. In statistical evaluation only complete deafness appears to be a significant factor testyfying a bad prognosis.

1. The main aim the work was to determine the usefulness BERA for localization of the lesion on the pathway. The results curves of BERA could be divided into three groups. In the first group the curves were normal in the second findings of the cochlear type and in the third group patients with retrocochlear lesion.

Individual types of brainstem responses and their representation in groups according to the result of treatment.are on table 1. :

TABLE 1

RESULTS OF TREATMENT ACCORDING TO TYPE OF BERA MEASUREMENT

Results of treatment	Type of Bera		
	normal	cochlear	retrocochlear
Without improvement (26)	0	13	13
Partial improvement (17)	2	10	5
Normal hearing (22)	7	7	8
Patients (65)	9	30	26

In statistical evaluation it is possible to show only a greater probability of improvement in patients with a normal BERA recording. With the given number of patients it was not, however, possible to show a statistically significant difference betwen the cochlear and retrocochlear type.

2. The comparison of the results evaluation of stapedial reflex with the results of the recordings brainstem potentials are on table 2.

TABLE 2
COMPARISON RESULTS IMPEDANCE AUDIOMETRY WITH RESULTS BERA

Diagnostics	Type of hearing loss	
	cochlear	retrocochlear
Impedance audiometry	50	15
BERA	39	26

The testing of provision with stapedial reflexes point to the provalence of cochlear pathology. 50 of the 65 patients were proveded with reflexes. In 15 patients was absence or decay reflex. The BERA method revealed retrocochlear pathology in a large number-in 26 patients. This method is, then, clearly more sezitive for the diagnostics of retrocochlear pathology. By a combination of both methods of testing it is, however, possible simultaneously to diagnose multiple defects of auditory pathway.

3. The third aim was the determination of a possible prognosis sudden hearing loss. The testing was carried out at the onset of the illness when there were still mainly serious hearing defects and it was not possible to carry out the usual conventional method of examination.

In statistical evaluation, however, there was not ascertained a prognostic diference between cochlear and retrocochlear pathology ascertained by means of brainstem potentials recording.

Prognosis according stapedial reflex evaluation is, however, possible. The probability of improvement in patients with discernable reflex is greater than in those without reflex. ($x2$ test = 12,1). For the determination of prognosis, then, testing with impedance audiometry is of greater significance than with brainstem acoustically evoked potentials.

TABLE 3

PREDICTABILITY THE RESULTS OF TREATMENT (P) ACCORDING TO IMPEDANCE AUDIOMETRY (STAPEDIAL REFLEX)

Results of treatment	Type of hearing loss	
	cochlear	retrocochlear
Without improvement (26)	14	12
Partil improvement (17)	15	2
Normal hearing (22)	21	1
Patients (65)	50	15

4. The fourth part of the work was the concerning of the stability of the brainstem potentials in connection with hearing improvement.

The picture of cochlear lesion according to the BERA test turned out to be a stable finding. In no case was there any change in control tests.

The situation was different in the group of 26 patients who were included among the retrocochlear lesions according to the first test. In 6 cases a change was always the same type of change : the original retrocochlear finding became a cochlear finding. Our opinion : cochlear lesion is stable, confirmation of retrocochlear lesion should be carried out by repeared tests.

5. The last aim of the work was confirmation of the usefulness Brainststem potentials for the diagnosis acoustic neurinomas which may appear at first to be a sudden hearing loss.

In the group of 65 cases this diagnosis was ascertained in two of them. In both testing showed retrocochlear lesion from the start. The suscipion was not, however, confirmed at first by CT examination including meatocisternography. Repeated CT after a period of time showed tumour. The finding was verified by surgery.

REFERENCES

1. Antonelli AR : Audiologic Diagnosis of Central vs. VIII.Nerve and Cochlear Auditory Impairment in Adults and Children, Human Comunnication, Canada, Vol.9, No.5., 1985, 137-143
2. Born JD et al. : Relative prognostic value of best motor response and brainstem reflexis in patients with severe head injury, Neurosurgery, 16/5, 1985, 595-601
3. Claussen CF : Neurootology, Senzory system analyzis by evoked potentials, Medical focus, 2/1986, 2-8
4. Friedrich G : Zur etiologie und Pathogenese des Hörsturzes, Laryngol. Rhinol.Otol., 64/2, 1985, 62-66
5. Lazsig R, Battmer RD, Hesse G : Reliabilityof audiological test methods in retrocochlear diagnosis, Audiology in practice V/2,1988, 6-8
6. Picton TW : Abnormal brainstem auditory evoked potentials. A tentative Classification. Frontiers of Clinical Neuroscience Vol. 3, 1986, 373-378

NEW IMPEDANCE MEASUREMENTS OF THE EAR

PROF. DR. HANS EUBE
7010 Leipzig, Philipp-Rosenthal-Strasse 66

THE PROBLEM

Acoustic immittance instruments and procedures are now commonplace not only in audiology clinics, but in ear-nose-and-throat clinics, public school audiology programmes and other diagnostic facilities.

(The term acoustic immittance refers to either acoustic admittance or acoustic impedance. Acoustic admittance, in turn, is a general term expressing the ease with which sound energy flows through a system and acoustic impedance represents the total opposition to the flow of sound energy. Acoustic admittance and acoustic impedance are reciprocal quantities.
- high acoustic impedance = low acoustic admittance)

MEASUREMENT REQUIREMENTS

All acoustic immitance measurements need a means to:
1. Ensure a hermetic seal of the probe unit in the ear canal.
2. Vary and monitor air pressure in the ear canal.
3. Introduce a probe phone in to the ear canal.
4. Monitor ear canal sound pressure level and
5. Display the results calibrated in acoustic immitance terms.

In contrast to most audiometric techniques, then, acoustic immitance measure are quite valuable in the audiological evaluation of infants, young children, the mentally retarded and other populations for which behavioral audiometry is not always a feasible or a reliable alternative.

MATERIAL AND METHOD

The stimulus was given by a positive and negative electrode (about 10 mm) applied to one external canal by means of the battery operated myostimulator "Jogger" (figure 1).

Stimulation parameters

Fixed parameters	Single pulse duration approx. 7µs (rectangle pulse)	
	Pulse interval approx.	14µs
Variable parameters	Pulse group width	10 - 1000 µs
	Pulse rate	01 - 0100 Hz
	Output voltage	00 - 60 V
	Output peak current	200 mA

The ear sensing element is fitted with electroconductive rubber at its expanding end. The rubber electrodes which are opposite each other are joined to the "jogger" via a cable. The ear sensing element is connected to the impedance meter via tubes in the usual fashion. The electrically induced impedance jumps are demonstrated in the following illustration.

THE AIM OF THE TOPIC

The aims of the present study were to demonstrate an isolated constraction of the stapes muscle. The impendance test battery, and especially acoustic reflex findings, demonstrate greater sensivity to middle ear pathology than traditional audiometric threshold tests.

The stapedius muscle is innervated by the facial nerve (cranial nerve VII), while the tensor tympani muscle is innervated by the trigeminal nerve (cranial nerve V). The neural network of the stapedial (acoustic) reflex is located in the lower brainstem and consists of both ipsilateral and contralateral routes During loud (about 65 - 80 dB) acoustic stimulation, impulses from cochlear sensory cells are transmitted by acoustic nerves to the ipsilateral ventral cochlear nucleus. The majority of axons from the ventral cochlear nucleus pass through the trapezoid body to the medial part of the facial motor nucleus, then down through the facial nerve to the ipsilateral stapedius muscle. Some nerve fibers pass from the ventral cochlear nucleus through the trapezoid body to the ipsilateral medial superior olivary complex. From the ipsilateral medial superior olive nucleus, impulses are transmitted to the medial part of the ipsilateral facial motor nucleus. Thus, the ipsilateral stapedius reflex consists mainly of three, but in some cases four, neurons. The contralateral acoustic reflex arc always contains four neurons. From the acoustic nerve and the ventral cochlear nucleus, impulses are transmitted to the medial superior olive and across to the contralateral facial motor nucleus. The specific site of pathological involvement within the acoustic reflex arc is determined by comparing stapedial reflexes between crossed and uncrossed stimulation.

In the demonstration of the acoustic reflex, the impedance meter measures the sudden change in ear canal sound pressure caused by the decrease in compliance of the middle ear system as the muscle contracts.

RESULTS SO FAR

1. Eustachian Tube Function (figure 2). In the case of a normal middle ear and Eustachian tube, the tympanogram peak will occur near ambient pressure. The normal opening and closing of the Eustachian tube maintains equilibrium between ambient pressure and the pressure in the middle ear space.

2. The acoustic reflex threshold (ART) is the lowest intensity of an acoustic stimulus at which a minimal change in middle ear compliance can be measured.

3. Otosclerosis. Patients with fixed middle ear disorders. such as otosclerosis, have only conductive hearing losses shown by normal tympanogrammes and absent reflexes.

4. Ossicular disruption. In most cases of ossicular disruption the reflexes are absent in all conditions, with the exception of normal reflexes being present with ipsilateral stimulation of the good ear. However, the reflex may be absent with stimulation of the impaired ear (due to the air-bone gap); but intact with the probe in the impaired ear if the discontinuity involes only the crus of the stapes.

5. Eustachian Tube disorder. A deviation from normal functioning and tympanometric peak pressure graeter than - 50 da Pa, low peak amplitude or a flat tympanogram.

6. Adhesion processes. The tympanogram is flat. The gradient, as the pressure interval required for a 50 % decrease in tympanometric peak on either side is greater than 3,4 da Pa.

7. Middle ear effusion. Otitis media with middle ear effusion in whole middle ear space shows positive tympanometric peak pressure.

8. Recruitment-Test for Loudness Recruitment. A positive Metz test result indicates that an acoustic reflex is observed when stimulating an ear at 60 dB or less above the puretone threshold. This is a strong indicator of a cochlear lesion.

9. Retrocochlear pathology. Reflex decay occurs when the amplitude of the acoustic reflex declines by more than half its initial magnitude. Reflex decay is determined by presenting the stimulus test tone at 10 dB above the acoustic reflex HTL for 10 sec at 500 Hz and 1000 Hz.

10. Facial nerve disorder. The acoustic reflex measurement is helpful in determining the site of lesion of the facial nerve disorder as either distal or proximal to the stapedial branch of the seventh nerve.

11. Nonorganic hearing loss. The presence of an acoustic reflex suggests that true hearing loss is no greater than 20 dB less than the reflex HTL.

12. The patulous Eustachian tube. If the passive tubel occlusion is too weak, then the Eustachian tube is open; the tube is patulous.

DISCUSSION

It seems obvious that acoustic reflex measurements provide valuable information concerning the nature of the patient's hearing loss when compared with the contribution of other audiometric techniques. In cases of conductive hearing loss the acoustic reflex has a 50 % chance of being present when the

Impulse structure of the "jogger"

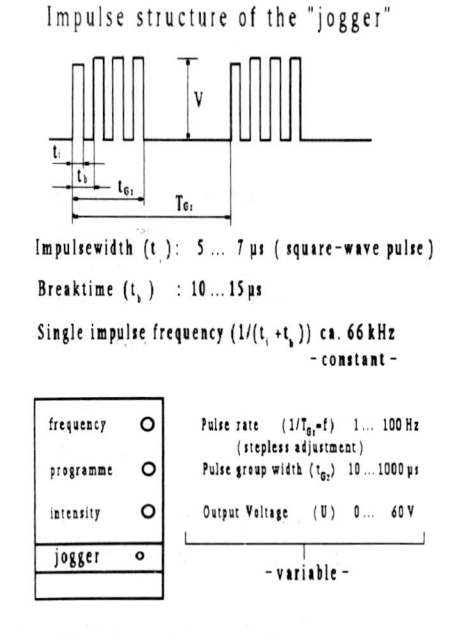

Impulsewidth (t_i): 5 ... 7 µs (square-wave pulse)

Breaktime (t_b): 10 ... 15 µs

Single impulse frequency ($1/(t_i + t_b)$) ca. 66 kHz
- constant -

frequency	○	Pulse rate ($1/T_{G_1}=f$) 1 ... 100 Hz (stepless adjustment)
programme	○	Pulse group width (t_{G_2}) 10 ... 1000 µs
intensity	○	Output Voltage (U) 0 ... 60 V
jogger	○	

- variable -

figure 1: Parameters of the impulse stimulation

Normal middle ear

Compliance

Electromyostimulation

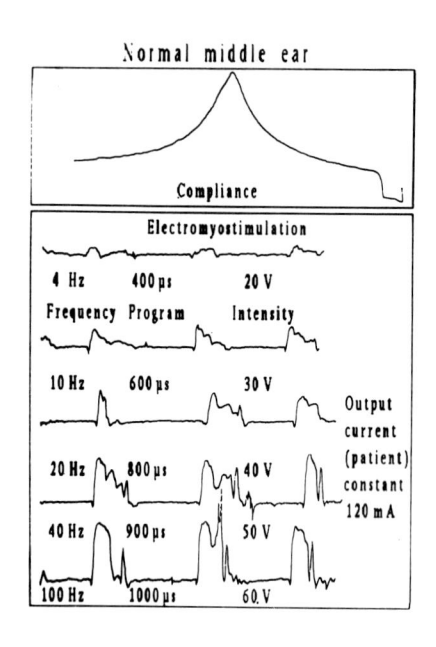

4 Hz	400 µs	20 V
Frequency	Program	Intensity
10 Hz	600 µs	30 V
20 Hz	800 µs	40 V
40 Hz	900 µs	50 V
100 Hz	1000 µs	60 V

Output current (patient) constant 120 mA

figure 2: Impedance measurements with electromyostimulation

probe is in the normal ear with a 27 dB unilateral air-bone gap in the conductive loss ear. With electrical stimulation we know that the stapedius muscle is functioning. In the same way, the important diagnostic patters of the acoustic reflex in sensory-neural differential diagnosis are based on the relationship of the acoustic reflex threshold level to the degree of hearing loss, the time course of the reflex to sustianed signals and the relationship of the ipsilateral to the contralateral reflex. We need analogous information to examine the cochlear pathology, retrocochlear pathology and facial nerve disorders and for further use of the acoustic reflex in hearing screening programmes. In all these cases we cut through the arc reflex pathway at a definable place.

ABR IN HIGH-RISK NEONATES

GÁBOR KATONA, TIBOR TIMÁR, ZSOLT FARKAS
Department of ORL, Heim Pál Hospital for Sick Children,
1089 Budapest, Üllői út 86. (Hungary)

INTRODUCTION

Audiological screening of high-risk newborns is an old problem that has not been solved. The methods that can be used in this group are subjective, not reliable enough and of questionable prognostic value. With the appearance of objective methods, among which ABR, these investigations have gathered more energy. Direct information can be obtained about hearing on the one hand and the functional integrity of the brainstem on the other. The test can be performed several times, is necessary.

MATERIAL AND METHODS

We examined 22 neonates during last year in our department of pedaudiology. The patients were being treated at the department of neonatal pathology of our hospital. Six of them were hospitalized for diseases not compromizing hearing ability, they served as normal controls. The rest of the patients (numbering 16) were categorized as "high-risk" infants, according to the 1982 American Academy of Pediatrics Joint Committee on Infant Hearing Screening Position Statement. All the infants had been born with a gestational age of at least 38 weeks and a birth weight of more than 2500 grams. Hereditary hypacusis did not have to be considered. The main diagnoses can be seen in table 1.

TABLE 1
MAIN DIAGNOSES OF PATIENTS

Hyperbilirubinemia	8
Bacterial meningitis	1
Perinatal cerebral lesion	4
Neonatal hypoxia	2
Neonatal acidosis	1
Bronchopneumonia (controls)	6
Total	22

After obtaining a thorough patient history we performed otoscopy (otomicroscopy) and hearing tests using subjective methods and reflex audiometry. This was followed by ABR, always performed after feeding, without sedation of the newborn.

The patients showing normal curves at the first examination were controlled after 3 to 4 months and declared intact in the case of normal results obtained several times. In the case if the ABR curves were pathological the newborns were followed up and reexamined at the age of 2, 4 and 6 months.

RESULTS

In 10 of the 16 high-risk neonates normal curves were obtained. The data of the other six are shown in Table 2.

TABLE 2

Patients	Diagnosis	ABR changes (1st examination)	Present status
1. T.F.	hyperbilirubinemia	elevated threshold	improvement, observation
2. T.T.	lasio perinat. cer.	elevated threshold increased interpeak latencies (I-V)	after 5 controls good hearing
3. F.M.A.	hyperbilirubinemia	no response	unknown (went abroad)
4. C.B.	neonatal hypoxia	absent waves, elevated threshold	improvement, observation
5. S.A.	hyperbilirubinemia	no response right side elevated threshold left side	observation mild improvement
6. T.R.	hyperbilirubinemia	no response	after 5 controls good hearing

In the case of two patients we could prove the reversibility of the damage caused by a perinatal noxa using multiple examination. None of them had to be supplied with a hearing aid, but we continue the follow-up.

DISCUSSION

The importance of connatal and first of all perinatally acquired hypacusis is great in the quality of life of the patient. The latter is the group in which the lesion can be reversible and the rehabilitation most successful.

Numerous technical problems arise in the examination of newborns. Due to somatic lability general anesthesia cannot be used in this age group. Neonatal ABR curves are different in several aspects to those of adults, and also less consistent. Some peaks (mainly the second and the fourth) are of low amplitude, sometimes even absent. It is difficult to tell an abnormal curve from that of a premature infant with incomplete myelinisation. There is much discussion about the importance of different perinatal factors. Some authors consider hyperbilirubinemia to be crucial, others believe that hypoxia and the perfusion by acidotic blood in the cochleovestibular system is more important. According to the majority of authors perinatal lesions are retrocochlear, mostly localized in the nuclei of the brainstem.

We tried to evade traps by cross-checking and multiple examinations. In two patients we could successfully prove the reversibility of perinatal hearing loss (with both subjective and objective methods), so that rehabilitation can be started early.

REFERENCES
1. American Academy of Pediatrics Joint Committee on Infant Hearing Screening Position Statement 1982. Pediatrics 70:496-497 (1982)
2. Holpern J, Hosford-Dunn H, Malachowski N (1987) Four factors that accurately predict hearing loss in "high-risk" neonates. Ear.Hear. 8:21-25
3. Galambos R, Despland P.A (1980) The auditory brainstem response (ABR) evaluates risk factors for hearing loss in the newborn. Pediat.Res. 14:159-163
4. Perlman M, Feinmesser P, Sohmer H et al (1983) Auditory nerve--brainstem evoked responses in hyperbilirubinemic neonates. Pediatrics 72:658-664

POSTTRAUMATIC AUDIOVESTIBULAR SYMPTOMS IN NEUROOTOLOGY

MIDDLE - AND INNER EAR HEARING DISORDERS DUE TO TRAUMA*

GAVALAS G, VATHILAKIS J, SFETSOS S, PASTIDIS L
Department of Audiology - Neurootology The Red Cross Hospital of Athens (Greece).

INTRODUCTION

In clinical practice, temporal bone fractures are classified in two main groups, the longitudinal and the transverse ones, although in most cases they are expressed in the mixed and not in the pure type.

Longitudinal fractures, which compose 70-80% of all temporal bone fractures, are caused by blows to the temporal - parietal region and are characterized by a fracture line running parallel to the long axis of the petrous bone. The fracture damages the conductive mechanisms of the middle ear and the bone canal of the external meatus.

Transverse fractures are caused by blows to the frontal - or occipital area and are characterized by a fracture line running perpendicular to the long axis of the petrous bone. As the fracture line passes through the labyrinth, it destroys the cochlear and vestibular end organs. Occasionally, it may cross the internal auditory meatus.

MATERIAL AND METHODS

During the last 8 years, 43 patients with hearing disorders due to head injury, have been examined in our department. Twenty five of them were male and 18 female. Their age ranged from 14 to 63 years. The audiological symptoms were hearing loss and/or tinnitus. The majority of them came for an audiological evaluation long after head injury, hospitalization and a detailed examination by other disciplines. Only few of them with mild head trauma and good state of consciousness came for consultation the first posttraumatic days. So, our audiological results are referred more or less to long term posttraumatic findings.

With the exception of 2 patients (4,6%) who suffered a pure transverse fracture and 5 cases without any evidence of a fracture all other cases were of the longitudinal-mixed type.

After a detailed history inquiry and an ENT examination, a complete audiological and vestibular examination was carried out.

AUDIOLOGICAL RESULTS

TABLE I
The time of the first ENT/Audiological examination in relation to the day of the trauma

Posttraumatic day	3-10	11-20	21-30	31-60	> 60
Patients	7	22	7	5	2

TABLE II
The causes of the head injury

Automobile accident	Work acc	Motorcycle acc	Tractor acc	Drop on the ground
18	10	7	5	3

TABLE III
The type of the damage

Transvese fracture	Longitudinal	Mixed	No fracture evidence	Skull fracture
2	35		5	1

TABLE IV
The findings of the otoscopy

Eardrum rupture	Hemotympanum	Deformity of the external auditory wall
17	11	3

TABLE V
The findings of audiometry

Conductive HL	Sensorineural HL			Mixed HL		Bilateral HL		Tinnitus		
18	8			17		4		31		
	Ac trauma	Severe	Sur	Mod	Severe	SN (R) Mixed (L)	Cond Acoustic trauma L	↓ F	↑ F	
4	2	2		15	2	3	1	5	26	

TABLE VI
The findings of tympanometry

Tympanogram	Normal	Type B	Type A_D (Ossicular discontinuity
	4	11	6

Stapedial Reflex	Elicited bilateral	Elicited ipsilateral
	2	12

DISCUSSION

The effect of a head injury on the mechanisms of hearing is very important. The otological findings varies in character and they are depending on the type, severity and direction of the blow to the head. Peripheral hearing disorders are related to the type of the temporal bone fracture. The conductive component of hearing is damaged by longitudinal types and the sensorineural by the transverse ones.

Tympanic membrane rupture, hemotympanum and ossicular chain discontinuity, alone or in combinations, result to conductive diminishing of hearing.

Traumatic injury of the inner ear may be caused by concussion or by a fracture line crossing the cochlea or the internal auditory canal. Nevertheless, the hearing disorder is not always associated with an evident fracture. It can be explained on the basis of concussion causing a microfracture, bleeding in the labyrinth or mechanical laceration of the organ of Corti (5 of our cases).

Although peripheral hearing disorders are dominant in head injuries, studies of Dieroff, Lehnhardt and Howe have shown that the central auditory pathway (lemniscus lateralis, colliculus inferior) can also be damaged. Especially damage of the brain stem area was demonstrated with the histopathologic work of Makishima and Snow and the registration of the acoustically evoked potentials by Howe and Miller.

Concerning our audiological findings, we must point out that they are related to the time of the patient's examination, which was performed in most of the cases in a late posttraumatic period. So, there is the possibility that some of them could have other audiometric findings during the first posttraumatic days. It is known that despite the sudden destruction of the conductive mechanism, a number of them recover spontaneously sometimes without functional defects (f.e. Restoration of previous incudostapedial joint separation). On the other hand, a progressive posttraumatic hearing deterioration, which happened in one patient with moderate sensorineural hearing loss 2 months after the injury, is also possible.

Perilymphatic fistel which was found in 2 cases and was manifested with fluctuating hearing and persistent vertigo, could be cured by surgical procedure.

A large number of our cases showed sensorineural hearing loss. The acceleration and the sudden deceleration which develops during the accident, leads to a violent displacement of the basic cochlear membrane damaging the organ of corti or the released mechanical energy creates microbleedings in the inner ear (Goodhill, 1979).

The cases with acoustic trauma can be explained by vibratory energy of high intensity which was transmitted to the inner ear and created damage of the high frequencies (Schuknecht, 1969).

We also consider the possibility that some cases of sensorineural hearing loss were resulted by an acute happening, because of the fear and stress the injury causes to the patient.

Two cases with total deafness were resulted by a transverse fracture whose line crossed the internal auditory meatus.

Tympanograms were indicative for middle ear fluid (11 cases) and ossicular chain disruption (6 cases). Four of them were normal and 5 others showed a slight anomaly of the curves.

Stapedial reflex was not elicited in some cases in which it should be present. It is perhaps explained by a loosening of the conductive mechanism of ear, a brain stem disfunction or an inhibitory action on the reticular formation of drugs patients received.

We didn't find any patient with known pretraumatic hearing disorder. Most patients were followed up for more than one year.

Patients with ossicular chain disruption were operated on. Three patients developed a labyrinthine hydrops 7-14 months after the injury.

We must point out that some patients simulate or aggravate posttraumatic hearing loss and/or vertigo or they try to present an old eardrum perforation as a new one in order to get financial profits. The detailed anamnestic injury, the repeated audiological examination using the special available tests and the collaboration with the other disciplines will establish the accurate diagnosis in order to avoid any medicolegal problem.

SUMMARY

Today a number some of hearing disorders result from head injuries. The damage of the auditory function can be (or not) connected with an obvious fracture of the petrous bone. Longitudinal fractures are the commonest and are usually caused by blows to the temporal - parietal area. They result more often in damage of the conductive mechanism in the middle ear. Transverse fractures are usually caused by blows to the frontal or occipital area. The fracture line is usually extended transversely across the petrous bone, occasionally though the internal auditory meatus and the labyrinthine capsule. It is damaging to the vestibular and cochlear system. In this paper, we present the obtained audiological findings of the patients with hearing disorders due to head injuries, who were examined in our department in the last eight years. Furthermore, we describe the clinical symptomatology and we discuss the mechanisms in regard to the posttraumatic hearing damage.

REFERENCES

1. **Dieroff HG**: Zentrale Horschaden bei frontobasalen Bruchen. Laryng. Rhinol. 54, 734-740, 1975.

2. **Goodhill V**: Sudden hearing loss syndrome. In: Doodhill, V (ed) Ear diseases deafness and dizziness, Harper and Row, Hagerstown, 1979.

3. **Howe JF and Miller CC**: Midbrain deafness following head injury. Neurology, 25: 286-289, 1975.

4. **Lehnhardt E**: Audiological characteristics of central deafness following head injuries. Vortrag auf dem XII. Congress of Audiology, Paris, 1974.

5. **Makishima K and Snow JB Jr**: Effects of hesd blow on the development of hearing loss. Laryngoscope, 86 (7): 971-978, 1976.

6. **Munker G**: Progrediente Innenohrschwerhorigkeit nach Schadeltrauma. Z. Laryng. Rhinol. 51, 506, 1972.

7. **Schuknecht HF**: Mechanism of inner ear injury from blows to the head. Ann. Otol. 78: 253-262, 1969.

DIAGNOSIS OF CENTRAL VESTIBULAR LESIONS AFTER HEAD INJURY

SÁNDOR SPELLENBERG and JUDITH LÁNG

János Hospital H N O Clinic Audiol. and Otoneurol. Department, Diósárok str. 1, 1125 Budapest, Hungary

INTRODUCTION

The majority of patients suffering from post-traumatic vertigo suffer from the "post concussion" syndrome. Some of these symptoms are undoubtedly due to psychological changes - the so-called "post concussion neurosis". When the patient is being examined for medico-legal purposes it can be difficult to judge which symptoms are caused by the accident and which symptoms are exaggerated by the patient to enhance his claims. Therefore it is necessary to perform a full neuro-otological examination.

MATERIAL AND METHODS

Patients complaining of vertigo due to brain-stem dysfunction after head injury rarely have any localizing neurological signs. Our patients (n=37) age from 18 to 67 years - 16 males, 21 females.

Spontaneous nystagmus (n=35). The commonest ENG findings in our cases were bilateral gaze nystagmus in the horizontal axis. The nystagmus was unaffected or even reduced by eye closure. Vertical nystagmus was strongly suggestive of a central disorder. So the down beating nystagmus, especially on lateral gaze, suggest a lesion of the lower brain-stem or cervico-medullary region. Lesion of the anterior vermis of the cerebellum are said to cause a large amplitude up beating nystagmus in the primary position, which is increased by upward gaze. The nystagmus decreases rapidly after a few seconds, both in velocity and frequency: although a few beats of increased amplitude may persist.

Derangements of optokinetic nystagmus (34 out of 37 cases!). In our cases a marked optokinetic asymmetry indicated the CNS lesion, apparent on ENG recordings if the slow phase velocity of the nystagmus in each direction differs by more than 30 degrees/second. Disorganized and disconjugated optokinetic responses are also suggestive of brain-stem post traumatic syndrome.

Derangements of smooth ocular pursuit (n=20). These are common in brain-stem concussion. The disorganized and disconjugated ocular pursuit may indicate brain-stem disease and shows that the patient has replaced smooth eye movements with a series of saccades.

Ocular dysmetria (n=26). These occur when the eye movement overshoots (hypermetric saccades) or undershoots (hypometric saccades) the target, also rapid, saccadic eye movement.

Positional nystagmus (n=29): Central disorders cause nystagmus, which is not associated with vertigo, and does not fatigue. In our cases the positional and positioning nystagmus was direction changing, present in both head down and head up positions, and were greater than 7 degrees per second on slow phase velocity. Therefore it could be accepted as due to central dysfunction caused by head injury.

The caloric test may reveal a directional preponderance and/or unilateral or bilateral weakness.

CONCLUSIONS

Trauma may cause vertigo due to injury to the peripheral labyrinth or due to disturbance of the central vestibular mechanisms. Unfortunately the prognosis is poor. 56% of minor and 68% of moderate head injury patients had persistent postural vertigo 5 years after the original injury. Only 12% of the patients were able to return to their pre-accident or equivalent work, and 43% never returned to any occupation. When clinical investigations reveal definite signs of a central vestibular derangement - following head injury - the prognosis should be guarded. Even when no vestibular abnormality can be demonstrated, it cannot be assumed that the patient's symptoms are non-organic, as a central disorder cannot be completely excluded using the presently available test battery.

REFERENCES

1. Barber, HO: Positional nystagmus, especially after head injury. Laryngoscope (1964) 74:891-944
2. Berman, JM and Fredrickson, JM: Vertigo after head injury - a five year follow-up. J. Otolaryngol. (1978) 7:237-244

3. Darroff, RB: Ocular oscillations. Ann. Otol. Rhinol. Laryngol. (1977) 86:102-107

4. Dix, MR and Hallpike, CS: The pathology, symptomatology and diagnosis of certain common disorders of the vestibular system. Ann. Otolaryngol. (1952) 61:987-1016

5. Harrison, MS: Notes on the clinical features and pathology of post concussional vertigo with special reference to positional nystagmus. Brain (1956) 79:474-482

6. Harrison, MS and Ozsaginoglu, C: Positional vertigo. Arch. Otolaryngol. (1975) 101:675-678

7. Láng, J: L'evocation du nystagmus optocinétique a l'aide d'un nouvel appareil et l'importance diagnostique de la méthode. Acta Oto-Laryngologica, Belgica. (1962) 16:5

8. Preber, L and Silferskiold, BP: Paroxysmal positional vertigo following head injury. Acta Otolaryngol. (1957) 48:255-265

9. Schuknecht, HF and Davidson, RC: Deafness and vertigo from head injury. Arch. Otolaryngol. (1956) 63:513-528

10. Toglia, SV: Acute flexion-extension injury of the neck: electronystagmo- graphic study of 309 patients. Neurology (1976) 26:808-814

11. Tuohimaa, P: Vestibular disturbances after mild head injury. Acta Otolaryngol. Suppl. (1978) 359:1-59

12. Walker, AE: Mechanisms of cerebral trauma and the impairment of consciousness. In: Neurological Surgery. Youmans, J. (Ed.), Vol. II (1973) 936-942. W.B. Saunders, Philadelphia.

TINNITUS AND HEARING REDUCTION AS A RESULT OF ACOUSTIC TRAUMA IN THE FEDERAL GERMAN ARMED FORCES

M. PILGRAMM

ENT Department, Federal Armed Forces Hospital, Detmold, Heldmannstr., 4930 Detmold, (Chief Physician: H.P.Weibel)

Acute acoustic trauma with its consequences of hearing reduction and tinnitus represents a problem in all armies that hold shooting practice. In the Federal Republic of Germany we find ourselves not infrequently confronted with this clinical picture,too. We thus conducted a study from 1979 to 1987 with 1182 patients to give more evidence concerning the epedemiology, the diagnosis, the therapy, the prophylaxis as well as the post-traumatic development.

1) EPIDEMIOLOGY

1a) Frequency

As no nation-wide statistics are kept as yet, the frequency of acoustic trauma within the Federal German Armed Forces can only be extrapolated from the regional statistics that are available. It is assumed that 30 to 50 acoustic traumas occur every working day. Of those patients who suffer acute damage, only about half report for medical diagnosis. The prime reason for this failure to report to unit medical officers is, firstly, the frequent lack of information provided to the young soldier and, secondly, the expectation of a spontanous recovery, which does indeed occur in some 50% of cases. As we can assume the additional complete spontaneous recovery of 50% of the rest, there are approximately ten acoustic traumas that require treatment in the Federal German Armed Forces every working day.

1b) Cause

As far as the cause of the acoustic trauma is concerned, the statistics all tally, with the G3 rifle ranking first with about 70%. The reason for that percentage may be that every soldier is trained to use that weapon and it often has to be fired whilst the soldier is moving. This, in turn, brings great problems when it comes to ear protection. Other weapons play a subordinate role.

2) DIAGNOSIS

2a) Typical audiogramm

The patient who has suffered the first acute acoustic trauma shows a damage in the high tone between 3 and 8 kHz, with a principal drop at 6 kHz. 500 patients who have suffered acute acoustic trauma and who showed no tendency towards spontanous recovery had the following average value:

2 kHz	−	5 dB	+	4 dB		6 kHz	−	56 dB	+	13 dB
3 kHz	−	24 dB	+	9 dB		8 kHz	−	46 dB	+	11 dB
4 kHz	−	44 dB	+	17 dB						

2b) Tinnitus

2% (10) of the patients we had evaluated (s.2a) did not show any tinnitus, 24% (120) showed tinnitus on the right ear, 49% (245) had tinnitus on the left ear and 25% (125) tinnitus on both ears. 98% (480) of the patients reported tinnitus in the 4 to 6 kHz range at 5 to 10 dB above the threshold.

2c) Relation

The results of 2b show that the left ear (49%) is most frequently affected. This is due to the fact that a large number of patients are right-handed, and hence during shotting the left ear is less well protected by the upper arm, the shoulder and the butt than the right ear.

3) STUDIES

Since unit medical officers in the Federal Republic of Germany are generally very young colleagues, many of whom have no experience, we attempted to develop a therapeutic scheme that can be applied rapidly and simply, and without any danger. An important point for us was to exclude patients from the studies who tended to spontanous recovery.

3a) Study exclusion criteria

Only patients who had suffered acoustic trauma within the previous 48 hours were included in the study. A hearing loss of 40 dB had to be attained at an individual frequency. Twenty-four hours following admission and without therapy, there still had to be a hearing loss of 40 dB and no hearing gain in excess of 20 dB at any individual frequency. It had to be the first time damage had been suffered and the middle ear system (with regard to the explosion trauma) was not to be involved.

3b) Methods

We conducted ten studies on 500 patients who suffered acute acoustic trauma. Nine studies were double blind, number ten (HBO-study) was a controlled randomised study. As a general principle, the reference substance was low-molecular dextran.

The following methods of therapy were tested:
NaCl, low-molecular dextran, low-molecular hydroxyethyl starch, Betahistin, Naphtidrofurylhydrgenoxalate, Vinpocetin, Pentoxifyllin, Fluranicin, Benzyclan, RNA, Hyperbaric oxygen (HBO).
Those vaso-active or metabolically-active substances were, as placebo or verum, added to the infusion therapy.
We measured the hearing gain after ten days, the period as an in-patient, and after 42 days, the end of the study.

3c) <u>Statistically significant results</u>

Due to the limited range of this article, we cannot present the detailed results here. They can be given on request.
If the main study results are assessed in statistical terms, four statistically significant results were obtained:
In terms of hearing gain and elemination of tinnitus, low-molecular dextran is superior to NaCl. Low-molecular dextran in conjunction with hyperbaric oxygen is superior to low-molecular dextran in isolation. There is no significant difference between low-molecular dextran and low-molecular hydroxyethyl starch. Vaso-active or metabolically active substances do not produce any significant difference when applied as an adjunctive therapy as compared with the hemodilutoric monotherapy.

4) SPONTANOUS RECOVERY

On the basis of the strict study exclusion criteria (s.3a) a tendency towards spontanous recovery was seen at 48% of the cases (568/1182).

5) PROPHYLAXIS

In the struggle against the acute acoustic trauma, a sufficient prophylaxis, which is offered by ear protection and in the form of information is as important as successful therapy.

5a) <u>Information</u>

Surveys of our patients have shown that only 48% (270/565) had been informed about acoustic trauma prior to their first shooting practice.
A survey conducted amongst young unit medical officers in the Federal Armed Forces Sanitary Academy shows that only 8% of the young unit medical officers questioned had been informed of the possibility of damage due to impulsive noise during their university education. This can be explained by the fact that acute acoustic trauma is not a clinical picture encountered by the university but a con-

dition met primarily in military medicine.

5b) Ear protection

If a study is conducted of the wearing of ear protection then it is seen, surprisingly, that 62% of the soldiers who suffered damage were not wearing ear protection. The ear protection in question was generally the familiar "Comfit" ear protection or the "Selektone" system.

If this surprising phenomenon is studied in great detail, it has to be ascertained that, in a large number of cases, the ear protection had fallen out during shooting practice, particularly during movement exercises and during shooting practice using guns. This happened in 57% of cases with "Selektone" ear protection and in 66% of cases with "Comfit" ear protection. If this result is taken into account, then it shows that more than 68% of cases were using ear protection after all.

6) THE POST-TRAUMATIC DEVELOPMENT

Since we in the Federal Republic of Germany are an army of conscripts and military service generally ends after 15 months, it was important for us to know whether there is any progression of the damage after an acoustic trauma has been suffered. We thus called in 60 soldiers one year after they had suffered acoustic trauma and received therapy in order to conduct a renewed diagnosis.

6a) Hearing

If the patient is excused from shooting and blasting for less than 12 months, after one year, the rate of improvement is equal to the rate of deterioration in audition (22%/22%). If, however, the patient is excused from any further shooting or blasting, and is also not given noisy work to do, then a statistically significant difference is seen between improvement and deterioration after one year (41%/22%).

6b) Tinnitus

If the patient is not exposed to shooting or deployed on noisy work for a lengthy period after suffering acoustic trauma, the tinnitus problem will have subsided by almost 20% after one year and, in the reverse case, increased by more than 20%.

7) SUMMARY OF THE RESULTS

The results of the treatment of 1182 patients who had suffered acute acoustic trauma at the Federal German Armed Forces Hospital in Ulm from 1979 to 1987 can be summed up as follows:

- The information supplied to the soldiers and the unit medical officers about traumatic damage to the inner ear needs to be improved within the Federal German Armed Forces.
- The ear protection "Selektone" and "Comfit" at shooting practice with the rifle is insufficient. That's why in the Federal German Armed Forces a new ear protection (EAR) has been introduced some months ago.
- The spontanous recovery rate for acute acoustic trauma is approximately 50%.
- The therapy of choice is low-molecular infusion solutions (Dextran or HAES), if possible in conjunction with hyperbaric oxygenation.
- There can, however, also be a deterioration in hearing over a period of a year following the acoustic damage, which would seem to be independent of the type of occupation taken up by the patient following the acute phase.
- Progessive deterioration of hearing cannot be predicted on the basis of the finding of acute damage.

References at the author.

**POSTTRAUMATIC VASCULAR PROBLEMS
WITH RESPECT TO NEUROOTOLOGY**

VESTIBULO-MOTOR REACTIONS DURING THE FREE FALL AND IN THE LANDING PHASE OF NORMAL AND PERINATALLY HYPOXIC RABBITS

THOMAS SCHWARTZE, HELMUT TEGETMEYER, HANNELORE SCHWARTZE
Institute of Pathological Physiology, Faculty of Medicine, Karl Marx University, 7010 Leipzig (G.D.R.)

SUMMARY

During sudden free falls and after landing the EMG activities were recorded from fully conscious rabbits using chronic electrodes implanted in limb flexor and extensor muscles (triceps brachii, brachialis, quadriceps femoris). The experiments were performed between the 8th and the 20th postnatal day (PD) in normal animals and in rabbits surviving a single severe hypoxia (5% inspiratory oxygen content over 3 hours) at the 1st PD. Using optimum combinations of various EMG parameters a significant discrimination between hypoxic rabbits and normal controls was possible at the 8th and the 20th PD, but not at the 14th PD.

INTRODUCTION

Perinatal complications accompanied by hypoxia may cause motor disorders [1] as well as behavioural disorders [2] and deficits of intellectual capacities [3] during the further postnatal development.

The neurons of the brain stem regions including the neurons of the vestibular nuclei are already high differentiated at the time of birth [4]. Therefore, these neurons are also especially susceptible to damages caused by oxygen deficit. The investigation and quantification of motor reactions to vestibular stimulation seem thus to offer suitable methods for the early diagnosis of the consequences caused by a perinatal hypoxia/asphyxia [5].

MATERIAL AND METHODS

Simultaneous recordings of the multiunit electromyographic (EMG) activity of the M. triceps brachii caput lateralis (MTB), the M. brachialis (MB), and the M. quadriceps femoris caput lateralis (MQF) were obtained from a total of 24 hare-coloured German giant rabbits between the 8th and the 20th postnatal day (PD). 12 of these rabbits (hypoxic rabbits, HR) were exposed to a normobaric hypoxic atmosphere with an oxygen content of 5% for 3 hours at the 1st PD [6]. The other unexposed 12 rabbits from the same litters were used as paired controls (control rabbits, CR). The EMG recordings were performed with pairs of fine wire electrodes chronically implanted at the 7th and the 14th PD, respectively.

The vestibulo-motor reactions were investigated in intervals of 3 days from the 8th PD to the 20th PD. The stimulation program consisted of 20 subsequent sudden free falls with covered eyes from a height of 50cm on a soft cushion. The EMG signals of the three muscles were simultaneously registrated during the free fall and during the landing period, stored on FM magnetic tape and afterwards high-pass filtered (100Hz/-3dB), full wave rectified, and electronically integrated with a time constant of 2.5ms. The resulting traces of integrated EMG activity were written down by a pen recorder (0-140Hz, 240mm/s) and analysed by hand at equidistant time intervals (Fig. 1).

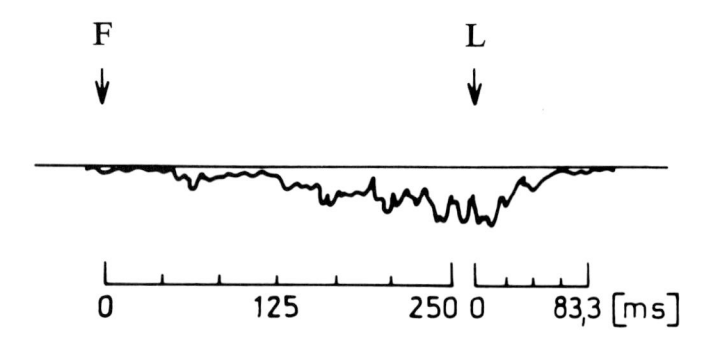

Fig. 1. Example (MTB, 14th PD, HR) of the course of integrated EMG activity (upper trace, arbitrary units) and the time scannig for activity measurements (below). The arrows indicate the begin of the free fall (F) and the begin (contact of the forepaw with the ground) of the landing reaction (L), respectively.

RESULTS

Until the 14th PD the EMG activity of the investigated muscles showed an irregularly fluctuating course during the free fall. This predominant phasic character of the muscle reactions and their great interindividual variability made it not possible to verify statistical significant differences of the EMG activity course from the mean activity level. However, at the 17th and the 20th PD the EMG activity increased significantly in all muscles during the fall up till the contact with the floor.

Though the EMG reactions of HR and CR were qualitatively similar, some of the EMG parameters differed significantly between the two rabbit groups. In the CR, but not in the HR, the proportion between the EMG activity during the fall and of the EMG activity during the landing reaction increased significantly in the MTB and the MB between the 8th and the 20th PD. Contrary to the HR, the CR were able to raise the fall activity of their MB during the subsequent 20 fall stimulations at the 20th PD.

A linear discriminant analysis (7) was performed in order to determine the EMG parameters suited to discriminate between the HR-group and the CR-group. The following nine parameters M were used for the analysis: Normalized EMG activity of the MTB (M1), the MB (M4), and the MQF (M7) 83ms after the start of the free fall. EMG activity during the first 10 fall reactions in proportion to the EMG activity during all 20 fall reactions of the MTB (M2) and the MB (M5). EMG activity during the free fall in proportion to the EMG activity during the landing reaction of the MTB (M3) and the MB (M6). Mean median values of the duration of the landing reaction in the MB (M8). Body mass (M9).

A significant discrimination between the CR and the HR was possible at the 8th and the 20th PD, but not at the 14th PD. Fig. 2 shows the optimum parameter combinations and the standardized discriminant values (ws) of the discriminant analysis for the 8th and 20th PD. It has to be emphasized that the discriminating parameters changed during this postnatal period.

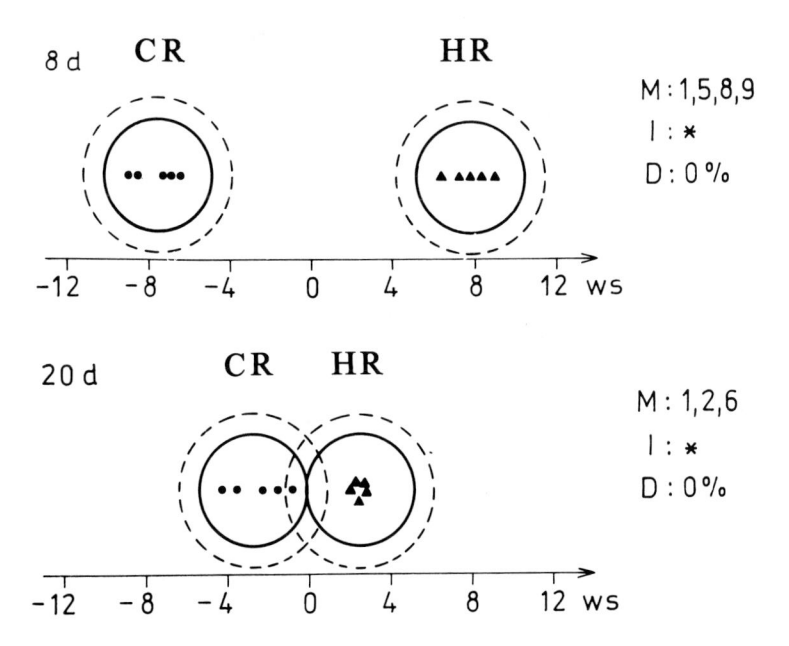

Fig. 2. Results of the linear discriminant analysis at the 8th PD (above) and the 20th PD (below) in form of standardized unidimensional discriminant values (ws) of the HR (triangles) and the CR (points). M: single parameters used for discrimination (see text). I: significance of group discrimination (*: p<0.05). D: discrimination error estimated by the cyclic exchange procedure. circles: variance ranges of 95% (continuous line) and 99% (interrupted line), respectively.

DISCUSSION

The differences in the EMG parameters observed at the 8th PD between CR and HR indicate that the single exposition to hypoxia applied at the 1st PD resulted in long lasting functional changes (8) or even in necrosis (9) of brain stem neurons responsible for the elicitation of vestibulo-motor reactions (10). During the further postnatal development up to the 20th PD the neuronal disturbances in the HR effect the formation of such EMG activity patterns which appear as a functional compensation of the initial hypoxic changes at the 8th PD mentioned above. However, these EMG activity patterns at the 20th PD are different from the reactions of the CR in their parameter structure and, contrary to the CR, the HR are not able to vary these activity patterns considerably with increasing number of subsequent free fall stimulations.

Further investigations are needed in order to show whether these experimental findings are suitable as a basis for clinical function diagnosis in human infants. However, in search of consequences caused by perinatal hypoxia, special attention should be paid to the analysis of movement structure and the EMG activity pattern of vestibulo-motor reactions as well as to the ability to adaptive changes and variations of these reactions (11) in the course of consecutive stimulations.

REFERENCES

1. Lou HC (1982) Developmental Neurology. Raven Press, New York
2. Gillberg IC, Gillberg C (1983) Dev Med Child Neurol 25:438-449
3. Paneth N, Stark RI (1983) Am J Obstet Gynecol 147:960-966
4. Jacobson M (1985) Annu Rev Neurosci 8:71-102
5. Vojta V (1984) Die zerebralen Bewegungsstörungen im Säuglingsalter. 4.Aufl. F Enke Verlag, Stuttgart
6. Schönfelder J, Tegetmeyer H, Woldag K, Woldag H (1989) Biomed Biochim Acta 48:S217-S220
7. Ahrens H, Läuter J (1981) Mehrdimensionale Varianzanalyse. 2.Aufl. Akademie-Verlag, Berlin
8. Dwyer BE, Nishimura RN, Powell CL, Mailheau SL (1987) Exp Neurol 95:277-289
9. Myers RE, Wagner KR, De Courten-Myers GM (1983) In: Mylunsky A, Friedman EA, Gluck L (eds) Advances in Perinatal Medicine. Vol. 3. Plenum Medical Book Co, New York
10. Wilson VJ, Peterson BW (1981) In: Brooks VB (ed) Handbook of Physiology. The Nervous System. Vol.2. Williams and Wilkins, Baltimore, pp 667-702
11. Touwen BCL (1978) In: Clinics in Developmental Medicine No. 67. William Heinemann, London

AUDIO-VESTIBULAR DISTURBANCES DUE TO ACUTE AND CHRONIC TRAUMAS OF THE CAROTID AND VERTEBRAL ARTERIES

HARALAN HARALANOV, PETER SHOTEKOV, LYUBOMIR HARALANOV
Institute of Neurology, Psychiatry and Neurosurgery, Medical Academy, Sofia, Bulgaria

INTRODUCTION

In literature there is very scanty information about purposive and comprehensive investigation of the auditory and vestibular systems when there is an insufficiency of blood supply in the region of the carotid and vertebral arteries in cases of acute and chronic traumas of the head and neck.

MATERIAL AND METHODS

The present study describes the results from the investigation of 75 cases of trauma and extravessel compression of the magistral cerebral arteries, selected from 690 patients with pathological angiographic results in the same arteries.

Complex clinical, sonographic, angiographic, otoneurological and electrophysiological investigations (EEG, ENG, BAEP, AEP, VEP) were carried out.

RESULTS

It is established that the carotid arteries can be compressed along their whole length: from their exit from the aortic arch to the intracranial part.

Compression and trauma of the common carotid artery are found in the following: malignant tumours in the mediastinum and in the lung apex, accessory cervical rib, fracture of the clavicular bone, struma maligna or strumectomy, covered or open traumas in the neck region, periarteritis after deep Röentgen therapy of the throat and other tumours, Behterev's disease, etc., Schaumann disease/lymphogranulomatosis.

Compression and trauma of the internal carotid artery in the neck region were established in the following cases: covered or open traumas of the neck, tumours in the epipharynx and larynx, periarteritis and enlarged lymph nodes, as well as lymph cancer metastases, gunshot damages through the mouth, compressions caused by exostosis of the hyoid bone, damages in cases of tonsilectomy or peritonsillar abscess, trauma of the artery in children having swallowed blunt voluminous objects, traumatic damage and thrombosis of the artery in cases of attempts for strangulation.

A case of interest is a 6-year-old child with needle damages through the mouth - traumatic thrombosis of the internal carotid artery. Another case, when a horizontally stretched cable stroke while travelling through an open railroad platform, caused a traumatic stenosis and an aneurysm of the artery.

It is rare that a compression of the internal carotid artery in the carotid canal is found. This part of the artery has its significance for the otorhinolaryngologists, because here the artery is right next to the internal ear. In this part part the artery can be damaged by: exostosis of the carotid canal, compression after fracture of the temporal bone, after head trauma, etc.

A few cases of compression of the internal carotid artery in the carotid canal after periarteritis after chronic otitis and fracture of the cranial basis, when the process has reached the more distal parts of the artery, are worth noting. The angiographic results in two of these patients are similar to those after hypoplasia of the internal carotid artery.

Compression and trauma of the internal carotid artery in the cavernosis were present in the following cases: periarteritis after sinuitis, damages through the eye-socket caused by sharp long objects, compression caused by tumours and cysts in the paracellar region, basilar meningeomes, damages after surgical treatment of Gasseri ganglioma, etc.

We observed a unique case of thrombosis of the internal carotid artery after trauma in the sinocavernous region after enucleation of the eyeball, caused by strong air and water flows. Retrogradically the thrombosis reaches the part of the neck of the internal carotid artery.

In its first and primary part the vertebral artery is most often compressed by the anterior scalenus muscle, as well as after fracture of the clavicular bone.

In its second part (the vertebral canal) the artery can be compressed in the following cases: osteochondrosis, trauma of the cervical vertebra, malformations, luxation and tumours of the vertebrae, etc.

We observed 4 cases of traumatic lesion of the cervical vertebra after car accidents, when there was a compression of the two vertebral arteries and the spinal artery by the 'drawer' mechanism. In such cases the lesion of the cervical part of the spinal cord is acquired. With two patients there was an improvement in the clinical status after a long treatment.

In a number of cases we established a bilateral compression of the two vertebral arteries at many levels after severe cervical osteochondrosis, which sharply decreases the lumen of the vessel. In some cases the compression of the vertebral arteries, caused by cervical osteochondrosis is combined with primary thrombosis of the carotid arteries.

The 3rd part of the vertebral arteries, which includes the curve round the atlas to its entrance in the posterior fossa is compressed in the following cases malformations of the atlas, platybasia, craniocervical malformations, contractions of the small muscles, situated over the atlas, etc. In four of the patients it resulted in transitory disorders of the vertebro-basilar blood circulation after fracture of the epistropheus on sudden falling in an iced-over place.

In the pathogenesis of the insultus, besides the decrease or the complete obturation of the lumen of the arteries, an immense part is played by the vessel spasm, which is caused by the compression of their neuro-vegetative fibers.

In cases of compression and traumatic damages of the carotid arteries, especially on the right side, disorders in the spatial hearing are observed: the patients localise hearing irritation applying in the left part of the hearing zone on their right side (acoustic alloesthesia) or the otolocalisation is strongly distressed; in cases of simultaneous hearing irritation from the left and the right hearing zones, the patients ignore the one coming from the left one. Observed are also difficulties in rhythm apprehension with the left ear and changes in the speech audiogram of the left ear.

The damages in the binaural hearing are accompanied by other disturbances in the spatial perceptions for the left part of the body and the surrounding space. We also observed a peculiar type of spatial acalculia in arithmetics of multinominal numbers in a vertical order. In more than 80% of the patients having compression of the vertebral arteries we observed transitory audio-vestibular disturbances, which are usually provoked by a twist of the head or hypertension of the neck, as well as by a sudden movement from a lying position or being long in a standing position. The otoneurological investigation shows very often labyrinthine lesion - complete or partial Meniere's disease. Two patients with a compression of the vertebral arteries, caused by neck osteochondrosis, showed Lermoyez' syndrome, which often changes with Meniere's syndrome. In one of these cases also brainstem symptoms from the region of the inferior anterior cerebellar artery were established. We found out that in this case, when the compression of the vertebral artery by osteophyte, at a certain position of the head is followed by a decrease in hearing and and noise in the ear. An improvement in hearing is acquired a few minutes after straightening the head and freeing the artery, which is accompanied by strong vertigo. It is evident that in this case the improved blood circulation of the labyrinth after the compression release of the artery leads to a vertigo and a consequent improvement in hearing.

In some cases the compression of the vertebral arteries causes focal ischemia in the brainstem. Most frequently the ischemic foci are in the region of the inferior posterior cerebellar artery (Vallenberg's syndrome) and rarely it is so in the region of the inferior anterior cerebellar artery.

In these cases it is useful to investigate the auditory brainstem evoked potentials. They are normal in cases of Vallenberg's syndrome, while in cases of Foville's syndrome they are changed.

BARO-TRAUMA OF THE INNER EAR AND ITS DETERMINATION WITH

NEUROOTOLOGICAL TESTS

GOTTFRIED AUST
Beratungsstelle für Hörbehinderte
Paster-Behrens-Straße 81, D 1000 Berlin 47 (West Germany)

INTRODUCTION

Diving has markedly increased during the last 45 years. While diving men come into contact with an environment unlike his normal living conditions. Therefore special requirements of the body and psychic functions of the organism arise. As a consequence borderline medical problems develop, which extend over different branches of medicine.

Besides barotrauma frequently caused by diving we know from occupational medicine of lesions in the middle and the inner ear in caisson-workers. Decompression sickness is one of the frequent problems in these patients.
Air-embolism leads to disturbances of the blood circulation in the brain stem and in the inner ear followed by ischemia and functional lesions.

Problems in the inner ear due to pressure changes are known in pilots. Furthermore it is also known that cochlear and vestibular dysfunctions arise after mild physical stress, e.g. gymnastics, forced blowing of the nose, or during child birth.
Head trauma with damage to the bony structures of the inner ear lead via fractures or fissures expose the middle and the inner ear or the spaces of the cerebrospinal fluids to the harmful substances in the environment.

Ventilation disturbances of the nasal sinuses and of the middle ear spaces play an important role in the ENT region. As a consequence of these ventilation disorders we can observe pressure peaks in the middle ear, which can be followed by ruptures of the tympanic membrane. The sudden pressure peaks - positive or negative - can also expand into the inner ear resulting in cochlear and vestibular sensory damage. Another mechanism is the development of a fistula between the middle and the inner ear. The leakage between these spaces is followed by injuries of the sensory epithelia of the inner ear.

Congenital malformations of the middle ear can also be the cause of abnormal communication between inner and middle ear and in these cases the sensory epithelia of the inner ear are highly sensitive to pressure changes. Mild distorsion of the inner ear might be expressed by alternobaric vertigo, repeated high pressure increase lead to inner ear lesion.

The influx of cold water into the middle ear spaces, caused by a tympanic membrane rupture, results initially in a caloric reaction with vertigo and nystagmus. Occasionally otitis externa or media can be a complication. In cases of a fistula the infection can reach the inner ear and cause labyrinthitis.

CLASSIFICATION OF BAROTRAUMA (after Molvaer & Natrud)

Barotrauma of the ear canal
        barotrauma meatus acusticus externus
        barotitis externa
        ear canal squeeze
Barotrauma of the middle ear
        barotrauma auris media
        barotitis media
        middle ear squeeze
Inner ear barotrauma with membrane rupture and/or bleeding
        barotrauma auris internae
Inner ear barotrauma with perilymph fistula
        fistula perilymphatica barotraumatica
Decompression sickness
Gas embolism
Counter diffusion

SYMPTOMATOLOGY OF BAROTRAUMA

The subjective symptoms of inner ear lesion are: hearing loss, tinnitus, instability during standing and walking, vertigo, and nausea. The symptoms become acute, in most cases during the pressure change. In other cases one can observe a prolonged

development of symptoms. We explain this by the altered barrier-
conditions between the middle and the inner ear, possibly following an infection with consequent labyrinthitis.

MIDDLE EAR FINDINGS

Barotrauma with perforation of the tympanic membrane is
diagnosed by otoscopy, possibly also by microscopy. Tympanometry
is important in many cases. Tympanoscopy is necessary in a few
cases to clarify the middle ear situation.

NEUROOTOLOGIC TEST RESULTS

Cochlear findings

Changes in the cochlear and vestibular functions can be
determined using neurootologic tests. Audiometric results show
in cases of isolated cochlear damage constant or fluctuating
hearing loss of pancochlear or apicocochlear type. In cases of
ruptures of the tympanic membrane and of bleeding or effusion
into the middle ear spaces additional conductional hearing loss
can be verified. In a few cases suprathreshold audiometry or
acousticly evoked potentials point to findings of retrocochlear
lesions.

Tinnitus is a frequent concomitant of barotrauma, its determination, however, is difficult or even impossible.

Vestibular findings

Frequent accompanying findings are spontaneous, position and
positioning nystagmus, although they are non defining symptoms.
The caloric reactions on the lesioned side can show inhibition or
total functional loss, in some cases directional preponderance
can be found.

All of these findings are typical but not characteristic and
do not lead to the diagnosis of barotrauma. In cases of perilymph
fistula and of alternobaric vertigo without fistula, however,
sometimes none of the above-mentioned findings appear.

In some cases the fistula test with application of positive
or negative pressure to the external ear canal confirm the presence of a fistula, in a few cases the Hennebert-sign is positive. Vertigo and nystagmus are discret signs during fistula test

using Frenzel glasses. Ear drum movements during controlled pressure changes can be observed with the help of the Siegle-lens, eye movements, however, can not be seen by the examiner simultaneously. Electronystagmography in combination with pressure application using the Politzer-balloon provides more information, the electronystagmographic traces, however, are superimposed on artifacts in many cases. These artifacts are caused by the patients' discomfort due to pressure to the external ear canal and vertigo or nausea.

Tympanometry in combination with recording of eye movements in the electronystagmogram and/or recording of the body sway by posturography is one of the best devices for the determination of a perilymph fistula. Controlled positive and negative pressure during a defined time can be applied by the tympanometric pump, recording of the pressure protocol is possible for documentation.

TREATMENT

The treatment of barotrauma - medication or operative - depends on the diagnosis. Conservatory means are bedrest with head elevation, avoiding straining (Valsalva maneuver) and violent blowing of the nose, and controlled sedation. Preventive antibiotic treatment might be indicated in cases of ear drum perforation with otitis of the external or the middle ear to avoid labyrinthitis or meningitis.
Exploratory tympanotomy in experienced hands is indicated, if 48 hours after conservative treatment no improvement of the hearing can be seen.

CONCLUSIONS

According to statistics, decompression sickness is not the main cause of fatal diving accidents. Exhaustion, embolism, and panic are the causes of death during diving in 76%, followed by accidents with excessive pulmonary pressure and by cardiac failure.

Barotrauma is a characteristic and frequent but not fatal accident in diving. The diagnosis of barotrauma is clear in cases of known history and typical findings. Difficulties arise under unclear conditions, and in these patients further diagnostic procedures, e.g. X-ray, CT-scan, and tympanotomy are necessary.

Prevention and specific training are of great importance. Divers, caisson-workers, pilots, and other involved in professions which entail pressure changes must be trained to detect the signs and symptoms of barotrauma. Early treatment is necessary to avoid deterioration and further inner ear damage. The knowledge of possible changes in hearing ability and equilibrium help the patient to react adequately and not to panic. These people should also be regularly examined by specially trained physicians.

REFERENCES

1. Bhansali SA (1989) Ear, Nose and Throat J. 68:11-28
2. Black FO, Lilly DJ, Nashner LM (1987) Otol. Head Neck Surg. 96 (2):125-134
3. Coles RRA (1976) Audiology 15:273-278
4. Ehm OF, Gerstenbrand F, Strutz I (eds) (1989) Tauglichkeitsuntersuchungen bei Sporttauchern. Springer-Verlag Berlin, Heidelberg
5. Ingelstedt S, Ivarsson A, Tjernström Ö (1974) Acta oto-laryng.(Stockh.) 78:1-14
6. Katsarkis A, Baxter JD (1976) J.Otolaryng. 5:24-32
7. Lang J, Rozsahegyi I, Tarnoczy T (1971) Mschr. Ohrenheilk. 105:9-12
8. Lansberg MP (1973) ORL (Basel) 35:184-188
9. Molvaer OI, Natrud E (1979) Acta Otolaryngol. Suppl. 360, 187-189
10. Tjernström Ö (1974) Acta oto-laryng. (Stockh.) 78:376-384
11. Moser M, Wolf G (1981) Laryng.Rhinol.Otol. 60:381-382

VERTIGO AND TINNITUS IN TRAUMATIC CERVICAL VASCULAR LESIONS

DECKER, I., OMLOR, A., SCHIMRIGK, K., HUBER, G., JÄGER, H.
Institut of neurology and Institut of neuroradiology, 6650 Homburg

We want to present you 3 cases of traumatic carotid dissection, which were diagnosed in our hospital in the years 1988-89:

Pat. no 1 was a 39-year-old woman. During an influenza she got fit of coughing and suddenly she felt a pulsating tinnitus in her right ear. She also compained of hedache floating from the occiput to the forehead and of vertignious attacks. 3 years ago the patient had a motoring accident with a whiplash injury of the cervical spine and a concursion of the brain. During the initial physical examination one could auscultate a pulsating sound over the right mastoid, the patient also had a gait deviation to the right side. The doppler sonography showed a constriction of the right internal carotid artery from the bifurcation to the angle of mandible, the quantity of internal blood flow, however, measured by MAVIS, was normal.

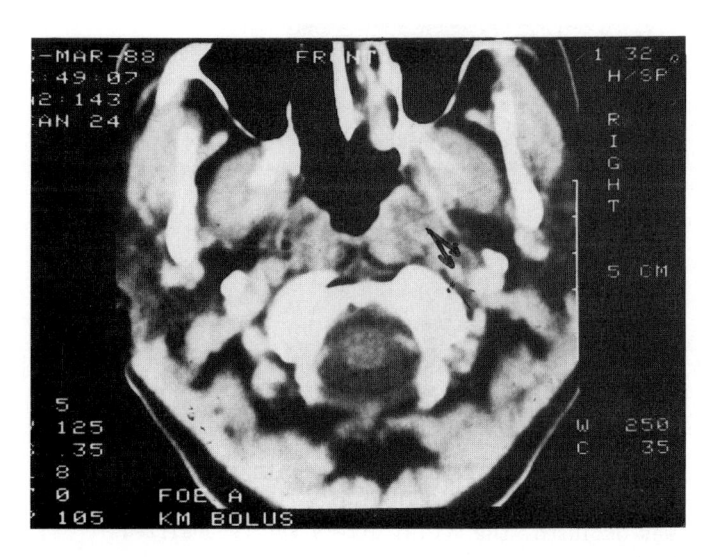

Fig. 1   Bolus-CT with the sickle shaped dissection of the internal carotid artery.

The brain CT was normal. The angiography showed an irregular constriction of the internal carotid artery from the bifurcation to the base of the skull.
Then we performed a CT of the upper neck with a bolus injection of contrast medium in mod-fast-technic. We could see the reduced lume of the right internal carotid artery with a sickle-shaped dissection (central and medial). The treatment was a follows: full-dose-heparinisation, then low-dose-heparinisation and the dissection becomes smaller.

The Pat. no 2 was a 22-year-old man who came to our hospital with a hemiplegia of the right side, a total aphasia and a Horner's Syndrome at the left side. 9 months before, the patient had a motoring accident with a whiplash injury of the cervical spine.
The initial CT was without pathological findings, the second CT two days later showed the big media-infarction on the left side. The extracranial doppler sonography was normal. The angiography showed an aneurysm of about 1,5 cm of the internal carotid artery in the middle between the bifurcation and the sinusoidal section.

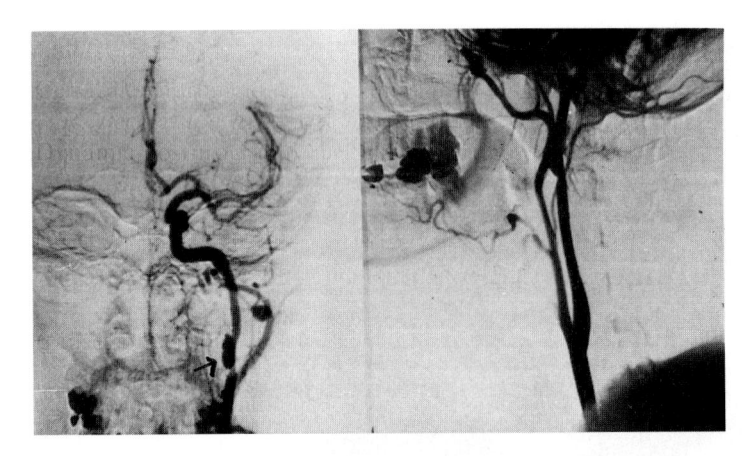

Fig. 2   Angiography of the right internal carotid artery with the aneurysm.

The left vertebral artery was occlused, the medial artery was recanalized. The therapy was as follows: rheological infusions, then low-dose-heparinisation. Full-dose-heparinisation was not possible because of the bleeding risk in the infarction. Moreover, the left internal carotid artery was occluded by the neurosurgery to provide further embolies.

Pat. no 3 was a 63-year-old woman who had a motoring accident with contusion
of the thorax and the neck, mainly in the region of the girdle. The patient
complained of hedache and pain of the neck. During the following day the
patient became more and more somnolent and got a hemiplegia of the left
side.
The initial CT was still without pathological findings, the following CT,
however, showed an infarction on the right side. The angiography showed an
incomplete occlusion of the right internal carotid artery. One could see the
typical moniliform vessel. A part of the middle cerebral artery was occluded.
The bolus-CT could not be performed because the patient was too restless.
But in the magnetic resonance tomography the partial thrombosis of the right
internal carotid artery could be seen above the bifurcation. The therapy
was rheological infusions and then low-dose-heparinisation.

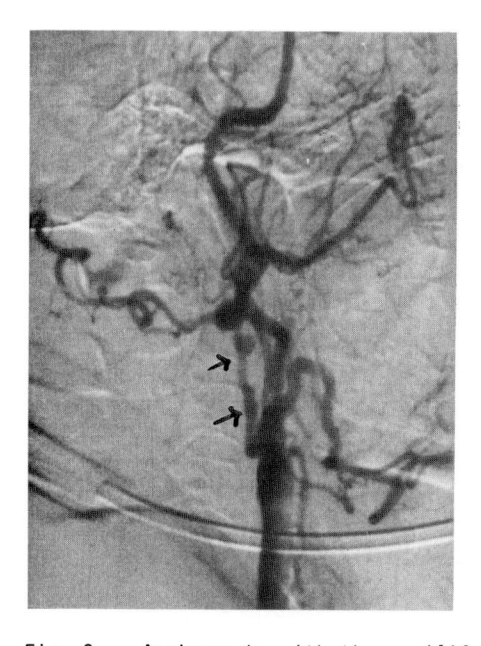

Fig. 3.   Angiography with the moniliform internal carotid artery.

The 3 patients described in the preceeding lines had a traumatic dissection
of the internal carotid artery. This disease does not occur very often.
But when studying the literature of the last few years we found out that it
is more frequent than generally assumed:

Bogousslavsky from Lausanne, for instance, found a dissection - but not only traumatically caused - of the internal carotid artery in 2,5 % of 1200 consecutive patients with a first stroke examined over a period of six years, which means 30 patients.
In 1983 Hart and Miller declared, that 5 % of all ischemic infarctions of younger adults are caused by dissection.
Most articles, however, were case reports of a few patients with this disease.

Etiology besides traumatic lesions:
- fibromuscular dysplasia
- atherosclerosis
- Marfan-Syndrom with cystic necrosis of the middle cerebral artery (mesenchymal disturbance with hyperplasia of the cartilage zone of growth)
- Ehlers-Danlos-Syndrom (in the cavernosus region)
- Moya-Moya

The pathogenetic mechanism is a follows:
As the result of chaps of the intima of the artery false aneurysms begin to develop. The other way are hemorrhages of the vasa vasonum. In this case there is no connection between the lumen of the vessel and the lumen of the dissection. In the other case there is a connection between the true and the false lumen.
Cerebral insufficient circulation - in most cases an infarction - can be caused ischemically by reduction of the blood flow through the constricted vessel. It can also be caused embolically by the thrombosed blood of the false lumen.

The symptoms leading to the diagnosis carotid dissection

1) sudden, quick increasing pain of face or head (90 %)
2) delayed symptoms of the correspondent hemisphere which are caused by a global ischemia (70 %)
3) partial Horner's Syndrome on the ipsilateral side (50 - 60 %)
4) ipsilateral pulsating tinnitus (40 %) with detached objective arterial murmur (30 %)
5) pain of the neck (20 %)
6) syncopes (10 %)
7) dysfunction of the lower cranial nerves (10 %)
8) amaurosis fugax (6 %)

The diagnosis can be made sure by doppler-sonography, angiography, CT of the neck with bolus CM or MRT. The prognosis is much better if the diagnosis is recognized during slight symptoms like tinnitus or Horner's Syndrom and if the treatment is started immediatly. The prognosis is worse if there is already an cerebral infarction. The treatment is a conservative one with full-heparinisation. If that is not possible because of contraindications one should apply rheological infusions, low-dose-heparinisation and then long time treatment with cumarin or acetylsalicylacid as long as neccessary. The control can be doppler sonography or, if neccessary, angiography.

REFERENCES

1. Andersen CA, Collins GJ, Rich NM, McDonald PT (1980) The american surgeon 263-265
2. Bogousslavsky J, Despland PA, Regli F (1987) Arch Neurol 44:137-140
3. Bradac GB, Kaernbach A, Bolk-Weischedel D, Finck GA (1981) Neuroradiology 21:149-154
4. Gee W, Kaupp HA, McDonald KM, Lin FZ, Curry LJ (1980) Arch Surg 115:944-949
5. Hart RG, Miller VT (1983) Stroke 14:110-114
6. Marx A, Messing B, Storch B, Busse O (1987) 58:8-18
7. Stillhard G, Waespe W, Germann D (1988) 118:1933-1940

CLINICAL AND INSTRUMENTED INVESTIGATIONS INTO VERTEBROBASILAR INSUFFICIENCY

B. FISCHER and H. VON SPECHT

Klinik für HNO-Krankheiten, Medizinische Akademie Magdeburg,
Leipziger Str. 44, DDR-3090 Magdeburg,

In his daily routine practice, the E.N.T. specialist is increasingly confronted with the clinical picture of vertebrobasilar insufficiency (VBI). This phenomenon is due to a relative increase in high-risk factors (luxuries, diabetes), mechanical traumatic causes (traffic accidents or other injuries, e.g. fractures of the cervical spine), vascular processes, etc.

This is why our branch has experienced a growing demand for making a differential diagnosis or giving a specialist opinion (e.g. in the field of diagnosing somebody an invalid; physical fitness for a particular job or for driving).

The vast clinical picture and the great variety of symptoms are due to the fact that 10 out of 12 cerebral nerves, all ascending and descending pathways, hearing and vestibular organ as well as parts of the cerebral cortex supplied by the vertebrobasilar system are subject to recurrent, transient local inadequate circulation.

A definite diagnosis of vertebrobasilar insufficiency is often difficult and can frequently be made after long-term observation only, since the present state of the art in diagnosing cerebral circulatory disturbances is limited.

Therefore, a total of 20 patients with clinically apparent VBI were examined at the E.N.T. Clinic and the Clinic for Neurology, both affiliated to the Magdeburg Medical Academy. In the case material studied, women in the age group from 46 to 65 years were prevailing, a finding consistent with data reported in the literature. Sixty-five percent of the patients complained of paroxysmal headache commencing in the occipital region in 62% of the cases. In addition to exhibiting a large number of neurological symptoms, 70% of the patients suffered from attacks of rotary vertigo. X-ray pictures of the cervical vertebral column revealed pathological changes in 55% of the patients.

When examined under the Frenzel glass, 20% of the case material showed horizontal spontaneous nystagmus.

Further meaningful evidence was obtained after thermal labyrinth stimulation by quantitative vestibular fine diagnosis using the 4-channel-PENG method according to Gestewitz and computer-aided analysis of the nystagmus parameters known at present.

At the beginning, 30% of the patients showed a small nystagmogram (petite écriture) in which the amplitude appeared to be approx. 30% lower and the total number of beats 30% higher (Fig. 1).

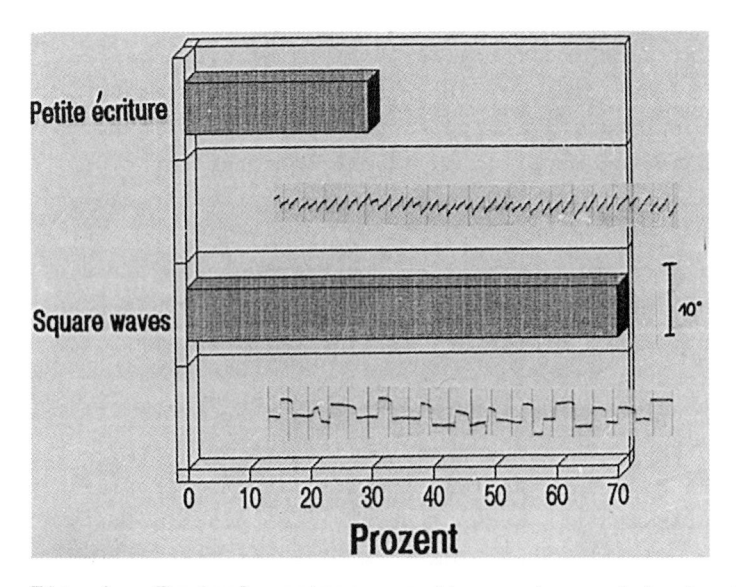

Fig. 1. Typical nystagmus patterns in vertebrobasilar insufficiency.

Excluding fixation in the dark, especially obvious and considered insignificant in former times are spontaneous eye movements, the so-called square waves [2,3]. These findings strongly correlate with the clinical picture of vertebrobasilar insufficiency as also proven by Gestewitz [4].

In 40% of the cases, evaluation of auditory evoked potentials revealed suspicious shape variations of waves III and V drifting widely with regard to their configuration (Fig. 2). Statistical evaluation made on the basis of histograms of the I-V interval showed a clear tendency of expansion without, however, exceeding the 4.6 ms limit which would be considered as a disturbance of generation fast auditory evoked potentials (FAEP) in the brain stem (brain stem weakness; see [2]).

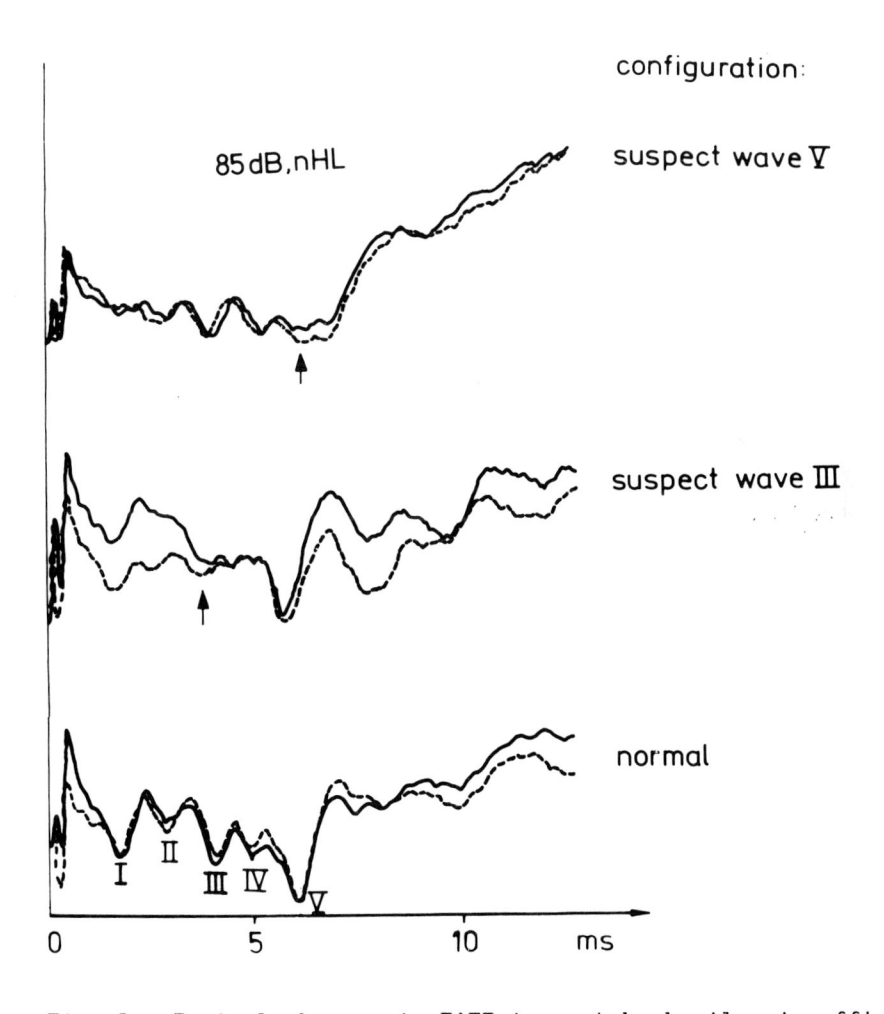

Fig. 2. Typical changes in FAEP in vertebrobasilar insufficiency.

After provoking the circulatory condition in the vertebrobasilar region by changing the head position (R.H. and L.H. positions and reclination of the head), many of the cases exhibited changes in wave III, altered interpeak latencies, and myogen components, and the entire curve pattern was not reproducible [5].

The electroencephalograms showed unspecific abnormal findings in 50% of the patients examined; these did not correlate with brainstem circulatory disturbances.

Different in 40% of the cases, the regional cerebral brain perfusion provided additional information to facilitate overall evaluation.

Cerebral computed tomography revealed a typical cerebral atrophy with hydrocephalus internus in 40% of our patients. Because of the limited resolving power, brainstem infarction was demonstrated in as little as 10% of the cases.

To summarize, the results of the present investigation showed that vestibular-acoustic functional disturbances were proved in one third of the patients with vertebrobasilar insufficiency. The otoneurological findings were found to yield useful diagnostic information facilitating evaluation of the course of cerebrovascular diseases.

REFERENCES

1. Fischer B, Freitag M (1990) Die vertebrobasiläre Insuffizienz – Diagnostik in der HNO. Paper presented at 14th National Congress of E.N.T. Society of the G.D.R. (Magdeburg, March 1990)
2. Claussen CF (1981) Schwindel. Leitfaden für Klinik und Praxis. edition m + p, Dr. Werner Rudat Co., Hamburg.
3. Gestewitz HR (1974) Z Wiss u Fortschr 24:416-421
4. Gestewitz HR (1988) Der Einsatz der PENG-Methode in der Oto-Neuro-Ophthalmologischen Diagnostik unter besonderer Berücksichtigung des Hirnstamm-Schwindels. Paper presented at the Symposium of the Oto-Neuro-Ophthalmologic Section (Budapest, April 1988)
5. Stoye U (1990) Frühe akustisch evozierte Potentiale und klinische Befunde bei Patienten mit vertebrobasilärer Insuffizienz. Dissertation A, Medizinische Akademie Magdeburg

VERTIGO AND NAUSEA IN PATIENTS WITH DIABETIC AUTONOMIC NEUROPATHY

W.BOSSNEV, M. DASKALOV, N.NIKOLOVA, S. GHIKOVA, ZL. STOYNEVA
Medical Academy - Sofia

INTRODUCTION

The most frequent etiology of polyneuropathy is diabetes mellitus. More realistic is the assumption that almost 20-50% of the patients with diabetes mellitus have polyneuropathy (2). The autonomic structures are frequently injured in diabetic neuropathy (3). The symptoms of the autonomic neuropathy are closely connnected with the tonus of the sympathetic adrenal and parasympathetic structures (especially the affection of n.vagus). The role of acute and chronic hypoxy should be underlined when speaking of the pathogenesis of cerebral disorders in patients with diabetes mellitus and hypoglycaemy (4).

The relationship between vestibular crisis and diabetes mellitus is not cleared in all aspects. The purpose of this study is the investigation of neuro- otologic syndromes in patients with diabetic autonomic neuropathy.

CLINICAL CONTINGENT AND METHODS OF INVESTIGATION

Fifty one patients (16 men and 35 women) with diabetic autonomic neuropathy and clinically confirmed neuro- otologic syndromes have been investigated. The age of the patients is between 20 and 69 years. According to the type of the diabetes they are distributed as follows: I type (insulin independent diabetes) - 18 patients (35%), II type (insulin independent diabetes) - 5 patients (10%), III type (insulin-exausted reserve) - 28 patients (55%). Most are the patients with duration of diabetic illness to 10 years.

A wide diagnostic complex of contemporary uninvasive methods are used including a directed anamnesis neurologic status, neuro-otologic investigation, frontal-mastoid and bimastoid rheoencephallography, biomicroscopy of the capillaries of eponichium, thermistor thermography, Doppler sonography of a. digitalis palmares propriae, and a. dorsales pedis and a. tibiales post.

RESULTS AND DISCUSSION

In all investigated patients with diabetes mellitus have been diagnosed diabetic autonomic neuropathy together with central, peripheral or combined neuroautologic syndromes. The neuro-otologic syndromes have been with a duration of 5 years. The distribution of vertigo and nausea is almost equal (table 1) and the central otoneurologic syndrome prevails (table 2). The patients are mainly with a bad metabolic compensation - 36 patients and 25 patients have an insulin need mainly from 40 to 80 units.

TABLE 1
VERTIGO AND NAUSEA IN PATIENTS WITH DIABETIC AUTONOMIC POLYNEUROPATHY

Sex	Vertigo	Vomiting	All
Men	10	6	16
Women	16	19	35
All	26	25	51

TABLE 2
NEUROAUTOLOGIC SYNDROMES

Sex	Central	Peripheral	Combined	All
Men	14	1	1	16
Women	23	6	6	35
All	37	7	7	51

TABLE 3
BAD METABOLIC COMPENSATION AND NEURO-OTOLOGIC SYNDROMES

Sex	Central	Peripheral	Combined	All
Men	8	1	1	10
Women	17	5	4	26
All	25	6	5	36

In all investigated patients with diabetes mellitus and vertigo an increased vascular resistence and decreased pulse blood filling are registered by means of bimastoid rheoencephalography. In some of the patients a moderate to greatly increased vascular restistence in the region of carotid arteries at fronto-mastoid rheoencephalography has been registered, Doppler sonography of the distal arteries of the four limbs shows in 13 patients greatly expressed circulatory disorders (fig. 1,2).

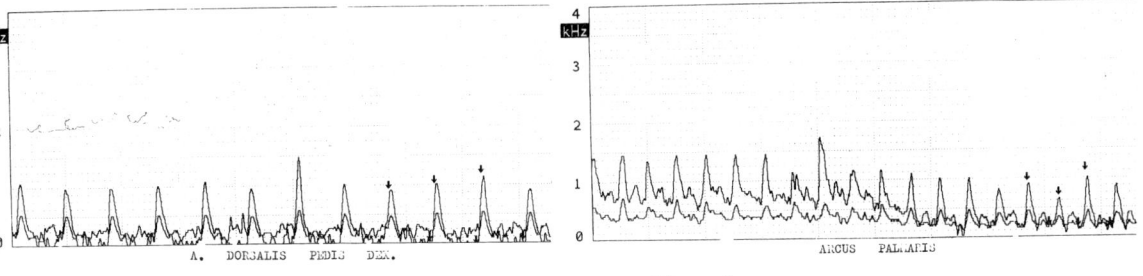

Fig.1

Fig. 2

Spastic capillaries and a palid phone of the microscopic field have been seen biomicroscopically in all investigated patients with autonomic diabetic neuropathy. The relative part of the patients with expressed distal hypothermy (20 patients to 25-23°C) predominates when measuring the superficial skin temperature of the limbs.

The presented results confirm the frequent development of neuro-otologic syndromes in patients with diabetes mellitus and diabetic autonomic neuropathy. The results of Doppler sonography, rheography and biomicroscopy of the capillaries of the hands prove micro- and macroangiopathy in a great part of the patients. They play an essential role in the etiopathogenesis of diabetic autonomic neuropathy and in the origin of the neuro-otologic syndromes. In this group of patients manifestations of greatly increased vascular resistance in the region of vertebro-basilar system have been established. The pathology of sympathetic vasomotor innervation plays an important role in the development of transit disorders of the brain blood circulation, based on the mechanism of circulatory insufficiency.

REFERENCES

1. Bossnev W., Daskalov M, Nikolova N (1990) Zirkulatorische Störungen bei der peripheren diabetischen Angioneuropathie. Ärztezeitschr. f.Naturheilverf. 31:22-27.
2. Brown M, Asbury A (1984) Diabetic Neuropathy. Ann.Neurol. 15: 2-12.

3. Krönert K. (1984) Die diabetische Neuropathie des autonomen Nervensystems aus internistischer Sicht. Internist. 25:607-612

4. Prichoschan V (1981) Porajenie nervnoi sistemi pri saharnom diabete. Moskva, Medizina.

DOPPLER SONOGRAPHICAL FUNCTIONAL TESTS AND OTONEUROLOGICAL
INVESTIGATIONS IN PATIENTS WITH CEREBRAL TRAUMA

PENKO SHOTEKOV, VANJA RAICHEVA*, GEORGI POPTODOROV, JULIA PETROVA,
NEVENA POPOVA
Department of Neurology, Medical Academy, 1431 Sofia,(Bulgaria)
United Research Institute of Aviation Medicine, 1431 Sofia*

It is known, that the traumatic lesions within the central nervous system produce various disturbances in vessel reactivity, which can be related with the mechanisms of postraumatic cerebrasthenic syndromes. The unstability of the cerebrovascular reactivity following traumatic injuries of the nervous system is in the basis of some neuroothological syndromes. Kuhl et al.(1980).

The introducing of the transcranial Doppler sonography by Aaslid et al.(1982) gave an opportunity for a noninvasive monitoring of the blood flow velocity (BFV) and application of tests for an evaluation of the cerebrovascular reactivity (CVR). Recently CO_2-test is the most popular one. It shows the dynamics of BFV in responce to the change of CO_2-blood contents. Markwalder et al.(1984), Widder (1985), Ringelstein et al.(1986, 1988). The parallel investigation of BFV changes in applying the CO_2-test as well as in the regional cerebral blood flow by Xenon-133 have shown correlations between the two parameters. Ringelstein et al.(1986), Bishop et al. (1986). The application of CO_2-test is connected with the use of an equipment for quantitative inhalation and transcutaneus analyser of CO_2-level in blood that can be provided only in specialised laboratories.

Therefore, we have introduce on simple and usefull complex of methods for vegetative exploration and medicamentouse testing of CVR, carried out on healthy persons in various age.

We have aimed in this report to investigate the pecualiarities of the CVR in persons, underwent cranio-cerebral traumas with consecutive cerebrasthenic and neurootological complications.

MATERIAL AND METHODS

Altogether 12 persons, who underwent brain commotional syndrome after cranio-cerebral injury were investigated - 8 men and 4 women. Their mean age was 37 $\pm$ 15 years. All the patients have suffering from expressed postcommotional syndrome and neurootological complains: dizziness, transient vertigo attacks(without dirrectional preponderance), sometimes nausea or vomiting, unstable gait, headache, fatigue ets.

The patients were investigated by means of routine neurootological tests. For evaluation of the CVR a complex of tests are used.

All the patients were investigated with extra and transcranial Doppler sonography to exclude a pathology in the cerebral arteries. The transcranial Doppler sonograph type "EME" TC-2 64 was used for the evaluation of the CVR. The patients were adapted to the conditions of the laboratory in lying position for 15 min. The middle cerebral artery was monitorized by means of a transtemporal approach in deabth of 50-55 mm. The spectral analysis of the BFV was registered on an "Epson" printer.

The following vegetological and medicamentous tests were performed:

1. Hyperventilation lasting for 3 min within evaluation of the restoration time;
2. Walsalva test;
3. Orthostatic test - the person was set upright following a 20 minute stay in a supine position. The changes of the BFV were evaluated for a period of 5 min and after that its restoration in a supine position was followed up;
4. Nitroglycerin test - sublingual admission of the drug (0,5mg) and successive registration of the BFV at 3-ed and the 5-th minute.

The normal changes of the BFV were investigated with 70 clinically healthy persons aged 10 to 80 years, aged averagely 44,9 years. They were subdivided into 7 age groups by step of 10 years.

RESULTS

Significant decrease of the systolic, diastolic and mean velocity of the blood flow velocity was established during the test with each control cases investigated (Fig. 1).

In all 12 patients with postcommotional syndrome a significant decrease (P/t/ <0,001) of BFV was established, valid for all tests used. However for the orthostatic test a markedly expressed reduction of the BFV can be observed (Table I).

No significant age-depending difference of the percentage velocity changes was established in the control groups investigated except in the group aged over 60 years for the hyperventilation test.

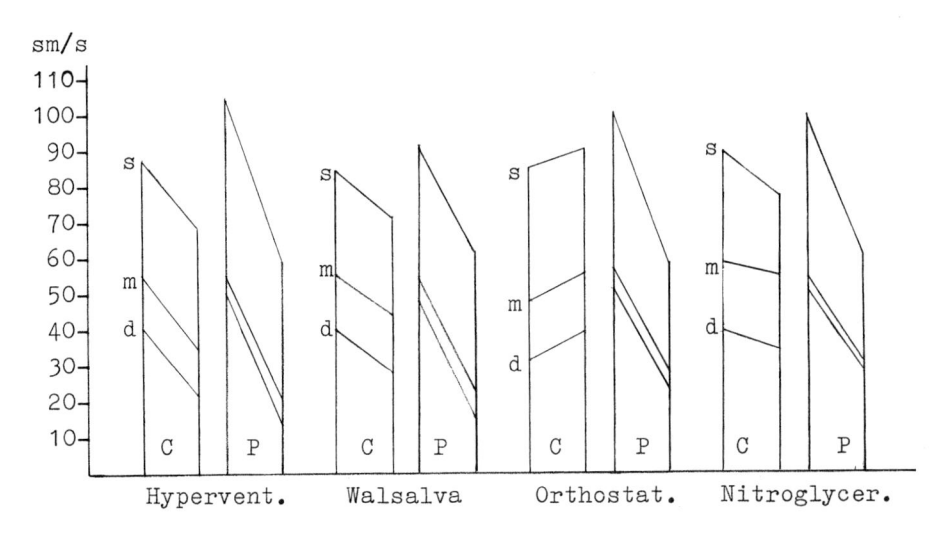

Fig. 1. Changes of the blood flow velocity before and after performing the tests in controls(C) and patients(P). s - maximal systolic velocity, m - mean velocity, d - diastolic velocity.

Table I
Percentage changes of the mean blood flow velocity after performing the tests in controls and in patients with cerebral trauma.

	CONTROL GROUPS	PATIENTS WITH A CEREBRAL TRAUMA
No CASES	50	12
AGE	10 -60	37 ± 14
	% CHANGE OF THE BFV (ml/s)	
HYPERVENTILATION	41,32	57,40
	$P/t/ < 0,05$	
WALSALVA TEST	23,1	62,11
	$P/t/ > 0,01$	
ORTHOSTATIC TEST	15,85	48,14
	$P/t/ > 0,05$	
NITROGLYCERIN TEST	19,16	45,28
	$P/t/ < 0,05$	

The functional tests produce demonstrative difference in percentage of mean velocity indexes with respect to control groups. The differences are significant for the orthostatic and Walsalva test. Table I.

The regresion analysis showed a linear negative interrelation between the initial mean BFV values and corresponding values after performing the tests by increasing the age. Fig. 2, 3, 4, 5.
It can be seen a marked shift of the regression curves for the patients outside of normal limits, with positive correlation index.

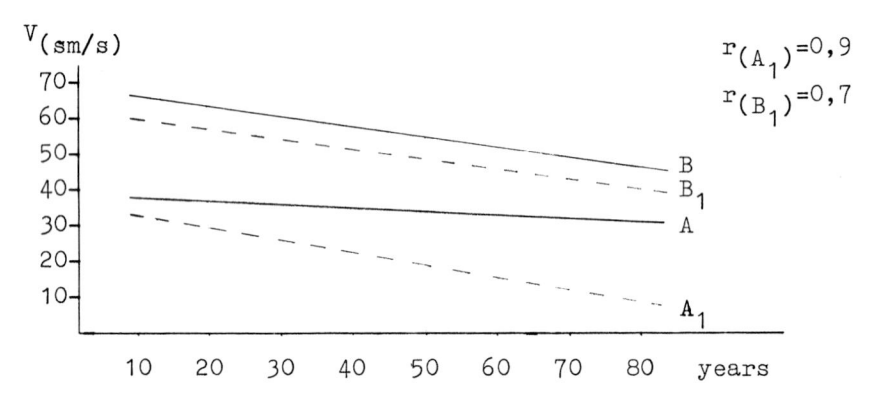

Fig. 2. Age depending changes of the mean blood flow velocity(V) in control groups before(B) and after(A) hyperventilation and the same changes in patients with a cerebral trauma (B_1, A_1).

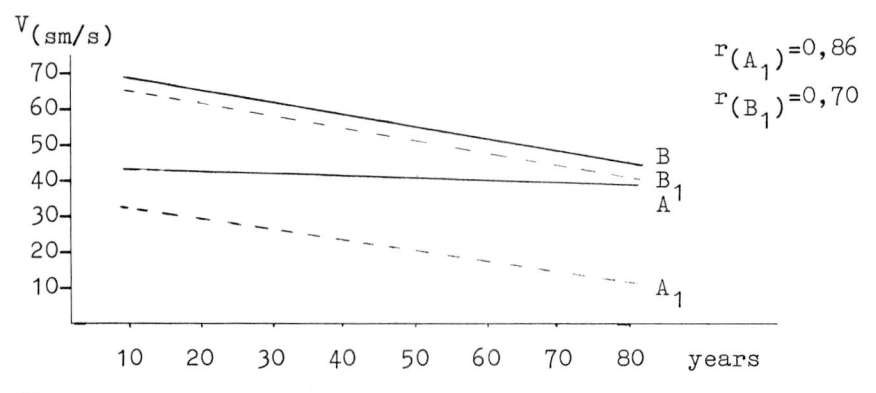

Fig. 3. Age depending changes of the mean blood flow velocity in control groups before(B) and after(A) Walsalva test and the same changes in patients with cerebral trauma (B_1, A_1).

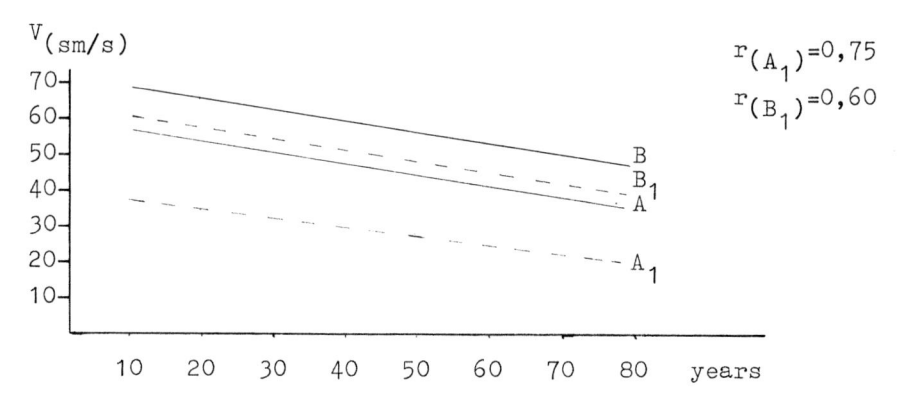

Fig. 4. Age depending changes of the mean blood flow velocity(V) in control groups before(B) and after(A) <u>orthostatic test</u> and the same changes in patients with cerebral trauma(B_1, A_1).

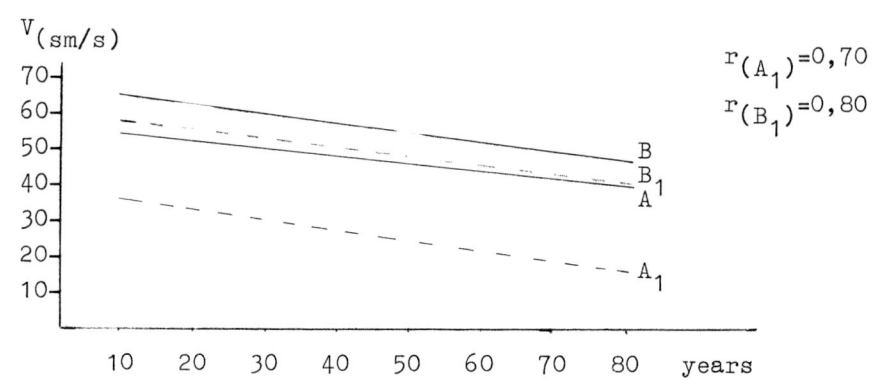

Fig. 5. Age depending changes of the mean blood flow velocity (V) in control groups before(B) and after(A) <u>Nitroglycerin test</u> and the same changes in patients with cerebral trauma(B_1, A_1).

The neurootological investigations reveal in 8 patients data for spontaneus nystagmus, most likely as a combined receptor--brainstem neurootological syndrome. In 4 patients there were not objective findings, however some subjective complaints of dyzziness and gait unstability existed.

DISCUSSION

The functional investigation on CVR of patients with postcommotional syndromes, following cranio-cerebral traumas have revealed the next findings:

Expressed dysautoregulation of the cerebral circulation by monitoring of BFV in the middle cerebral artery. There is significance for the data obtained by Walsalva and orthostatic test.

Despite the fact that this dysautoregulation concern the area of the middle cerebral artery, it should be considered as a valid fact for the general brain circulation, including the vestibular analyser. It can explain the part of the subjective and objective neurootological symptoms and signs.

The present complex of tests can be of value in the investigation of the vascular mechanisms, taking participation in the appearance of neurootological syndroms after cranio-cerebral traumatic injuries.

REFERENCES
1. Kuhl DE, Alavi A, Hoffman J, Pheleps ME, Zimmerman RA, Obris WD, Bruce DA, Joel CB, Greenberg HJ, Uzzell B (1980) J Neurosurg 52:309-320
2. Aaslid R, Markwalder TM, Hornes H (1982) J Neurosurg 57:769
3. Markwalder TM, Grolimud P, Sailer R, Roth F, Aaslid R (1984) J Cereb Blood Flow Metab 4:368-372
4. Widder B (1985) DMW 110:155
5. Ringelstein EB, Otis SM, Grosse M (1986) First international conference of transcranial Doppler sonography Rome, 6-8 November (Abstract)
6. Ringelstein EB, Sievers G, Eacker S, Shneider P, Oyis SM (1988) Stroke 19:963-969
7. Bishop CR, Powell S, Brewse R, (1986) First international conference of transcranial Doppler sonography Rome, 6-8 November (Abstract)

**PSYCHOLOGICAL FEATURES
IN HEAD AND NECK TRAUMA**

VEGETATIVE RESPONSES DUE TO POSTTRAUMATIC NAUSEA REACTIONS

CV.POPIVANOVA, L.NAKOVA
Institute of Hygiene and Occupational Health,
Medical Academy, 15,Dimitar Nestorov str.,Sofia 1431,Bulgaria

INTRODUCTION

The posttraumatic cerebral syndromes with frequently met nausea symptom, on the basis of general vegetative disfunction in patients,undergone cranium-cerebral trauma (CCT), put a number of problems of pathogenic, differential-diagnostic, prognostic etc. aspects, which have to be solved.

The present study aims at determining the type, rate and dynamics of the vegetative and vestibulo-vegetative manifestations in patients with CCT and present posttraumatic reaction of nausea, according to age, sex, limitation of CCT, localization of the otoneurological disturbance - central, peripheral and combined. On the basis of complex results we shall try to explain some pathogenic moments, stipulating the rich vegetative and vestibulo-vegetative symptomatic.

MATERIAL AND METHODS

Studies are carried out on 61 patients undergone CCT. Age and sex groups are formed of 32 men and 29 women from 20 to 65 years old. In order to compare the data a control group of 52 healthy persons, age 20 to 65 years with normal neuro-vegetological and otoneurological status and with no data for undergone CCT in the anamnesis is used. A complex of methods is used: directed vegetological anamnesis, coordination of tests of Römberg, Babinsky-Weil, nose-index test, ortho-clinostatic test, clinical test - eye-cardiocerebral reflex of Ashner-Danini, response test of Barany with angular acceleration of $90°/sec^2$ (Kehaiov,A.,1982), caloric test with cold water $20°C$ after the method of Barany, (Kehaiov,A.,1982) tracing before and after vestibular provocation the hemodynamic indices - pulse rate, systolic and diastolic blood pressure.

RESULTS AND DISCUSSION

The results show, that in the structure of the anamnestic data the posttraumatic symptoms of nausea and vomiting are accompanied most frequently by headache - 80%, and by disturbances in the balance - giddiness,vertigo,sinking,gate instability - 67%.The symptoms of nausea and vomiting are met in all age and sex groups; relatively prevail in women - 71,4% to 42,7% in men.Usually they are reported during the first year after CCT - 54,8%, after the 10th year they decrease, and after the 20th year reach 25%.The complex of leading subjective complaints - nausea,balance disturbance, headache is most frequently met in 36-50 years old women (56,7%) to 28,4% in men ($p < 0,05$), probably because of unstable neurovegetative background in relation to eventual endo-crinic age readjustment (Vantov,M,1987).With advance of age the coordination tests, orthoclinostatic test and eye-cardiac reflex of Ashner-Danini turn positive usually, but with no statistical significance ($p > 0,05$).The vegetative syndrome, in rotatory and caloric vestibular tests abounds in amphotonys, mainly sympathicotonic manifestations (tremor, sparkling glance,turning pale, feeling cold,anxious) - 68%. Only in 20,4% of the vegetative disturbances have compound character, and in 12,0% - prevail the parasympathicotonic manifestation (nausea,vomiting,hypersalivation,perspiration,etc.).In most patients the vegetative disturbance contrast with the vestibular hyporeflexia 63,5%,areflexia - 19,2% and in 17,3% with hyperreflexia. The vestibulovegetative reactions are more frequent in patients over 55 years old(86,1%), most probably because of the addition of age-depending vascular-cerebral changes (Blagovestenskaja,N.S.1976). Most significant are the vegetative disturbances with dominating sympathicotonic character in patients with diagnosis central otoneurological syndrome - 78,4%, followed by patients with peripheral otoneurological syndrome - 57,0% and at the end those with combined otoneurological syndrome - 47,4% ($p > 0,05$).The provocation of the vertical vestibular substrates most frequently determines the vegetative symptomatic - 87,3% in central and peripheral otoneurological syndrome ($p < 0,01$).These data have to be specified in order to clarify the role of the vertical semicircular ducts in the pathogenic mechanism of the vegetative syndrome. The general vegetative reactivity is studied by tracing the hemodynamic indices - pulse rate and arterial blood pressure before and after vestibular provocation. In the group of patients with cranium-cerebral trauma the prevailing time reaction is the hypertensive - rising of the systolic and diasystolic blood pressure and pulse rate - 74,1% ($p < 0,01$). Only in 10,3% is registered a light decrease of the arterial pressure on the background of accelerated pulse, and in 15,6% there are fluctuations of the hemodynamic indices, but with tendency towards high values. The time for recuperation after provocation varies from 4 min. to several hours, as in some patients the high values remain for a long time. In the group of healthy persons the hemodynamic changes show no significant differences ($p > 0,05$). Similar results are established also by other authors who studied the dynamics of the hemodynamic indices in patients with diencephalic syndrome (Zaprjanova,L., Iv.Ivanov, N.Beshkov, 1989). Approximately the general sympathicotonic type of response to the vegetative nervous system in patients with different diagnosis and different etiology of the suffering certifies for certain unspecificity in the functioning of the pathogenic mechanism.

All mentioned up-to now data show, that the vegetative changes due to posttraumatic reaction of nausea have mainly sympathicotonic character, they are relatively resistant, unsignificantly affected by sex, more by age, with tendency for more frequent manifestation before the end of the first year after the cranium-cerebral trauma and in the presence of central otoneurological disturbance.The sympathicotonic type response is accepted as timely neurophysiological reaction,satisfying the extremely increased necessities at the stressogenic influence of the CCT. The parasympathic display of nausea and vomiting as physiological balance to the sympathic reaction appears as expedient adaptive reaction,directed towards maintaining the biochemical homeostasis. By means of nausea followed by vomiting during the vestibular crisis is restored the alkaline-acidic and ionic balance, and is normalized the level of K and especially the interrelation K, Ca and Mg, which is in

relation with the excitability of the central nervous system,
the endocrine glands, the cardio-vascular system, etc (Kehaiov,
A. 1978, et al.). The inclusion of the vestibular formation
in the pathogenetic mechanism of the vegetative reactions, as
data point out, plays powerful stressogenic effect, expressed
by various vestibulo-vegetative and hemodynamic changes. The
comparative stability and persistence in the time of advantageous
sympathicotonic manifestations is a prerequisite for comparative
loss of vital importance energy, decrease of the compensatory
and reserved possibilities, decrease of the stressogenic
threshold, respectively increase of the danger from risk
situations. The dynamic and the character of the vegetative
and vestibulo-vegetative disregulatory deviations can have
diagnostic and prognostic value.

REFERENCES

1. Blagovestenskaja N S (1876) Clinical otoneurology in cerebrum damages, Medicina, Moscow, pp 154-156 (in Russian)
2. Vantov M (1867) Diseases of the vegetative nervous system, Medicina i Fizkultura, Sofia pp.171-172 (in Bulgarian)
3. Zaprjanova L, Iv Ivanov,Beshkov N (1983) Changes in the hemodynamic indices under the influence of the vestibular provocation in patients with diencephalic syndromes. Otorhinolaringology, XXVI, 2, Medicina i Fizkultura,Sofia pp 1-7 (in Bulgarian)
4. Kehaiov A (1978) Space, time, movement. Vestibular, visual and auditory perceptions.Medicina i Fizkultuta, Sofia, pp 139-141 (in Bulgarian)
5. Kehaiov A (1982) Mannual on otoneurology. Medicina i Fizkultura, Sofia pp. 135-152 (in Bulgarian)

THE SUBJECTIVE SYMPTOMS COMPARED WITH ELECTRONYSTAGMOGRAPHIC FINDINGS IN VESTIBULAR NEURONITIS

PEKKA SILVONIEMI, EERO AANTAA

Turku University Central Hospital, ENT Clinic, SF-20520 Turku, Finland

INTRODUCTION

Vestibular neuronitis is a disease with acute intensive rotatory vertigo, spontaneous horizontal nystagmus to the healthy ear and totally extinguished or markedly diminished caloric response on the affected side. Hearing is normal (1-2). Intensive symptoms relieve gradually in a week and most of the cases are able to work after one month. In this study special interest was paid to the disabling symptoms, to the correlation of the subjective symptoms with electronystagmographic findings during the follow-up period and to the subjective sensation of vertigo caused by the caloric irrigation during the recovery phase.

MATERIAL

Thirty-three successive cases with vestibular neuronitis, mean age 42.3 years, range 12-67 years, 13 females, 23 males were examined. The diagnostic criteria were a sudden intensive vertigo, spontaneous horizontal nystagmus to the healthy ear and a total loss of the caloric response of the affected ear with 44 and 30°C water irrigations recorded with electronystagmography (ENG).

METHODS

The acute stage examination was performed 1-5 days after the onset of symptoms and the follow-up examinations on the average 1 month and 1 year afterwards. Thirty-three subjects took part in the first, 29 in the second and 32 in the third examination. Special attention was paid to the analysis of the vertiginous symptoms. A clinical neuro-otological examination was carried out. Spontaneous, positional and provoked nystagmus were observed with Frenzel's glasses in a dark room. Nystagmus was recorded with ENG in supine, right and left lateral positions first with eyes closed and then open in the darkness. The caloric tests with 44 and 30°C water were carried out with open eyes in darkness.

The subjective sensation of vertigo during the caloric test was estimated from 6 to 0 according to the following scores:

6 A very strong sensation of rotatory vertigo, falling down and vomiting
5 A strong sensation of rotatory vertigo
4 A moderate sensation of rotatory vertigo in a specific direction
3 A mild sensation of rotatory vertigo
2 No evident rotatory vertigo, a sensation of swaying or swinging
1 An unspecific sensation of swaying or swinging
0 No subjective sensation of vertigo at all.

RESULTS

The sudden onset and the intensity of the vertiginous symptoms compelled most of the cases to medical examination during the first two days. Seven subjects suffered from a mild prodromal sensation of unsteadiness during 1-7 days before the onset of vigorous vertigo. Intensive symptoms lessened gradually during the first week in most cases.

TABLE I
THE DURATION OF DISABLING VERTIGO. THE SUBJECTIVE EVALUATION OF THE PATIENTS.

	No	%
1-7 days	23	69.7
8-14 days	9	27.3
15-30 days	1	3.0
total	33	100

The recovery period was characterized by vertigo during fast head movements or while predisposed to optokinetic stimulus or moving in darkness. The analysis of the symptoms during the follow-up period proved of the benign course of this disease.

TABLE II
COMPLETE SUBJECTIVE RECOVERY OF VERTIGO (CUMULATIVE FIGURES)

	No	%
Symptomless after		
1 month	12	37.5
2 months	17	53.1
3 months	22	68.8
4 months	28	87.5
12 months	29	90.6

The abnormal ENG-findings were abundant also in the follow-up examinations. The incidence of nystagmus lessened during the follow-up period and the speed of the slow component decreased. The direction of nystagmus was changed in some subjects to the diseased ear during the follow-up period and these cases had also more subjective vertigo or the vertigo had begun again after a short symptomless period.

TABLE III
THE INCIDENCE OF SPONTANEOUS OR POSITIONAL NYSTAGMUS IN ELECTRONYSTAGMOGRAPHY

Nystagmus	Follow-up 1 month No	%	Follow-up 1 year No	%
to the healthy ear	15	51.7	15	46.9
to the diseased ear	5	17.2	5	15.6
direction changing	2	6.9	2	6.3
no nystagmus	7	24.1	10	31.3
total	29	100	32	100

The abnormalities of the caloric responses were characteristic of the follow-up findings. Also totally extinguished responses were observed at the second follow-up examination. The number of diminished caloric responses is remarkable and probably permanent.

TABLE IV
THE RESULTS OF THE CALORIC TESTS WITH 44 AND 30°C WATER IRRIGATION

	Follow-up 1 month No	%	Follow-up 1 year No	%
No reaction	14	50.0	3	9.4
Diminished reaction	6	21.4	11	34.4
Normal reaction	8	28.6	18	56.3
Total	28	100	32	100

The subjective sensation of vertigo during the caloric tests follows well the intensity and symmetry of the caloric responses. The subjective sensation of vertigo on the diseased side during the caloric tests was decreased compared with the result of the healthy side and with the healthy controls ($p<0.001$).

TABLE V
THE MEAN VALUES OF THE SCORES OF THE SUBJECTIVE SENSATION' OF VERTIGO DURING THE CALORIC TESTS

	Acute stage 1-5 years mean	SD	No	Follow-up 1 month mean	SD	No	1 year mean	SD	No
Healthy ear	4.1	1.1	33	3.8	0.9	28	3.8	1.8	32
Diseased ear	0.0	0.0	33	1.2***	1.6	28	2.6***	1.4	32

'Scores from 6 to 0 are explained on page 2.
*** $p<0.001$

DISCUSSION

The intensity of the symptoms compelled the patients immediately to medical examination. In spite of the intensive symptoms the habituation diminishes the vertigo during the first two weeks. The results of the follow-up examinations strengthen the earlier conclusions of the benign nature of this disease.

The correlation of the numerous abnormal findings in the ENG-recordings was not very good compared with subjective symptoms except in the very first days. Some subjects with recovery nystagmus to the diseased side expressed increase of the symptoms for some time possibly due to the recovering function of the diseased labyrinth (3-4). In most subjects abnormal caloric responses did not cause any difficulties to the balance in the first and second follow-up examination. The incidence of nystagmus is great during the follow-up period as a sign of the imbalance between the vestibular nuclei. The situation is probably permanent for these subjects. The central mechanisms compensate well this disbalance.

The subjective sensation of vertigo during the caloric response completes very well the objective measurable nystagmic response. It is in good correlation with objective measurements and also helps to distinguish the caloric response from the spontaneous nystagmus.

REFERENCES

1. Dix MR, Hallpike CS (1952) The pathology, symptomatology and diagnosis of certain common disorders of the vestibular system. Ann Otol Rhinol Laryngol 61:987-1016.

2. Aschan G, Stahle J (1956) Vestibular neuronitis. A nystagmographical study. J Laryngol Otol 70:497-511.

3. Aantaa E, Virolainen E. (1979) Vestibular neuronitis. A follow-up study. Acta Otothinolaryngol Belg 33:401-404.

4. Haid T, Mirsberger J. (1985) Die periphere Neuropathia Vestibularis und ein zentral-vestibuläres Äquivalent. HNO 33:262-270.

VERTIGO, TINNITUS AND HALLUCINATIONS DUE TO HEAD TRAUMA

SVETLOZAR HARALANOV, LYUBOMIR HARALANOV

Institute of Neurology, Psychiatry and Neurosurgery, Medical Academy, Sofia, Bulgaria

INTRODUCTION

Together with the objectively establishable symptoms, head trauma (HT) can provoke different subjective symptoms too. In the field of Neurootology such subjective symptoms are vertigo (V) and tinnitus (T). In their essence these are sensory experiences with no corresponding external stimulus at the moment of their appearance. From this point of view V and T answer the criteria, given by the classical Esquirol definition (see 1) of hallucinations (H). That is why, according to us, V and T can be accepted as H (i.e. as perceptions without object) or to be more exact as "organic hallucinations" (see 2), due to direct stimulus in the region of the respective sensory system - vestibular or auditory.

The present work is dedicated to clinical observations which verify the close interrelations between V and the vestibular H, as well as between T and the auditory H in patients with HT. Our observations were realised in the emergency psychiatric unit and in the neurological intensive care unit, with consultations between the authors - one of them a psychiatrist and the other - a neurologist.

MATERIAL AND METHODS

Two groups of patients were investigated: a) mentally ill patients after HT (29 schizophrenics) with no hallucinatory symptoms before the trauma and, b) patients with neurological symptoms after HT (21 patients with commotio and contusion). The schizophrenics have no focal neurological symptoms and the post-traumatic manifestations limit themselves to cerebrasthenic complaints. The idea was to compare the experiences diagnosticated as V, T and H respectively, having as a background the neurological symptoms on the one hand, and the psychopathological symptoms on the other. In all cases in the investigation the appearance of V, T and H (both isolated and in different combinations between one another) the causal connection with the HT is evident, because the symptoms have appeared immediately after the trauma or a few days later.

Basically the clinical method was used, which includes a complete neurological and psychiatric status, while the latter also includes a special interrogation for the subjective aspects of the perceptive pathology.

RESULTS

The results of the investigation can be systematised and summarised in the following way:

a) from clinical point of view, the differentiation of V from the vastibular H and of T from the auditory H is sometimes very difficult. In fact the appearance of a subjective noise in the ear of patients with neurological symptoms after HT is taken for T, while in psychic cases the principally analogous phenomenon is categorised as "elementary auditory hallucinations" or "acousmae". At the same time, the abnormal perception of one's own body in relation to the surrounding objects of patients with neurological symptoms after HT is taken for a neuropathological symptom and is noted as V, while in cases of mental illness the same phenomenon is categorised as a psychopathological symptom and is noted as "vestibular H".

b) the more elementary the structure of the respective pathological perceptive phenomenon (subjective noise or fake movements of the surrounding objects, accompanied by a feeling of falling into a precipice), the more probable it is that it would be categorised as T or V, and vice versa; the more complex and non-typical it is (bell ringing, cart noise, wind whistle, unclear voices, shouts, melodies, etc., as well as an appearance of moving images of objects, a feeling for a swinging bed, experience for flying, earthquake, etc.), the more probable it is to be taken as H - respectively auditory or vestibular.

c) not infrequently, even with one and the same patient, one and the same phenomenon is defined as V or T if the doctor is a neurologist, while the more complex of them - as "vestibular hallucinations" or "auditory hallucinations" if the doctor is a psychiatrist.

d) dynamic transitions are observed (in one or the other direction) between phenomena, which have characteristic features of V and phenomena, having characteristic features of vestibular H, as well as between phenomena, which have characteristic of T and phenomena, having characteristic features of auditory H. For example, a patient with neurological symptoms after HT complains from a feeling of instability and a sense of moving surrounding objects on a turning of the head which is categorised as V. After a while, the patient says that the floor on which he walks seems to be swaying, the walls too, and the ceiling seems to fall down on him. The patient is convinced that there is an earthquake and starts to shout. This condition is judged as hallucinatory. We can give an analogous example concerning the auditory modality: one of the patients with neurological symptoms after HT complains at the beginning from a monotonous permanent noise in the right ear, which is categorised as T. After some time, the same patient says that he hears a soft voice in his right ear, which calls him by his name. These complaints are categorised as hallucinatory.

CONCLUSION

According to us, the results show that between V and the vestibular H, as well as between T and the auditory H their pathogenesis is common. The clinical evaluation of the concrete perceptive phenomenon (i.e. its categorisation as V or T on the one hand, or as the vestibular or auditory H on the other) depends basically on three factors: a) the type of accompanying symptoms - neuropathological or psychopathological, b) the complexity of the respective phenomenon and, c) the speciality of the doctor - neurologist or psychiatrist.

The observed dynamic transitions from V to vestibular H and from T to auditory H should not be regarded as some kind of transformations of neuropathological to psychpathological symptoms, but rather - as a transition from a less complex to a more complex hallucinatory experience due to pathological changes in the brain after the trauma. On the one hand, the reverse transitions - from vestibular H to V and from auditory H to T - can be explained with a reverse development of the pathological changes in the brain, which is connected to the recovering adaptive compensatory processes, helped on by the carried out therapy. It is no coincidence that the transitions from more complex to simpler hallucinatory experiences are usually observed when there is an improvement in the condition of the patient, while the complications of the pathological perceptive phenomena are usually observed when there is worsening of the condition.

Summarising, we can conclude that as V and T, the respective vestibular and auditory H should be taken as pathological pathogenetically connected perceptive phenomena of a hallucinatory nature, caused by processes of excitement in the frames respectively of the vestibular and auditory sensory systems, causal connection of the HT. From this point of view the difference between V and the vestibular H is of degree (quantitative) and not qualitative. The same thing is relevant for the difference between T and the auditory H in cases after HT. Additional arguments in this direction can be found in the results of the pathophysiological mechanisms of V and T on the one hand and of H on the other. In 1933 Hautant points out that at the basis of both V and T lies the hyperexcitation in the analyser. Almost in the same period Tamburini summarises the classical neurological attitude towards H with the following: "hallucinations are the epilepsy of the sensory centers". Our own investigation of the pathophysiologic mechanisms of the hallucinogenesis also established data for excitational processes in the respective sensory systems when hallucinating.

That is why we think, that the role of HT is most probably brought to the cause of such damages in a certain sensory system, which lead to an appearance of an excitatory focus in it. According to the localisation extensiveness of this excitatory focus, T and V can subjectively be defined as pathological perceptive experiences in some cases, while in others - as vestibular or auditory H resp.

The practical conclusion which can be drawn on the basis of the established principal similarity between V, T and H, according to us, is that V and T, like H, can be treated with neuroleptics and tranquilisers. Of course, such symptomatic treatment does not cancel the necessity for causal treatment of brain damages due to head trauma.

REFERENCES

1. EY H. - Traité des hallucinations. Paris, Masson et Cie, 1973;

2. HARALANOV SV. - Methods and Apparatus for Provoking and Investigating Hallucinatory Experience: Possibilities and Perspectives. Dissertation,Sofia,1987;

3. HAUTANT A. - Le Vertige. Ann. d'O.R.L., 1933,1;

4. TAMBURINI A. - Sulla Theoria delle Allucinazioni. Rev.Sci., 1881,27:138-142;

5. HARALANOV SV., SCHKODROVA D., HARALANOV L., HARALANOV H. - Auditory Evoked Potentials in Cases of Verbal Hallucinations - In: 10th Joint Annual Meeting of EEG and Clinical Neurophysiology. Budapest, 1987;

6. HARALANOV SV., HARALANOV L. - Auditory and Visual Evoked Potentials in Patients Suffering from Hallucinations - In: 9th Joint Meeting of EEG and Clinical Neurophysiology. Varna, 1986;

7. HARALANOV SV., HARALANOV H. - Influence of Vestibular and Auditory Irritation on Hallucinatory Processes - In: 14th International Scientific Meeting of the NES. Sao Paolo, Brasil. Acta AWHO, 1987, 1:60;

DYNAMIC POSTUROGRAPHY IN PSYCHO-ORGANIC SYNDROME

T LEDIN, E JANSSON, C MÖLLER, LM ÖDKVIST.

Dept of ENT, University Hospital, S-581 85 Linköping, Sweden.

ABSTRACT

Seven patients previously exposed to industrial solvents and diagnosed with psycho-organic syndrome (POS) aged 38-69 years (mean 56 years) have been investigated by dynamic posturography and results were correlated to static posturography performed earlier. The patients were compared to healthy, age-matched controls. Dynamic posturography comprises a sensory organization part with either stable or sway-referenced support surface and visual surround, with included or excluded vision, in which the patient group showed significantly worse equilibrium performance compared to the control group in most test conditions. In the movement coordination part, where the platform makes active movements, no differences were found between groups. A relation between the sway area in static posturography with eyes open and sway in the simplest sensory organization test condition was found ($r=-0.79$, $p<0.05$), otherwise no correlations between static and dynamic posturography could be demonstrated. It is concluded that in addition to previous findings of pathology in visual suppression of the VOR, static posturography and some audiometry variables, patients with POS show an impaired equilibrium in the dynamic posturography.

INTRODUCTION

Solvents are known to cause central as well as peripheral nervous system damage (Begleiter et al 1981, Barregård and Axelsson 1984, Hogstedt et al 1980, Larsby et al 1976, 1978, Ledin et al 1989, Ödkvist et al 1982a, 1982b). One possible outcome is a psycho-organic syndrome (POS), characterized by several of the symptoms neurasthenia, personality changes, reduction of intellectual capacity, vertigo, dizziness and unsteadiness (Axelsson et al 1976).

In a previous study Möller et al (1989) studied audiological and otoneurological function in a group of nine men with POS compared to nine healthy age-matched controls not exposed to solvents at work. The results showed that central auditory tests and balance functions, clinical testing with the Romberg test as well as computerized static posturography, were significantly worse in the POS group, and that ocular smooth pursuit testing with randomized stimulation as well as the visual suppression of the vestibuloocular reflex (VOR) were significantly abnormal. The conclusion was that solvents caused disturbances of cerebellar and brainstem functions as well as CNS auditory mechanisms.

The present study is a three years follow-up of these patients with a clinical check-up and investigation by a new method, dynamic posturography, in order to study the dynamic balance performance in POS.

MATERIAL AND METHODS

All nine workers (Möller et al 1989) investigated in 1986, were contacted and asked to participate in the study. One refused to take part and one could not be reached. Thus seven patients aged 38-69 years (mean 56 years) were included in the study. They had been exposed to mixtures of alcohol, aromatic and aliphatic industrial solvents ranging between eight and thirty years (mean 21 years). All had a previous diagnosis of POS syndrome made in the Department of Occupational Medicine based on case history, neurophysiology and psychological testing (Hogstedt et al 1980). Since 1985, none of the subjects had been working with solvents. As control group, the nine age-matched (range 39-66 years, mean 56 years) non-exposed healthy controls used by Möller et al (1989) were used.

Dynamic posturography (Equitest, Neurocom Int Inc, Clackamas, Oregon, USA) was performed as described by Nashner (1987) and Cyr et al (1988). In the dynamic posturography, the subject is standing on a dual forceplate enclosed by a visual surround. Both the forceplate and the surround can be made to move with the person's antero-posterior (AP) sway or independent of the sway, thus enabling programmed disturbances of the equilibrium. The dual forceplate records the forces between feet and ground as well as shear forces, thereby allowing estimation of the position of the swaying body as well as the pattern of sway in terms of hip or ankle strategy.

The investigation is divided into two main sections: sensory organization test (SO) and movement coordination test (MC). The SO part is divided into six separate tests (see Ledin et al 1990 for figure), lasting 20 seconds each with test 4, 5 and 6 repeated three times. SO 1 is a quantified version of Rombergs test. The subject stands with eyes open and the surrounding as well as the ground is stable. SO 2 is equal to SO 1 except that the eyes are closed. In SO 3, performed with eyes open, the surrounding moves in response to the body sway. In test SO 4 the platform is sway referenced and the surrounding stable. In test SO 5, with eyes closed, the platform is sway referenced, and in test SO 6 both the platform and surrounding are sway referenced. Note that in SO 3 and SO 6 the tested subject might have some orientation information from the surrounding as it is only moving in the AP direction and not in the lateral direction.

From each test an equilibrium score is computed. The score is 100 for absolutely no sway, decreasing with increasing sway amplitude, and zero in case of falling. A strategy score is computed expressing the degree of ankle or hip movements- 100 means solely ankle and no hip movements and zero means exclusively hip movements. These calculations are related to the amount of shear force exerted. Alignment data is also calculated showing the angle between body and earth vertical during the trial. Initial alignment describes the conditions before the start of the each test and dynamic alignment is the angle during the test.

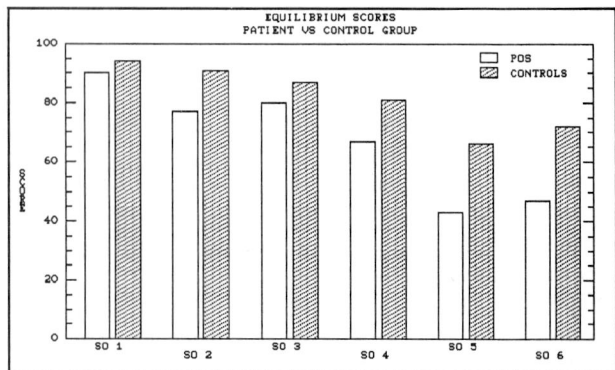

Figure 1. Equilibrium scores.

The movement coordination (MC) part is divided into eight separate tests: Small, medium and large backwards and forwards translation perturbations of the platform are repeated three times each to simulate falling forwards and backwards, respectively, and furthermore the platform is tilted toes-down and toes-up five times each.

From the translation perturbations the force response of each foot is evaluated to yield force symmetry scores between right and left foot. The slope and latency of force recruitment for each foot is also assessed to give estimations of the reaction of each foot separately. A strategy score is used to estimate the degree of hip vs ankle strategies. Finally the toes-up and toes-down tiltings are evaluated using an energy function to estimate the adaptation of the responses to the stimuli.

The results of static posturography performed in the patient group in 1986 were correlated to the results in dynamic posturography. Static posturography comprises upright standing in a darkened room for 60 seconds on a stable force platform with eyes closed and open. The center of pressure location is measured and a confidence ellipse area is computed estimating postural sway (Sahlstrand et al 1978).

Groups were compared using Student's t-test. Correlation analysis was used to assess relations between static and dynamic posturography in the patient group. The probability of correlation coefficients equalling zero was computed. A probability level of 5% was considered significant.

RESULTS

Comparing the results in the patient group with the control group in SO part of dynamic posturography revealed lower patient equilibrium scores in all test conditions (figure 1), yet not significant in test conditions SO 1 and SO 3. No significant differences were found in the MC part.

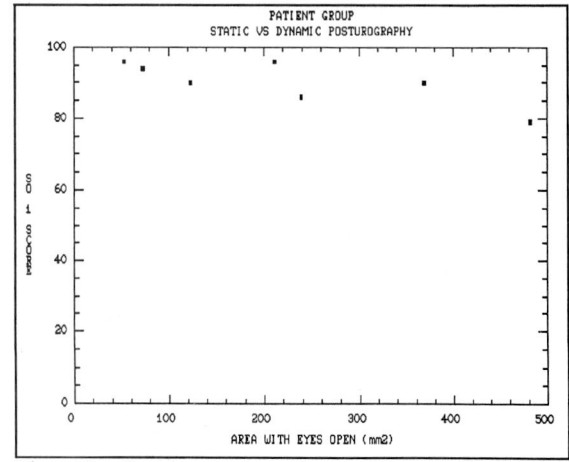

Figure 2. Static vs dynamic posturography.

There was a significant correlation between the area with eyes open in static posturography and the equilibrium score in SO 1 in dynamic posturography ($r=-0.79$, $p<0.05$). The corresponding relation between area with eyes closed and SO 2 was not significant.

DISCUSSION

Plastics and solvents are important parts of everyday life in a modern society. In a recent study Möller et al (1989) presented results on POS, indicating disturbances in the vestibulo-oculomotor system, auditory functions and equilibrium performance caused by industrial solvent exposure. The present study is a follow-up using a new equilibrium estimation method, dynamic posturography.

In the dynamic posturography the patients exhibited a worse equilibrium performance compared to controls, in agreement with the results in static posturography presented by Möller et al (1989). The patients with POS obviously have a deteriorated balance performance, even after five or more years of abstinence from exposure. The introduction of dynamic posturography in the test battery increases its sensitivity, which is shown by the positive findings on the movable platform. In all testing of solvent induced CNS lesions it is important to find the right level of test difficulty, may it be the vestibulo-oculomotor conflict tests or disturbed auditory tests.

Concerning balance it is concluded that the dynamic posturography is valuable in the investigation of patients with POS, presumably also for screening purposes.

REFERENCES

Axelsson O, Hane M, Hogstedt C. A case-referent study on neuro-psychiatric disorders among workers exposed to solvents. Scand J Work Environ Health 1976: 2: 14-20.

Barregård L, Axelsson A. Is there an ototraumatic interaction between noise and solvents? Scand Audiol 1984: 13: 151-155.

Begleiter H, Porjesz B, Chou CL. Auditory brainstem potentials in chronic alcoholics. Science 1981: 211: 1064-1066.

Cyr DG, Moore GF, Möller CG. Clinical application of computerized dynamic posturography. Ear, Nose and Throat Journal (suppl) 1988: Sep: 36-47.

Hogstedt C, Hane M, Axelsson O. Diagnostic and health care aspects on workers exposed to solvents. In: Zenz C, ed. Developments in occupational medicine. Chicago: Medical Year Book Publishers, 1980.

Larsby B, Ödkvist LM, Hyden D, Liedgren SRC. Disturbances of the vestibular system by toxic agents. Acta Physiol Scand 1976: Suppl 440: 157.

Larsby B, Tham R, Ödkvist LM, Norlander B, Hyden D, Aschan G, Rubin A. Exposure of rabbits to metylchloroform: Vestibular disturbances correlated to blood and cerebrospinal fluid levels. Int Arch Occ Env Health 1978: 41: 7-15.

Ledin T, Ödkvist LM, Möller C. Posturograpy findings in workers exposed to industrial solvents. Acta Otolaryngol (Stockh) 1989: 107: 357-361.

Ledin T, Möller C, Möller M, Ödkvist LM. Dynamic posturography and aging. Proceedings Neurootological and Equilibriometric Society 17th Congress, Bad Kissingen, 1990 (this volume).

Möller C, Ödkvist LM, Thell J, Larsby B, Hyden D, Bergholtz LM, Tham R. Otoneurological findings in psycho-organic syndrome caused by industrial solvent exposure. Acta Otolaryngol (Stockh) 1989: 107: 5-12.

Nashner LM. A systems approach to understanding and assessing orientation and balance disorders. Advances in diagnosis and management of balance disorders conference, Boston, MA, Oct 1987).

Sahlstrand T, Örtengren R, Nachemsson A. Postural equilibrium in adolescent idiopathic scoliosis. Acta Orthop Scand 1978: 49: 354-365.

Ödkvist LM, Bergholtz LM, Åhlfeldt H, Andersson B, Edling C, Strand E. Otoneurological and audiological findings in workers exposed to industrial solvents. Acta Otolaryngol (Stockh) 1982: Suppl 386: 249-251.

Ödkvist LM, Larsby B, Tham R, Åhlfeldt H, Andersson B, Eriksson B, Liedgren SRC. Vestibulo-oculomotor disturbances in humans exposed to styrene. Acta Otolaryngol (Stockh) 1982: 94: 487-493.

Acknowledgements: The technical assistance by Mr Johan Deblen and Mrs Lisbeth Noaksson and the financial support of the Swedish Work Environmental Fund are gratefully acknowledged.
Correspondence to: T Ledin, Dept of ENT, University Hospital, S-581 85 Linköping, Sweden.

CHANGES IN EVOKED POTENTIALS AND EEG DUE TO TRAUMA

AUDITORY EVOKED RESPONSES IN PATIENTS SUFFERING FROM DIABETES MELLITUS

IVAN CHROMEJ, JANA JAVORKOVA[+]
ENT Clinic and [+] Clinic of Paediatrics, University Hospital, Kollarova 2, 036 59 Martin, (Czecho-Slovakia)

INTRODUCTION

More than 100 years there is a controversy and the question remains unresolved whether or not diabetes may cause a CNS damage and whether a central equivalent of diabetic neuropathy really exists. Jordano as a first, reported in 1857 a case of a diabetogenic deafness and that idea was supported by Marchal in 1864 with his concept of diabetogenic encephalopathy, which may manifest itself with a laesion on the acoustic pathway, too. Then vast literature followed dealing with hearing level estimation in diabetics, but hasn't succeeded to bring some typical pattern of auditory deficit, mainly due to a technical barrier. A new approach started when Barjon et al. (1) added new features to the list of heritable disorders where diabetes is accompanied with ocular and hearing defects (Alström's Syndrome, DIDMOAD, Bujara-Bruck's Sy., Van den Eeckhaut-Mangen's Sy., Friedreich's Syndrome). One year later, Zelenka and Kozak (2) have proved there is a correlation between diabetic angiopathy and vestibular and hearing deficits.

Highly relevant findings were from Reske-Nielsen et al. (3), Olsson et al. (4), Kam-Hansen and Sorensen (5), who systematically studied histomorphology of CNS specimens from cadavers of young diabetics and found vascular stria angiopathy, endolymph haemorrhagy, spiral ganglion atrophy, leptomeningeal fibrosis, demyelination of acoustic nerve, brain-stem nuclei haemorrhagy, diffuse angiopathy of brain-stem, cerebellar and cortical nervous degeneration.

A real break-through has ensued from Donald et al. (6) first report on the prolongation of slow cortical vertwx-potentials and the supression enhancement of this response if the rate of stimulation has been increased. Martini et al. (7) have proved the prolongation of BAEP waves latencies in normal hearing diabetics and this anomaly was in correlation with occurence of diabetic autonomic neuropathy and with decrease of motor conduction velocity at the peroneal nerve.

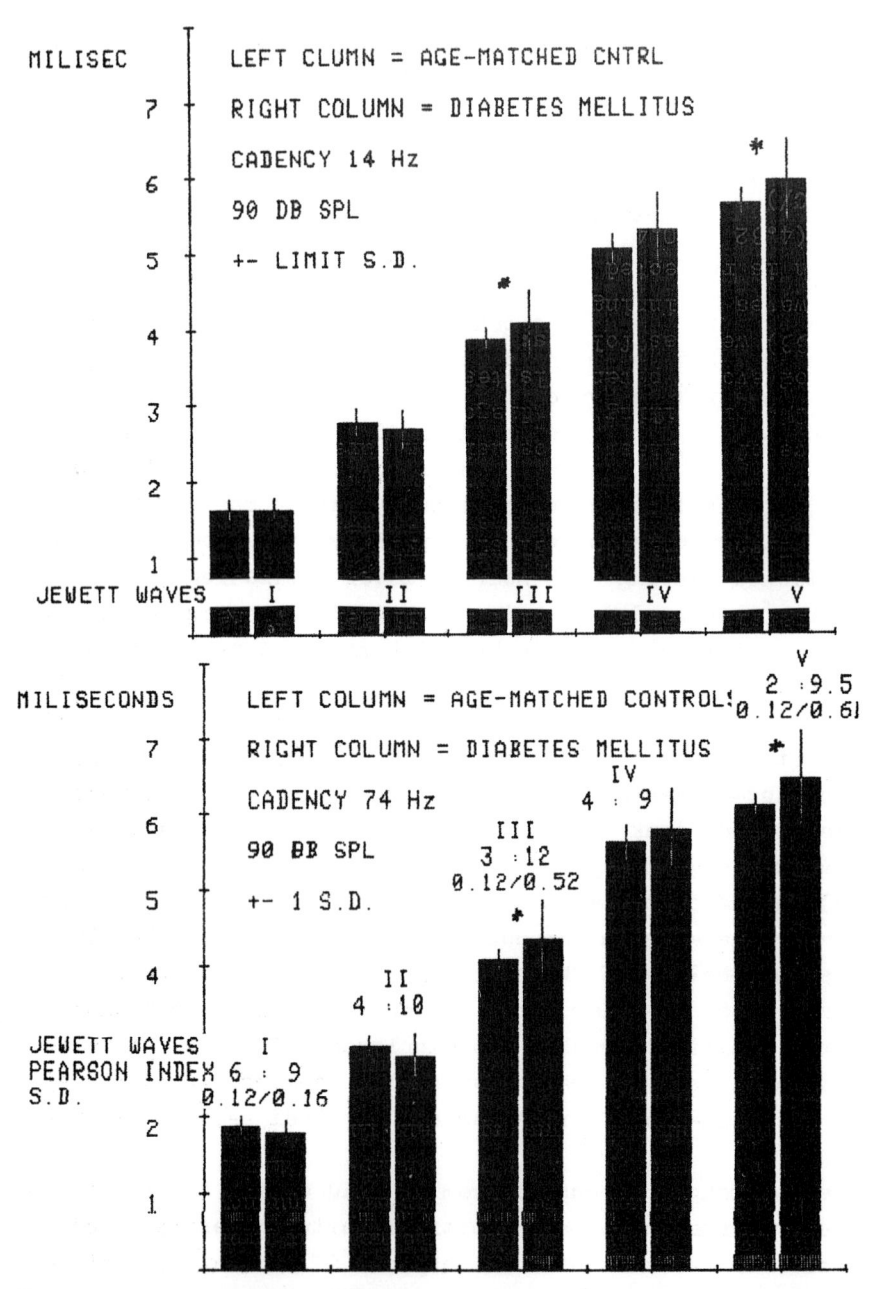

Fig. 1. Latencies of BAEP components related to the various rate of stimulation (cadency) in comparison with AMC (age-matched controls). Common parameters: click 0.1 ms duration unfiltered, time window 10 ms, 2000x averaged response, filters analog. LP 2kHz, vertex positivity upwards. Significancy: *p < 0.01 (t-distribution).

MATERIAL AND METHODS

Our patient group consisted of 170 diabetics collected since 1985. In this group the conventional audiometric pure tone thresholds were stated. Then the subgroup of 33 patients was defined consisting only of the patient with normal hearing thresholds, not older than 40 years, with normal levels of plasma lipids and without an exposure to chemical surdogens or noise never in the past. These patients have undergone the auditory evoked potentials test battery comprising brainstem and cortical modalities, frequency and binaural supression tests /Nicolet Pathfinder I/. The data were collected both in native form and as a frequency spectra using Fast Fourier Transformation analysis (FFT).

RESULTS

The incidence of manifest hypoacusia in pure tone audiometry amounts to 20%, prevailing the diagonal threshold decrease pattern. The results of evoked potentials test battery in normal hearing subgroup (n=33) were as follows:

1. All the waves beginning from J-III exert prolongation of latencies which is reflected in prolongation of central transmission time I-V dT (4.32 SD 0.45 versus 4.04 SD 0.14 ms in aged-matched controls /AMC/) using the rate of stimulation 14 Hz in BAEP.

2. The central auditory transmission delay was increased using the higher rate of stimulation 74 Hz (4.69 SD 0.54 versus 4.25 SD 0.16 in AMC) in BAEP. See Figure 1.

3. The abnormalities had a complex structure, being able to distinguish 4 essential types of: distortion only in 74 Hz (15%), distortion in 14 Hz, but not further enhanced in 74 Hz (9%), distortion in 14 Hz enhanced in 74 Hz (9%) and global deterioration (6%). No abnormalitiy, i.e. the results in the range of 2 SD of AMC were found in 61%.

4. The most salient feature of diabetic patient group there is a presence of higher frequency total power in frequency band 0.7-1.2 kHz instead of a greater power in band 0.25-0.4 kHz in AMC. Incidence of this fast generator was apparent in 25% of diabetics. Compare Figures 2 and 3.

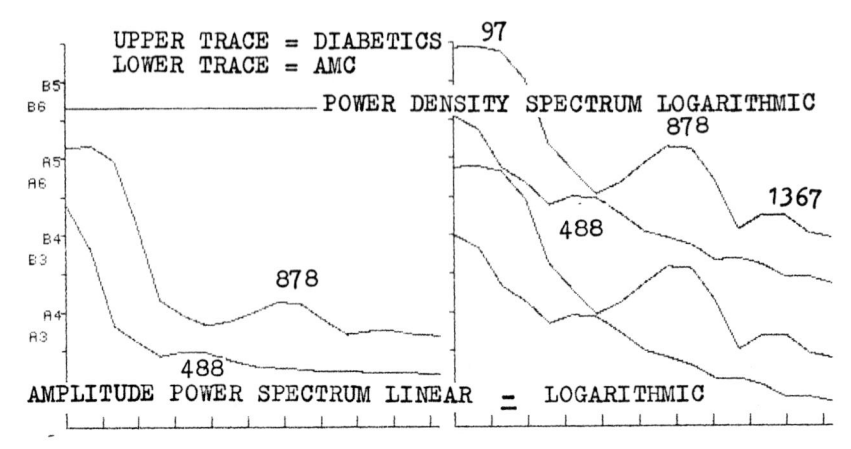

Fig.2. Frequency analysis of BAEP. Peak components are labeled. X-axis = 152 Hz/div.

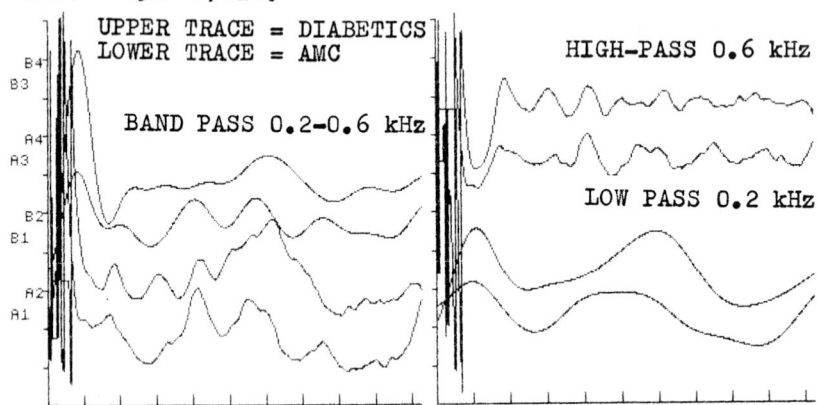

Fig. 3. Digital filtration of BAEP. Note the variable frequency composition of wave I-III e.g. X-axis = 1 ms/div.

LITERATURE

1. Barjon P, Labauge R, Cazaban R, Fabre S (1963) Diabete 11:331-337
2. Zelenka J, Kozak P (1965) J Laryng 79:314-319
3. Reske-Nielsen E, Lundbaek K, Rafaelsen O (1965) Diabetologia 1:233-241
4. Olsson Y, Säve-Soderberg J, Sourander P (1968) Path Europ 3:62-9
5. Kam-Hansen S, Sorensen H (1978) J Laryngol Otol 92:505-10
6. Donald M W, Bird C E, Lawson J S, Letemendia F J J, Monga T N (1981) J Neurol Neurosurg Psych 44:641-644
7. Martini A, Comacchio F, Fedele D, Crepaldi G, Sala O (1987) Acta Otolaryngol (Stockh) 103:620-627

BRAINSTEM AUDITORY EVOKED POTENTIALS IN PATIENTS WITH SUBDURAL HAEMATOMA

LYUBOMIR HARALANOV, SVETLOZAR HARALANOV
Institute of Neurology, Psychiatry and Neurosurgery, Medical Academy, Sofia, Bulgaria

INTRODUCTION

The investigation of the auditory afferent brainstem system by the method of brainstem auditory evoked potentials (BAEPs) of different diseases of the central nervous system is widening its application increasingly. Highly informative and sensitive are the interpeak latencies (IPL) between the three best expressed waves - I^{st}, IIIrd and V^{th} - in cases of brainstem and peripheral damages. Some amplitudinal ratios (AR) are also used, such as the amplitudinal ratio I/V.

The aim of this investigation is to study the changes in the IPL and AR of the BAEPs at different stages of the postoperative period in patients after evacuation of the unilateral subdural haematomae (USH), displaying severe preoperative dislocation of the brain.

MATERIAL AND METHODS

Three patients /male, from 22 to 66 years of age/ with different in size and period USH and two patients in the preoperative period with clinical and CT data for a dislocation of the medial brain structures were investigated. The BAEPs were studied our own original equipment; after click audiometry the normal hearing threshold was established. Then click stimuli of 80-90 dB above hearing threshold, a click rate of 12 Hz and 100 microsec duration were consecutively applied ipsilaterally and binaurally. The analysis time was 12 msec and the sensitivity - 30 microV/div. Needle electrodes were placed on vertex (+) and mastoids - (references). In order to establish the normal IPL I-III, III-V and I-V, as well as the most informative AR, 10 people with normal hearing were investigated. The mean values and standard deviations (SD) were found by the variational analysis, while the normal limits are established using a double-standard deviation.

All patients had a CT investigation of the brain beforehand. A worked-out by us method for establishing the subjective localisation of the binaural stereo click stimulus, applied with the same parameters as in BAEP investigation, was used before and after operative intervention. Through this method the patient gives the deviation of the binaural stimulus laterally from the middle line, left or right, without a receptory auditory damage.

VALENTIN K.R. 22 yrs
CT before operation

LEFT   RIGHT

90 dB
12 Hz

BINAURAL CLICK STIMULATION

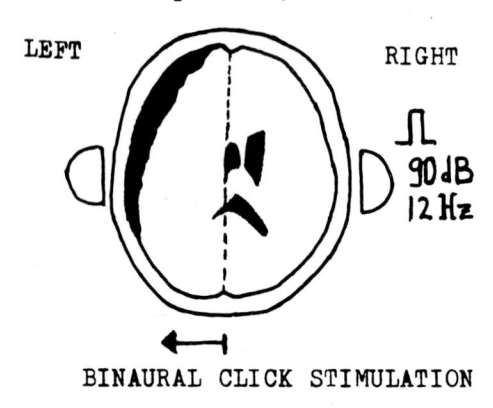

Fig. 1.

RESULTS

In neurosurgical practice during operative tratment of acute and chronic USH the influence of the microvessel circulatory system of the brainstem after acute decompression on the haematoma side, leading to back dislocation of the upper parts of the brainstem, is rarely accounted for.

We tried to preoperatively investigate 2 patients with chronic USH, proved by CT, with clinical data for quantitative disturbances of the consciousness and periods of psychomotor restlessness. In these cases it was not possible to read the changes in BAEPs, because of the provoked by the sound irritation jactitation during the investigation, which strongly changed the configuration of the BAEPs causing a multitude of artefacts by uncontrolled movements of the head.

One of them localised the sound laterally of the middle line, on the side of the haematoma, when he was investigated by our method.

This necessitated a postoperative investigation of the patients.

The first case (V.K.R., a 22-year-old man) had a subacute USH on the left frontal temporal side and clinical data for divergent congenital strabismus, anisocoria with wider pupil on the right side and light left-sided hemiparesis. There were also initial meningeal signs and somnolency in the preoperative period. During the binaural test the patient lateralised the stereo signals 3 cm away from the middle line in the left occipital side. After the evacuation of the haematoma the frontal part of the brain at the end of the operation remained exfoliated with 1.5 cm, while the back parts of the brain restored their normal position.

```
V.K.R. 22 YRS, INV-I/11.XII.87
N:79,80/10,80DB,F:156-2031HZ
GLS-19 POINTS
FIRST DAY AFTER OPERATION
```

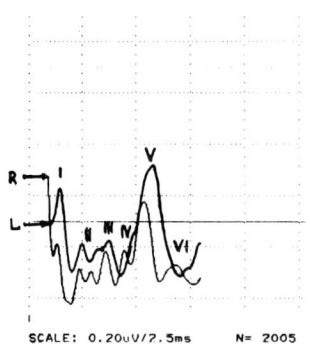

	LEFT	RIGHT	DEFFERENS
I - III :	2.35	2.30	- 0.05 = N
III - V :	2.00	1.75	- 0.25
I - V :	4.35	4.05	- 0.30
I/V :	0.75	0.74	N
III/V :	0.32	0.41	N

SCALE: 0.20uV/2.5ms   N= 2005

Fig. 2.

In the first 12 hours after the operation BAEPs show that the IPL I-V is shorter by 0.30 ms on the right side compared to the same index on the left side as in ipsi- and binaural stimulation. The configurations are normal, which is supported by the ARs of the main waves, as I/V and III/V. On control investigation after 7 days, when there is a complete disappearance of the above clinical symptoms, the results show an equalisation of the IPL on both sides. The binaural stimulus test did not display a lateralisation of the sound, i.e. it was perceived on the middle line.

The second patient (G.S.V., a 66-year-old man) had a chronic USH on the left frontal parietal side. Clinically the patient showed a double vision on looking down, a right-sided hemiparesis and a bradypsyche. He localised the binaural click stimulus on the left side of the mid-line. On the 18th day after the evacuation of the haematoma the postoperative left-sided latent hemiparesis continued to persist, while the double vision had gone. BAEPs showed equal bilateral IPLs, while the AR I/V was disturbed on left ipsilateral stimulation, because of a relatively lower amplitude of the Vth wave.

```
G.S.V. 66 YRS. INV-18 DAYS AFTER EVACUATION
IPSILATERAL STIMULATION      HEMISPHERE-LEFT
80 DB, 30MKV, F: 156-2031HZ
```

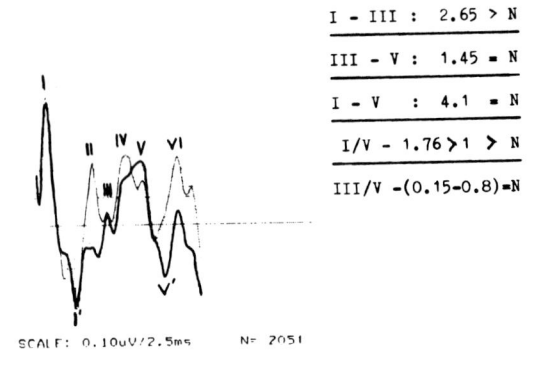

```
I - III  :  2.65 > N
III - V  :  1.45 = N
I - V    :  4.1  = N
I/V - 1.76 > 1 > N
III/V - (0.15-0.8) = N
```

Fig. 3.

The 3rd case with USH on the right side did not establish a lateralisation in the binaural stimulus test and the BAEPs were bilaterally normal after operation.

Analysis of the results shows that in V.K.R.'s case the lateralisation of the click stimuli is probably due to lack of symmetry when transpassing the afferent auditory impulses on brainstem level, caused by paradoxical decrease in the brainstem transmission time on the right side (opposite the side of the haematoma). As a result from the changes in the microcirculation, caused by brainstem dislocation, a change in the phase type conductance appears on the right side. In support of this is the fact that in the period of clinical normalisation the right IPL equalise with those of the ipsilateral side of the haematoma.

The next case: the changes are basically in the configuration as a result of disturbed generation of the Vth wave on the side of the haematoma. Probably the changes are due to damage after evacuation of the haematoma due to acute decompression and microcirculatory disturbances on this side.

CONCLUSION

In an attempt to investigate the BAEPs before operative evacuation of the USH with subacute or chronic behaviour in the stage of mental derangement the interpretation of the results is rather complicated, because artefacts caused by uncontrolled movements of the patient's head. Sedation is contraindicative because of the unclear clinical signs, whose control is extremely important until the operation. Cases of acute decompression caused by evacuation of chronic USH there are conditions for back dislocation of the brainstem structures and disturbance in the microcirculation of the brainstem blood circulation.

BRAINSTEM AUDIOMETRY IN PATIENTS WITH HEAD TRAUMA

YASUKO IMASATO ITO, TEOTONIO T. COSTA NETO, FABIO AKIRA SUZUKI,
RICARDO GALVANI FELIPE, HELOISA H. CAOVILLA, MAURÍCIO M. GANANÇA
Dept. of Otorhinolaringology, Escola Paulista de Medicina,
Rua Botucatu, 740-3º andar, 04023, São Paulo, Brazil

INTRODUCTION

Structural abnormalities like tumors, multiple sclerosis, infarction can be detected with radiologic techniques while functional anomalies caused by head injury are mor difficult to be assessed.

The sensory evoked potential studies have been most often used for clinical help for the localization of the dysfunction and thr prognosis for recovery in cerebral concussion (Pauline et al, 1984).

Among the auditory evoked potential, the "early" or brainstem responses elicited by clicks have been of relevant importance in the clinical setting. This electrical response can be recorded from the sclps of humans using computer averaging techniques (Rosenberg et al 1984).

The noninvasive nature, the technical ease of this testing procedure and the response stability in the presence of attention changes, light sleep, mild sedation, consciousness level, metabolic disturbances or drug make the use of auditory brainstem evoked potential (BAEP) quite feasible.

The peak latencies of I, III and V waves and the interpeak latencies (I-III, III-V and I-V) did not practically vary if the features of the stimulus were always the same (Davis, 1976). The clinical value of this evoked potential is based upos the measure of these latencies.

Schoenhuber et al (1983) examined 37 patients within 48 hous after a mild head injury. About half of these patients showed signs of cerebral dysfunction at the BAEP. The authors have seen that there is a great evidence of BAEP alteration if the patients were examined in the first 2 days after the head trauma.

Rowe & Carlson (1980) and Benna et al (1982) have found similar results in patients evaluated in a period of more than 1 month later, 41% and 44%, respectively. And according to Benna et al (1982), in a few patients retested after some months there was a tendency to recover.

On the other hand, in cases of severe head injury, in coma, the survival was related to the simultaneous preservation of long and middle latency and brainstem evoked potentials. The preservation of just middle-latency and/or brainstem components did not correlate with survival. In patients who survived, there was no pattern of evoked potential preservation that related to the quality of survival (Rosenberg et al, 1984; Karnaze et al, 1985).

Scherg et al (1984) have detected BAEP abnormalities in only 2 patients of 35 post-comatose patients evaluated after severe closed head trauma. These abnormalities consisted of lateral asymmetries, but not prolonged interpeak latencies or abnormal amplitude ratios. The investigators concluded that the BAEP does not sufficiently reveal brainstem lesions expected to persist after severe closed head trauma.

The BAEP of 35 patients with post-traumatic coma within the first 4 days following head injury, assessed by Cant et al (1986) showed an increase in the wave I-V interval or the loss of any all of its 3 most atable components (waves I, III and V). Although abnormal BAEP were associated with an unfavourable outcome in almost all patients (6 of 7), only 19 of 28 patients with normal BAEP had a favourable outcome. The finding of normal BAEP was therefore of little prognostic significance.

The objective of this present study was to analyze the presence of BAEP abnormalities in 8 patients after mild head injury in order to detect some organic affection in the Central Nervous System.

MATERIAL AND METHODS

BAEP studies were performed in 8 mild head injured patients admitted to the Neurosurgery Department of Escola Paulista de Medicina. They came to the Otorhinolaryngology Department within 1 week to 3 months after the trauma.

Their age ranged from 6 to 55 years. Five males and 3 females. Six patients had got headache, 2 presented complains about hearing loss. All the patients complained about difficult in the maintenance of balance, which had disappeared when they were examined in our Department. Five of them lost consciousness for a short time without posterior repercussion.

None of them presented neurological damage during the otorhinolaryngologic assessment. Only one patient showed blood in the middle ear. This patient was examined 2 months later again after the remission of middle ear damage.

All the patients were submitted to the otoneurological examination pure tone audiometry, impedance test, BAEP and vectornystagmography (Mangabeira Albernaz et al, 1986).

BRAINSTEM AUDITORY EVOKED POTENTIAL

The BAEP recordings were made in a shielded, sound attenuated room under standard conditions using Amplaid-MK10 clinical averaging system. The rate of stimulation was set at 11/s. Percutaneous silver electrodes were placed at the vertex (Cz) and both earlobes with the common reference electrode being placed on the earlobe contralateral to the estimulated ear, the amplifier band width was 50-2500Hz. A total of 2000 responses collected in the first 12ms duration were averaged. Latencies of individual and interpeak latencies in miliseconds were studied.

RESULTS

Six patients presented normal audiograms and the 2 patients who complain about hearing, showed audiological tests results, as following:

PATIENT A

PURE TONE AUDIOMETRY

	250	500	1K	2K	3K	4K	6K	8K Hz
Right ear								
AC	70	65	65	50	55	55	55	50 dB
BC		15	15	20	20	20		

Left ear: normal

PATIENT B
right ear
AC	10	15	10	50	70	70	70	60
BC				50	70	70		

left ear
AC	10	15	30	70	80	95	90	85
BC			30	70	↓	↓		

BRAISTEM AUDITORY EVOKED POTENTIAL

The BAEP results were compared to the control group obtained from 50 normal sublects, 25 males and 25 females (Costa Neto, 1990) showing normal BAEP recordings in 6 patients. The 2 patients with hearing loss presented BAEP recordings as following:

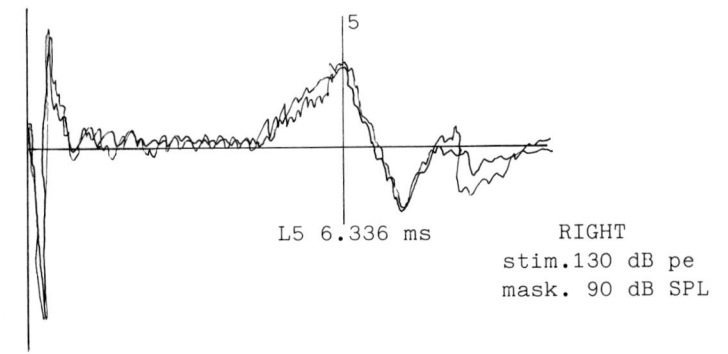

PATIENT A

L5 6.336 ms   RIGHT
                     stim.130 dB pe
                     mask. 90 dB SPL

PATIENT B: abscence of the responses bilaterally.

DISCUSSION

The assessment of the brainstem auditory pathway in mild head injured patients examined within 1 week to 3 months after cerebral concussion did not reveal alterations showing Central Nervous System damage in BAEP recordings in 8 post trauma patients.

These findings quite disagree with that found in severe head injured patient, which showed lots of abnormalities in mild, moderate, darked and severely abnormal levels (Karnaze et al, 1985).

We can say that our results were normal, because the only 2 BAEP recordings showing abnormalities, one with a long V peak latency and the other one with response abscences are in agreement with the hearing loss detected by pure tone audiometry in these 2 patients.

On the other hand, Schoenhuber et al (1983) have found abnormal BAEPs in almost half of post cerebral concussion patients examined within 2 days after light head injury. These abnormalities seen within 48 hours of post trauma may suggest that the BAEP assessment made within 1 week to 3 months with normal patterns are showing that the damage caused by trauma is reversible.

CONCLUSION

From the results obtained in our present investigation in 8 mild head injured patients, we would like to make the following comments:
1. the abnormal BAEP recordings were in agreement with the hearing loss detected by pure tone audiometry,
2. there was no abnormality in the brainstem auditory pathway.

REFERENCES
1. Benna R, Bergamasco B, Bianco C, Gilli M, Ferrero P, Pinessi L- Brainstem auditory evoked potentials in postconcussion syndrome. Ital. J. Neurol. Sci., 4:281-7, 1982.
2. Cant BR, Hume AL, Judson JA, Shaw NA - The assessment of severe head injury by short latency somatosensory and brainstem auditory evoked potentials. Electroenceph Clin Neurophysiol, 65:188-95 1986
3. Costa Neto TT- Influência do sexo e do tamanho da cabeça nas latências da audiometria de tronco cerbral. São Paulo, 1990. 56p. (Tese-Mestrado-Escola Paulista de Medicina)
4. Davis H - Electric response audiometry eith special reference to the vertex potentials. In: Nelf WD, Keidel WD - Handbook of sensory Physiology. Berlin, Heidelberg, New York, Springer-Verlag, 1976.
5. Karnaze D, Weiner JM, Marshall LF- Auditory evoked potential in coma after closed head injury. Neuroloy,35:1122-6, 1985.
6. Mangabeira Albernaz PL, Ganança MM, Caovilla HH, Ito YI, Novo NF Juliano Y- Aspectos clínicos e terapêuticos das vertigens. Acta AWHO, ! (Supp 2):49-109, 1986.
7. Newlon PG, Greenberg RP- Evoked potentials in severe head injury. J trauma, 24:61-6, 1984.
8. Rosenberg C, Wogensen K, Starr A- Auditory brain-stem and middle and long-latency evoked potentials in coma. Arch Neurol,41:835-8, 1984.
9. Rowe MJ, Carlson C- Brainstem auditory evoked potentials in post concussion dizziness. Arch Neurol, 37:679-83, 1980.
10. Scherg M, Cramon DV, Elton M- Brain-stem auditory-evoked potentials in post-comatose patients after severe closed head trauma. Neurology, 231:1-5, 1984.
11. Schoenhuber P, Bortolli P Malavasi P, Marzolini S, Tonelli L, Merli GA- Brainstem auditory evoked potentials in early evaluation of cerebral concussion. J Neuros Sci, 27:157-9, 1983.

TREATMENT

INFUSION THERAPY IN POSTTRAUMATIC HEARING DEFECTS AND DISORDERS OF BALANCE

STEFAN SPITZER, HANS-JÜRGEN WILHELM, HOLGER KIESEWETTER, FRIEDRICH JUNG, AND HERMANN-JOSEF SCHIEFFER

Medical and Outpatient Hospital, Internal Medicine III (Cardiology), [1]Dept. of Otorhinolaryngology, [2]Dept. of Clinical Haemostasiology and Transfusion Medicine, University Hospitals of the Saarland,
6650 Homburg-Saar (West-Germany)

INTRODUCTION

Hearing defects and disorders of balance after mechancial traumas such as commotio labirinthi or fractures of the petrous bone with delayed paresis of the facial nerve can be produced by the direct alteration of the censory cells or by vascular occlusions caused by swellings and bleedings or in connection with a consumptive coagulopathy. An acute phase reaction which often is characterized by an increase in fibrinogen, α1-antitrypsin, ceruloplasmine and haptoglobin[1+2], can also lead to hyperviscosity finally resulting in a rheological vascular occlusion[3]. Another possible lesion of the organ of hearing can be caused by an acoustic trauma leading to specific lesions of the hair cells, i.e. swelling[4], microbleedings in the cochlea and vestibular organ as well as a rupture of the tympanic membrane in some cases[5+6]. For this reason, it seems to be useful to increase the perfusion therapeutically in case of posttraumatic hearing defects and disorders of balance.

FLUIDITY OF BLOOD

The fluidity of blood is a complex parameter which cannot be clearly determined by physics. Blood is not a Newton's fluid such as water, oil or alcohol the viscosity of which is temperature dependent. It is a suspension of 40-50% of cells in a Newton's fluid, that is the blood plasma. The viscosity of blood does not only depend on the temperature but also on the velocity with which it passes through the vessels. Besides, the blood segregates on passing through the vessels. In the central flow the red blood cells are more concentrated than in the peripheral flow.

Furthermore, the cells are not equally distributed within the singular capillaries of the capillary system, the arterioles, capillaries and venules. The haematocrit in the so-called nutritive capillaries (also called supply capillaries) is about only 15%, in the shunt capillaries, however, this value can be more than twice as high.

Therefore, it is not relevant for the clinician to determine the so-called whole blood viscosity by means of plate-conic viscosimeters. The measurement of influence parameters, however, reveals clinically important data. The fluidity of blood depends on the following rheological parameters: the viscosity of plasma, haematocrit, thrombocyte aggregation, erythrocyte aggregation, erythrocyte rigidity and leucocyte adhesivity.

In addition to anamnesis and clinical examination for the determination of the patient's condition the most important rheological parameters should be measured in order to optimize therapy. These parameters are haematocrit, plasma viscosity, and thrombocyte aggregation. The methods of measurement and reference ranges are given in Table I.

TABLE I

PARAMETERS OF MEASUREMENT, METHODS AND REFERENCE RANGES

Parameter	Symbol	Method	Reference range		
Plasma viscosity	PV	Capillary tube plasma viscosimeter[7]	1.14-1.34	mPa.s	8
Haematocrit	Hct	Impedance method[7]	m: 39-52 f: 34-50	% %	8
Thrombocyte aggregation index	TAI	Cell count[9]	1.0-1.05	-	9

RHEOLOGICAL THERAPY

In addition to the basic therapy and after checking of the surgical possibilities, a hypervolaemic haemodilution with hydroxyethyl starch should be made. On haematocrit values above 42% the haemodilution should be combined with venesections of 250 ml. The procedure should be executed as described in the following: rapid infusion of 250 ml hydroxyethyl starch (within 20-30 minutes), then venesection of 250 ml blood (10-15 minutes), finally infusion of the remaining 250 ml within 15 to 20 minutes. The whole procedure should not exceed one hour. The most suitable starch in patients who are not tolerating too much volume or with a rather low hyperviscosity (plasma viscosity below 1.4 mPa.s) is Haes 200/0.5 10% (Haes steril®, Fresenius AG). Only if spontaneous thrombocyte aggregation is increased pathologically and if the risk of bleeding can be excluded 2x2 ampoules of Prostaglandin E1 (Prostavasin®) should be administered daily every 12 hours. The effect of the thrombocyte aggregation inhibition should be tested according to Grotemeyer[9]. If the acute phase reaction is considerable with fibrinogen values over 600 mg/dl a bag plasmapheresis is recommended[10], that is on haematocrit values equal to or less than 42% 500 ml blood are withdrawn after the administration of 500 ml hydroxyethyl starch. Erythrocytes are re-infused after sedimentation or centrifugation and the plasma collected is substituted for hydroxyethyl starch. This procedure can be applied every day; it should be tried to achieve a hypervolaemia of 250-500 ml. A combination therapy with a rheologically active substance such as naftidrofuryl (600 mg Dusodril® per day) oder pentoxifylline (1,200 mg Trental® per day)[11] is also useful in order to decrease plasma viscosity (by inhibition of the fibrinogen synthesis and intravascular accumulation of fluid due to the rheoregulation), erythrocyte aggregation, erythrocyte rigidity, and to inhibit leucocyte adhesivity. In case of consumptive coagulopathies it is necessary to heparinise with a low dose (4 U/kg body weight/h). The concentration of antithrombin III must be controlled, it should be greater than 80%. Otherwise, it must be substituted. It may also become necessary to substitute fresh plasma in case of a disturbed endogenic coagulation system and Prothrombin Proconvertin Stuart Prower Factor (PPSB) if the exogenic system is disturbed.

Immediately after trauma it is also possible to give cortisone in an established dose of 250 mg per day over four days and then a continuously decreasing dose over a period of ten days.

The intensive rheological therapy should be continued over a period of at least ten days but not longer than a fortnight. Own experiences concerning patients suffering from a posttraumatic loss of hearing show that it is possible to regain about 50% of the ability to hear.

REFERENCES
1. Jung M, Koppensteiner R, Graninger W, Minar E, Kretschmer G, Ehringer H (1988) Klin Wochenschr 66: 379-384

2. Mozes G, Friedman N, Shainkin-Kestenbaum R (1989) The Journal of Trauma 29 (1): 71-74

3. Kiesewetter H, Radtke H, Jung F, Schmid-Schönbein H, Wortberg G (1982) Biorheology 19: 363-374

4. Liberman MC, Dodds LW (1987) Hear Res 26 (1): 45-64

5. Lenarz T, Guelzow J (1983) Laryngol Rhinol Oto 62 (2): 58-61

6. Ylikoski J (1989) Scand Audiol 18 (3): 161-165

7. Kiesewetter H (1988) In: Kriessmann A (ed), Meßmethoden für die Blutfluidität. Aktuelle Diagnostik und Therapie in der Angiologie, Thieme Verlag, Stuttgart, pp. 66-72

8. Jung F, Kiesewetter H, Roggenkamp HG, Nüttgens HP, Ringelstein EB, Gerhards M, Kotitschke G, Wenzel E, Zeller H (1986) Klin Wochenschr 64: 375

9. Grotemeyer KH, Viand R, Beykirch K (1983) Dtsch med Wschr 108: 775

10. Kiesewetter H, Blume J, Jung F, Gerhards M, Spitzer S, Leipnitz G, Wenzel E (1988) Klin Wochenschr 66: 284-291

11. Pilgramm M, Schumann K (1986) HNO 34 (10): 424-428

TRANS-ETHMOID DECOMPRESSION OF THE OPTIC NERVE FOR POST-TRAUMATIC BLINDNESS

M. V. KIRTANE, S. R. NAYAK, M. V. INGLE
E.N.T. DEPTT. K.E.M. HOSPITAL, PAREL, BOMBAY 400 012, INDIA

INTRODUCTION

The incidence of visual impairment following closed head injuries is reported to vary from 2% to 5%. Compression of the optic nerve is one of the causes which may be reversible if timely decompression surgery is performed. The trans-cranial route for decompression of the Optic Nerve is not popular due to relatively poor results compared to the risk and morbidity of an intra-cranial surgery. The trans-ethmoidal route popularized by Miwa and Fukado[1] offers a relatively safe extra-cranial route, for decompressing the Optic Nerve Canal. This presentation discusses our experience with this technique used in 76 patients over the past 13 years.

CLINICAL PRESENTATION

The diagnosis of an optic foramen fracture is suggested clinically by the presence of an injury in the temporal region, with associated epistaxis, and an absent or sluggish direct pupillary reflex[1,2]. A consensual pupillary reflex elicited by stimulation of the opposite eye is usually present. The vision may be completely lost, or perception of light may be present in one or more of the quadrants. Plain X-rays delineating the optic foramen may show the fracture; however, tomograms or CT Scan may sometimes be necessary. At times a fracture may be missed even on tomography and the only certain way to detect the fracture is at surgery.

It is our contention that, in view of the relative safety of the operative procedure and the improbability of spontaneous recovery, suspected cases should be subjected to decompression of the optic foramen, even in the absence of positive radiological findings.

CLINICAL DATA

Seventysix cases of post-traumatic blindness with suspected compression in the region of the optic canal were seen by us over a thirteen year period from 1977 to 1989. Seventy patients were male while six were females, the youngest being 10 years old and oldest 45 years old. The 76 cases which were explored had suffered the injuries in vehicular accidents. Each of these cases had unilateral involvement only, the other eye being unaffected.

Of the 76 patients who underwent surgery 20 patients were seen within the first two days, 18 between the 2nd and 4th day, 12 within 4th to 7th day while the remaining 26 came after one week was over. All them were examined in detail by an ophthalmololgist before being referred to us. Any other serious intracranial pathology was excluded.

OPERATIVE PROCEDURE

The operation is performed under general anaesthesia(3,4). An incision is made which extends from 0.5 cm. medial to the medial canthus of the eye, and then curves laterally, parallel to and about 0.5 cm. below the eyebrow. The medial palpebral ligament is exposed and divided and the underlying periosteum of the medial wall of the orbit is elevated as widely as possible. The superior oblique muscle is displaced off the trochlea. The eyeball is gently retracted laterally. Sometimes, when needed, a Killian's long-bladed self-retaining nasal speculum may be used to achieve this retraction. The anterior and posterior ehtmoidal vessels are diathermized and divided. Adrenaline-soaked gauze strips are packed into the depth of the dissection, as required, to achieve haemostatis during the procedure. At a depth of about 4.5 cm. to 5 cm, in the same straight line as the anterior and posterior ethmoidal vessels, the prominence of the medial margin of the optic foramen is seen.

For better visualisation and greater clarity we use the operating microscope with a 300 mm. objective lens. The microscope is brought into use once the ethmoidal vessels are visualised. From here onwards all dissection is done under microscopic vision. The last step, viz. decompression of the optic nerve, is achieved by removing any fractured fragments of bone. Further decompression may be achieved by removing the medial lip of the optic foramen with the help of a curette or a small elevator or forceps. The sheath of the optic nerve is not opened. A soft rubber drain is retained for 48 hours. The periosteum of the maxillary and nasal bones and the medial palpebral ligament are sutured together with 3-0 catgut. The skin is sutured with prolene. A padded eye-dressing is applied. The patient is prescribed antibiotics post-operatively for one week, and the sutures are removed on the fifth post-operative day.

The commonest finding at surgery was a fracture of the ethmoids with a fracture of the inferomedial wall of the optic canal with a haematoma compressing the optic nerve (57 patients). A fracture of the thick ring of the optic foramen was seen in 21 patients with a distinct abrasion/laceration of the nerve in 17 patients. We have operated on 76 cases during the past 13 years and of these, 21 have shown improvement of vision, varying from perception of light to normal vision. None of the patients had any serious or significant post-operative complications.

DISCUSSION

Fukado(2) who reported 400 cases of surgical decompression of the optic nerve, found a remarkably high incidence of recovery of vision especially in those patients who were operated upon very early. He followed up these patients for a period of one year without any deterioration in the vision regained. This prompted us to operate on the cases of traumatic blindness referred to us by our ophthalmologist colleagues who from past experience felt that spontaneous recovery was unlikely.(4)

The operation of optic nerve decompression has in the past been performed by the neurosurgeon via a frontal craniotomy. The exposure was limited and the results unsatisfactory. The operation carried the risks associated with a craniotomy and hence the procedure is not often practised.

The transethmoidal route as described by Fukado is totally extracranial and therefore devoid of any complications. The area of operation, viz. the posterior ethmoidal region, is familiar to the oto-rhino-laryngologist and the use of an operating microscope ensures good illumination and adequate visualisation of the various structures in that area.

The radiographic demonstration of a fracture in the optic foramen is not an absolute pre-requisite to surgery.(4) One of our cases that showed complete recovery of function had a fracture in the posterior ethmoid region without any fracture in the optic foramen. Evacuation of the posterior ethmoidal haematoma which was pressing on the optic nerve led to complete recovery.

On the other hand, fragments from the fractured margin of the optic foramen tend to lacerate the nerve and thus worsen the prognosis. This makes us feel that the cases which carry the best prognolsis are those with haematomas without fractures of the optic foramen.

One point that required deliberation was whether the sheath of the nerve should be incised as for the facial nerve in Bell's paralysis.

Theoretically, an intraneural haematoma or oedema would be decompressed by such a manoeuvre. However, as the nerve sheath in this region consists of the layers of the meninges and the pia mater carries the vascular supply to the nerve (which is considered to be an extension of the brain itself), incising the sheath would jeopardize the blood supply to the nerve. Hence we desist from incising the sheath.

CONCLUSION

Blindness following injury around the eye may result from compression of the optic nerve in its canal. A transethmoidal approach to this region allows an easy and satisfactory decompression of the nerve. Since it is the general experience that such traumatic blindness almost never recovers spontaneously, surgery seems to be the only answer.

Surgery in this region is not new to the oto-rhino-laryngologist and his familiarity with the operative field, coupled with the use of an operating microscope, make the procedure very safe.

Though in our series of 76 operated cases only 21 showed recovery of vision, we strongly advocate surgery in such cases as the procedure is safe and spontaneous recovery unlikely.

REFERENCES

1. Miwa, T., and Fukado, Y. (1967) Industrial Health (Japan), 5, 50.
2. Fukado, Y. (1973) Proceedings of the 2nd International Symposium on Orbital disorders, Amsterdam, 1973, Vol. 14, pp. 474-484 (Karger, Basel, 1975).
3. Strohm, M. (1979) Personal communication.
4. Karnik, P.P., Maskati, B.T., Kirtane, M.V. et al (1983) Optic nerve decompression in head injuries. The Journal of Laryngology and Otology, 95 : 1135-1140.

Address for correspondence

Dr. M. V. Kirtane
Gokul, 3, Tejpal Road,
Bombay 400 007
INDIA

SELECTIVE CHEMICAL VESTIBULECTOMY FOR THE SURGICAL TREATMENT OF INTRACTABLE MENIERE'S DISEASE

CHARLES H. NORRIS, PH.D., RONALD G. AMEDEE, M.D.

Department of Otolaryngology-Head and Neck Surgery, Tulane University Medical School, 1430 Tulane Avenue, New Orleans, Louisiana, 70112, U.S.A.

INTRODUCTION

Vertigo attributable to Meniere's disease is managed successfully medically in 75% to 80% of affected patients through psychologic support, salt restriction, systemic diuretics, and when necessary, labyrinthine sedatives. The remaining 20% to 25% of the patients not responsive to medical therapy are usually offered a surgical alternative which involves unpredictable results in the case of endolymphatic sac decompression,[7,8,9,10,11] difficult surgical techniques with vestibular nerve section,[3,4] and profound hearing loss in labyrinthectomized patients.[12] An alternative procedure has been developed in our laboratories[12,13] that can diminish these complications by introducing streptomycin directly into the lateral semicircular canal of the involved labyrinth resulting in selective chemical destruction of the involved vestibular labyrinth (balance organ) while preserving the cochlear division (hearing organ) of the inner ear.

In 1956 Schuknecht reported on the treatment of bilateral Meniere's disease using intramuscular streptomycin to selectively destroy vestibular function in both ears and at the same time conserve hearing.[5] It should be noted that in five out of eight such cases, sustained improvement in auditory thresholds was observed. However, the importance of frequent auditory and vestibular testing associated with the patients prolonged periods of ataxia must be considered. More recently attempts have been made to titrate the streptomycin dosage in such a way that the symptoms of the Meniere's syndrome are ablated while hearing as well as some vestibular function are conserved.[6] It should be emphasized that great caution and supervision must be exercised in the use of this therapy. First, one must be very careful to get enough of the streptomycin effect to at least eliminate the vertiginous episodes but at the same time keep the dosage low enough to prevent deterioration of hearing. Secondly, systemic streptomycin affects both ears and therefore the therapy is not indicated in unilateral cases (the majority of the initial presenting cases).

We have developed a procedure using streptomycin which is simple, eliminates the episodes of vertigo, potentially conserves hearing, does not affect the uninvolved ear, and can be done as a "short-stay" surgical procedure. With this procedure patients experience a rapid recovery from initial postoperative vertigo and ataxia. It is analogous to a vestibular neurectomy in that its goal is to permanently block sensory information (originating within the involved vestibular end organs) from ever reaching the central nervous system. Preliminary animal and patient data from our laboratories were first reported at the Spring 1987 meeting of the American Otological Society.[12,13]

METHODS

Under general anesthesia, a postauricular approach is made to the horizontal semicircular canal. Bone is gently drilled away from a small area over the canal revealing the membranous duct. A small hole is made in the membranous duct and endolymph is allowed to mix with perilymph. A solid flake of streptomycin is absorbed onto a tiny piece of moist gelfoam. The gelfoam is placed between the bony canal and membranous duct on the end of the fenestration nearest the cristae ampullaris. The flake of streptomycin is formed in the following manner: 1 mg of streptomycin powder is weighed out in a sterile dish. This is then divided into eight equal separate and distinct piles of powder. A very small drop of absolute alcohol is added to each pile. After three to five minutes, the alcohol has completely evaporated leaving a firm flake of 125 micrograms of streptomycin in the place of each pile of powder. During surgery this flake is easily transferred on a piece of saline moistened gelfoam. The defect in the bony canal is then covered with gelfoam and fascia while the mastoid cavity is closed in a usual manner.

The patient selection criteria used in our procedure is:

1. Male or female adult patients of age 18 years and older.
2. Presence of intractable Meniere's disease documented by a thorough otolaryngologic history, physical exam, audiometric evaluation, and electronystagmographic analysis.
3. Presence of intractable Meniere's disease in patients who have received accepted medical treatment (e.g. low salt diet, diuretics, and vestibular suppressants).
4. Ability to tolerate general anesthesia.
5. Patients who have failed endolymphatic sac decompression surgery or retrolabyrinthine vestibular nerve section were not excluded from consideration.
6. Patients who have failed previous surgery which resulted in a postoperative CSF leak requiring surgical repair were excluded.
7. Patients with other forms of labyrinthine dysfunction may also be considered provided they meet the above criteria.

During the procedure, the cochlear compound eighth nerve action potential is monitored to assure that hearing is not compromised. Monitoring is done by means of an electrode placed in a mastoid air cell near the cochlea. Also vestibular and cochlear functions are periodically monitored pre- and postoperatively. In our patients pure tone and speech discrimination audiometric tests and a standard ENG test employing the Hallpike bithermal, binaural calorics are used.

RESULTS

After three years of animal research, 14 patients in our clinic have received this procedure as treatment for intractable Meniere's Disease which has failed accepted medical therapy. The initial 7 patients had 250 ug of streptomycin placed in the lateral semicircular canal and only 2 of the 7 had a hole made in the membranous labyrinth. The other 7 patients received 125 ug of streptomycin and all 7 had holes made in the membranous labyrinth. The longest postoperative follow-up is only one year, and most of the initial 7 patients in the 250 ug group sustained a 20-30 db loss of hearing loss with time. Many of these initial patients had pure tone thresholds near the 50-70 db level with very poor discrimination scores. In the second group of 7 patients treated with 125 ug of streptomycin, hearing levels were actually improved postoperatively except in one patient where technical problems at the time of surgery were felt to contribute to hearing loss. Within two weeks after surgery, all 14 patients enjoyed complete remission of their vertigo and ataxia. None of the patients in this series to date has had their vestibular symptoms recur. ENG results in all 14 have confirmed no response to calorics in the operated ear. In all patients the tinnitus levels have fluctuated but in none has it been made subjectively worse by the surgery. All patients who had a sensation of fullness in the ear pre-operatively reported relief of that symptom post-operatively.

CONCLUSION

Selective chemical vestibulectomy of the peripheral vestibular organ destroys the vestibular receptors and prevents further vertiginous episodes. Preservation and/or improvement of hearing appears obtainable with the correct dose of streptomycin. The fact that some patients did lose hearing was not acceptable to us and this is the reason for continued research with smaller doses of streptomycin. This procedure is not necessarily the final solution to problem patients with intractable Meniere's Disease, but this type of research and clinical application appears to be a step in a new and correct direction.

REFERENCES

1. Pulec JL (1974) Labyrinthectomy: indications, technique and results. *Laryngoscope* 84:1522-1573.
2. Kemink JL, Telian SA, Graham MD, Joynt L (1989) Transmastoid labyrinthectomy: reliable surgical management of vertigo. *Otolaryngol Head and Neck, No. 1, 101:5-10.*
3. Fisch Up (1973) Excision of Scarpa's ganglion. *Arch Otolaryngol* 97:147-149.
4. McDaniel AB, Silverstein H, Norrel H (1985) Retrolabyrinthine vestibular neurectomy with and without monitoring of eighth nerve potentials. *Am J Otol* November:23-26.
5. Schuknecht HF (1956) Ablation therapy for relief of Meniere's disease. *Laryngoscope* 66:859-870.
6. Graham MD, Sataloff RT, Kemink JL (1984) Titration streptomycin therapy for bilateral Meniere's disease: a preliminary report. *Otolaryngol Head and Neck,* No. 4, 92:440-447.
7. Portmann G (1927) Vertigo: surgical treatment by opening the saccus endolymphaticus. *Arch Otolaryngol,* No. 4, 6:309-319.
8. House WF (1964) Subarachnoid shunt for drainage of hydrops. *Arch Otolaryngol* 79:338-354.
9. Smith WC, Pillsbury HC (1988) Surgical treatment of Meniere's disease since Thomsen. *Am J Otol,* No.1, 9:39-43.
10. Thomsen J, Bretlau P, Tos M, Johnsen NJ (1981) Placebo effect in surgery for Meniere's disease. *Arch Otolaryngol* 107:271-277.
11. Bretlau P, Thomsen J, Tos M, Johnsen NJ (1989) Placebo effect in surgery for Meniere's disease: nine-year follow up. *Am J Otol,* No. 4, Vol. 10.
12. Norris CH, Brocato GD, Sawatsky SL, Tabb HG (1988) Application of streptomycin to the lateral semicircular canal. *Transactions of the American Otological Society* 75:84-88.
13. Shea JJ (1988) Perfusion of the inner ear with streptomycin. *Transactions of the American Otological Society* 75:89-91.

POST-OPERATIVE VERTIGO IN CHRONIC EAR SURGERY

GAVALAS G., PAPAMICHALOPOULOS M., DOKIANAKIS G., PAVLOPOULOS A.
ENT-Department and Department of Audiology/Neuro-otology
The Red Cross Hospital of Athens (Greece).

SUMMARY

Vertigo after chronic ear surgery mainly occurs in patients with vertebro-basilar insufficiency, functional disorders of the eustachian tube and in the cases of expansive and infected cholesteatoma with labyrinthine fistula. It can also occur, in a few cases of iatrogenic labyrinthine trauma, vestibular neuronitis, labyrinthitis, after the use of local anaesthetics and other reasons as well. Although we have operated on 5230 ears in the last 10 years in our department, post-operative vertigo remains a rare manifestation. In our presentation, we want to emphasize the significance of the pre-operative study, of the deep knowledge in the otosurgical techniques and of the post-operative care, for the avoidance of the patient's mismanagement. Finally, we stress the importance of the neuro-otological control in the differentiation of the post-operative vestibular disorders.

INTRODUCTION

Post-operative vertigo in chronic ear surgery constitutes a rare manifestation although the number of operations has enormously increased in the last years. The fact that otosurgeons are more numerous and more experienced, surgical techniques have improved and the surgical instrumentation has been completed and perfected, is a clear indication that vertigo after chronic otitis media is not exclusively related to surgery, but also to other factors. Nevertheless, after the appearance of vertigo, the following questions have to be answered by the surgeon:
1. What is the real cause of vertigo?
2. Is vertigo closely related or not with the surgical technique?
3. Which therapeutical management has to be followed?
As in the world literature vertigo is of multifactorial origin, we have tried to present in this paper the experience of our department.

MATERIAL

In the last 10 years, more than 5.000 operations have been performed for chronic ear disease in the E.N.T. department of the Red

Cross Hospital of Athens. Most of the patients with cholsteatoma (60%), presented a chronically discharging ear, eroded ossicles and granulation tissue. The majority of the patients were operated on under general anaesthesia, by 9 different otosurgeons, using the following surgical methods:
- Radical mastoidectomy in 39% of the cases
- Mastoidectomy with tympanoplasty (type III, IV) in 24%
- Myringoplasty and tympanoplasty in 21%
- Myringotomy in 8%
- Modified radical mastoidectomy in 8%

It is remarcable to say that in 10% of the patients with mastoidectomy, an otic capsule fistula caused by an expanding cholsteatoma, was discovered intraoperatively. Analysing the cases of post-operative vertigo, the following etiological factors were determined:
1. Myringotomy
2. Functional disorders of the eustachian tube
3. Local anaesthesia
4. Expansive and infected cholsteatoma
5. Labyrinthine trauma
6. Labyrinthitis
7. Removal of ear packing
8. Cold ear drops post-operatively
9. Miscellaneous causes:
    a. Vertebro-basilar insufficiency
    b. Psychological factors
    c. Meniere disease
    d. Vestibular neuronitis due to a post-operative viral infection
    e. Post-operative bedrest

By every patient, pure tone audiometry, tympanometry in some cases and fistula test in cholsteatomatous otitis media were performed. The vestibular examination which was carried out mainly constituted of:
- Search for spontaneous nystagmus
- Headshake nystagmus
- Positional tests
- Pendular tests
- Vestibulo-spinal reflexes

DISCUSSION

Through our discussion we will try to reveal the etiological factors of post-operative vertigo, in order to prevent the symptom and to treat the cause wherever possible.

1. Myringotomy: A direct damage to the round window is not possible even with an incorrect myringotomy incision if the round window is anatomically normal. There are two possible explanations for a perilymph fistula caused by rupture of the round window membrane:

   a. An indirect damage to the round window caused by a violent force acting directly on the tympanic membrane and the ossicles.

   b. Direct damage from suction on the round window.

The treatment consists in repairing the fistula with fascia temporalis. This should be done after observation of the severity of the symptoms and the degree of improvement (vertigo does not exceed 5 to 7 days). Vertigo responds satisfactorily to closure of the fistula whereas the results regarding hearing and tinnitus are more dubious.

2. Functional disorders of the eustachian tube the first days after surgery, caused by injury, blood clots or gelfoam. An overpressure is created in the middle ear by sudden Valsalva manoeuvre; this will cause laterosuction of the tympanic membrane and thereby of the stapes. The result is an inward movement of the round or/and the oval window membrane. The treatment is the same as in the case of fistula caused by myringotomy.

3. Local anaesthesia in the area of the external meatus can sometimes cause the acute diminishing of the vestibular function, which is followed by total recovery 24-36 hours later. We consider that lidocaine 2% (xylocaine) is incriminated more often. Another hypothetical factor could be adrenaline which we use in a ratio 1:100.000 (Gavalas et al., 1982).

4. Expansive and infected cholosteatoma is always a good reason to suspect a fistula. When the fistula is small it does not communicate with the perilymph, but in the course of time it enlarges, the endosteum disappears and the membranous canal comes in contact with the cholosteatoma matrix. When the cholosteatoma is infected, the inflammation can diffuse into the labyrinthine contents. Sometimes the epidermal lining of the advancing cholosteatoma sac covers the fistula and protects the labyrinthine contents from inflammatory involvement. In these cases, the cholosteatoma matrix is gently rolled off, in the medial direction, until the first sings of the membra-

nous canal are seen. Dissection is continued at a slow pace and the membranous canal is gently detached from the matrix. The fistula is then covered by fascia and bone chips. This technique does not cause the appearance of a more severe post-operative vertigo than routine stapedectomy (Palva et al., 1983)

5. Labyrinthine trauma: Iatrogenic trauma of the membranous labyrinth occured in a very few cases (0,2%). Trauma is inflicted either at the oval window by subluxation of the footplate from overzealous cleaning of disease about the stapes, by inadvertent uncovering of a labyrinthine fistula, or by fracture of the lateral canal (mainly) or the vertical canal with the drill or chisel. In all these cases, both the location and size of the fistula were important in the creation of vertigo. The prognosis is better, when the injury occurs away from the ampullary end of the canal, when no preceding ear pathology is present and when infection is prevented. Vertigo is likely due to haemorrage and serous labyrinthitis rather than to significant endolymph-perilymph intoxication. Management should include intra-operative cultures, closure of the open canal with bone chips and temporalis fascia graft. In all these cases we could have transient cochlear depression with normalisation within 5-6 weeks of trauma occured in most instances (Jahrsdoerfer et al., 1978).

6. Labyrinthitis: Post-operative diffuse serous induced labyrinthitis, sometimes follows a mastoid operation, espacially when the patient has had a previous circumscribed peri- or paralabyrinthitis. The symptoms appear from the $1^{st}-5^{th}$ day after the operation and the mechanism is either due to a direct injury of the labyrinth intra-operatively (symptoms appear at once), or by the absorption into the labyrinth of toxic products from bacterial activity in the middle ear and mastoid. Antimicrobial therapy included penicilline, gentamycin and metronidazole in i.v. administation.

7. Removal of ear packing: The improper removal of a compressive ear packing, especially in patients with radical mastoidectomy without tympanoplasty, may be another cause of post-operative vertigo.

From the miscellaneous causes of post-operative vertigo it is significant to mention the vertebro-basilar insufficiency, which was observed very often. The coexistence of chronic otitis media with a mild vertebro-basilar insufficiency, could be a serious reason of post-operative vestibular symptoms, usually in patients over 60 years old, after the prolonged hyperextension of the head and neck on the surgical table. The symptoms disappear after a few days bed rest.

CONCLUSIONS

Post-operative vertigo is a rare manifestation which mainly occurs in patients with vertebro-basilar insufficiency, functional disorders of the eustachian tube and in the cases of expansive and infected cholosteatoma with labyrinthine fistula. It can also occur in a few cases of iatrogenic labyrinthine trauma, vestibular neuronitis, labyrinthitis, after the use of local anaesthetics and other reasons as well. We want to emphasize that the preoperative study, the deep knowledge of the otosurgical techniques and the post-operative care, are necessary to avoid the patient's mismanagement. An important element for the Otosurgeon is the knowledge of the origin of vertigo. The study and the differentiation of the vestibular disorder is the duty of the Neurootologist, who provides significant help in such instances.

REFERENCES

1. Gavalas G., Papazoglou G., Chatzimanolis E., Dokianakis G.: Vestibular disturbances after local anaesthesia of the external meatus. Archieves of the 13th Greek-Jugoslav. Congress on ONON, p. 141-143, 1983.
2. Jahrsdoerfer R., Johns M., Cantrell R.: Labyrinthine trauma during ear surgery. Laryngoscope 88:1589-1595, 1978.
3. Palva T., Karja J., Palva A.: Immediate and short-term complications of chronic ear surgery. Arch. Otol. 102:137-139, 1976.
4. Mc Cabe Br.: Labyrinthine fistula in chronic mastoiditis. Symposium "Histopathology of the ear and its clinical implications" in honor of Schuknecht H.F., Boston, Aug. 1983
5. Canalis R., Gussen R., Abemayor E., Andrews J.: Surgical trauma to the lateral semicircular canal with preservation of hearing. Laryngoscope 97:575-581, 1987.
6. Cullen J., Kerr A.: Iatrogenic fenestration of a semicircular canal: a method of closure. Laryngoscope 96:1168-1169, 1986.
7. Palva T.: Treatment of ears with labyrinth fistula. Laryngoscope 93:1617-1619, 1983.
8. Palva T.: Surgery related to histopathology in chronic inflammatory middle-ear desease. Journal of Laryng. and Otol., 102:851-856, 1988.
9. Pratt L.: Complications associated with the surgical treatment of cholosteatoma. Laryngoscope 93:172-174, 1983.
10. Paparella M. et.al., Meniere's syndrome and otitis media. Laryngoscope 93: 1408-1415, 1983.

THERAPEUTICAL CONCEPTS IN POSTTRAUMATIC VESTIBULAR LESIONS

DIETER FUTSCHIK

Medical Academy Dresden "C.G.Carus"
Fetscherstr. 74, 8019 Dresden (Germany)

Due to central compensation mechanisms, vestibular disorders after craniocerebral traumata are of secondary importance in their clinical relevance compared to posttraumatic hearing disorders despite of the often considerable subjective annoyance. This is the reason why investigations have been carried out in conjunction with studies about the therapeutic possibilities with respect to vestibular disorders after craniocerebral traumata. Influenced by the still inadequate therapeutic efforts in the case of vestibular disorders, and stimulated by studies about the effect of nootropics on the vestibular reaction carried out by Oosterveld and Boniver, the first investigations were made on healthy probands without any other medication. In Europe, nootropics were first introduced into therapy about 18 years ago but not widely accepted. Above all, it is the following effects that render the nootropics potentially valuable also for a case material with craniocerebral traumata, viz:

1. Metabolic improvement by increasing the ATP/ADP ratio, the glucose consumption, and a reduction in the lactate/pyruvate ratio
2. Increase in oxygen consumption in the sense of a better utilization combined with an increase in the arteriovenous oxygen difference and in the clucose consumption
3. Promotion of the regional cerebral perfusion up to 20 % by a high dosage with normalizing tendency
4. Easing of the information exchange between the hemispheres in the region of the commissural systems and of the cortical control of subcortical functional circuits
5. Protective action against hypoxiah, intoxication (also with haematoma decomposition), trauma and infection
6. Strengthening of learning capability and memory in the rehabilitative phase

The photoelectronystagmography was used to record the vestibular reaction of healthy probandś after 20 seconds thermal stimulation with water of 20 °C and the sensation of vertigo scaled from 1 (none) to 5 (very pronouced). At random allocation, the probands orally received over 7 days either the agent or placebo in each case. Placebo tablets or dragèes were chosen so that their appearance and taste did correspond to the verum. The medication-free interval of 7 days was followed by a second application phase of 7 days with crossover medication. These investigations were designed as a double blind study.

Because like inbibitory effects on the vestibular reaction were described for central stimulants and antihistaminic agents, it was the further concern of our studies to check whether the occurring effects allow for a mutual demarcation or not.

Tested were piracetam, pyritinol and centrophenoxin as nootropics as well as amphetaminil as a central stimulant and tripelenamine as antihistaminic agent. The effects of each drug group were determined in 11 probands.

Under the action of piracetam and centrophenoxin we noticed a shortening of the nystagmus duration whilst this duration remained unchanged after the administration of pyritinol, amphetaminil and tripelenamine.

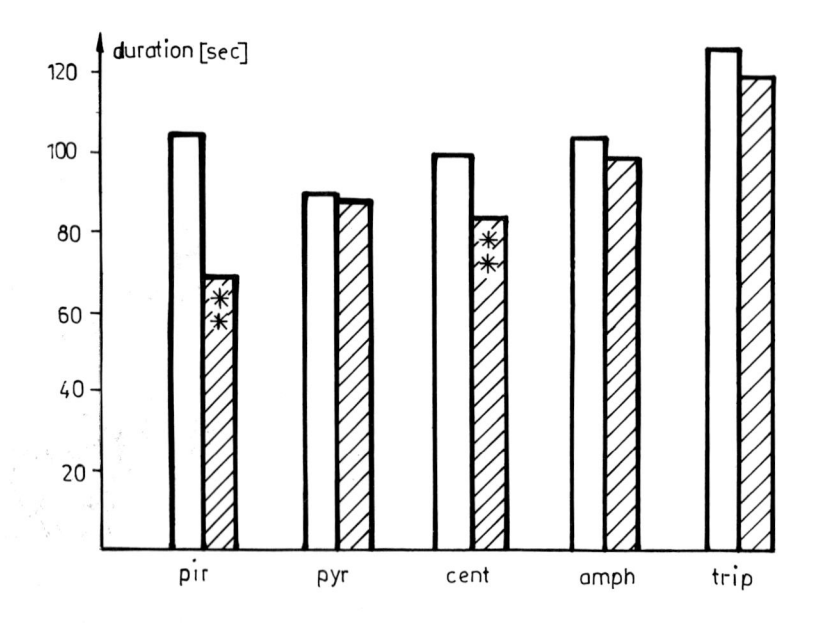

Fig. 1. Nystagmus duration prior to (□) and after (▨) repeated administration of piracetam (pir), pyritinol (pyr), centrophenoxin (cent), amphetaminil (amph) and tripelenamine (trip)
** $p<0,01$

Analogously to this reacted the latency and angular velocity of the slow phase as nystagmus parameters. After administration of piracetam and centrophenoxin we found a latency extension and a reduction in the angular velocity of the slow phase. The vertigo occurring after thermal stimulation became noticeably reduced with both the nootropics and amphetaminil as stimulant. But tripelenamine as antihistaminic agent proved to be inefficacious. Moreover, a comparison was made with respect to the value prior to repeated application becauses the vertigo always resulted in substantially higher scores at the first thermal stimulation.

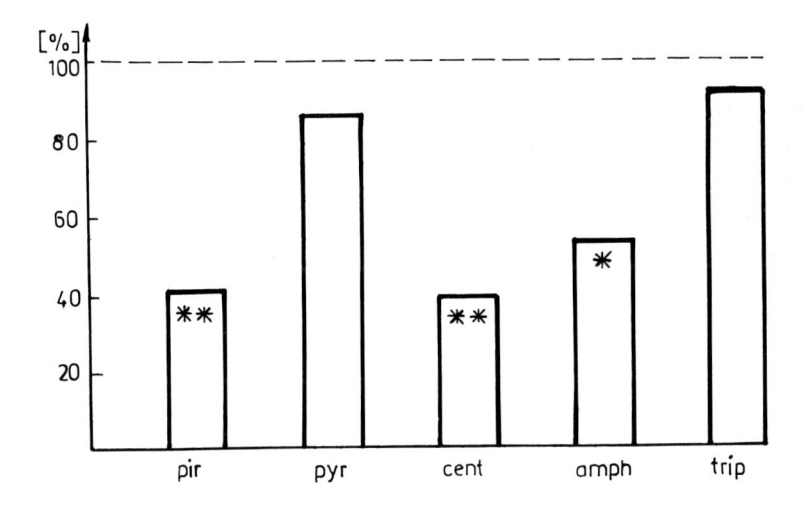

Fig. 2. Vertigo prior to and after repeated taking of the drugs
(for details, see Fig. 1.)
* p<0,02, ** p<0,01 compared to previos value (= 100 %)

The application of placebo exerted no significant effect on the criteria of the photoelectronystagmogram and on the vertigo. Seven days after the discontinuation of the drugs all changes observed were receded. But what are the clinical experiences gained up to now?

In the reports about the efficacy found with craniocerebral traumata the statements about a quick recovery compete with those of a freedom from complaints on the understanding that significant changes cannot be ascertained. Own examinations in 31 patients with otobasal skull fractures and typical nystagmus defunctionalization showed an observation time for spontaneous nystagmus and therefore an onset of freedom from complaints that, compared to a like untreated population with like traumatic aftereffects was shortened by 55 %.

Our findings emphasize that the known inhibiting effect of piracetam on the nystagmus is a characteristic of other nootropics as well. Of particular interest is the fact that even a single administration of centrophenoxin resulted in a distinct nystagmus reduction that became manifest with other nootropics only after repeated application. Because similar nystagmus-suppressive effects were described for some antihistaminic agents also we have used tripelenamine for comparison. But there was no influence on the nystagmus.

From our studies it is evident that nootropics can be clearly demarcated from central stimulants and antihistaminic agents. This is of significance insofar that an increase in vigilance is known for stimulants and for nootropics. This increase may also act on the nystagmus because a cortico-subcortical interaction modifies the nystagmus.

Since the effect of nootropics on nystagmus and vertigo occurred after a very short-term administration of low doses we think that our test assortment is suitable for the clinical use of potential nootropics. A plausible explanation of the nystagmus-reducing effect of the nootropics, however, cannot be found yet because their action mechanism is still somewhat obscure and irregular.

NEW CONCEPTS IN THE TREATMENT OF POSITIONAL VERTIGO

CESARANI A., ALPINI D., BAROZZI S., MINI M.
Institute Audiology University Milan
ENT departement Hospital Busto Arsizio (VA)
Istituto Don C. Gnocchi

INTRODUCTION

Positional nertigo (PV) is usally considered to have a peripheral origin and the specific treatment is physical rehabilitation.

The best known PP is the so-called bening faroxistic PY (BPPV) usually considered to be consed by cufololithiasis and usually treated by semont monouvre.

But vertigo is not always typical as in BPPV and Semont manonvre is not always so effective.

The aim of this paper is not to propose a new etiopathogenetic classification of PV but to show a personal "treatment low-chart" based on "functionaldiagnosis".

METHODS OF EVALUATION

In our opinion a lot of PV are consed either by central vestibular dysfunction or peripheral postural alterations and in all cases is it possible to modify central vestibular function by the mean of peripheral postural modifications. So the evaluation of pt with PV must be as complete as possible:
VOR: spontaneous ny with and without fixation positional and positioning ny caloric and roto-acceleratory ny
EOG: horizontal and vertical saccades and smooth pursuit
VSR: Romberg and Fukuda tests with and without shoes and on a soft carpet woth and without fixation, posturography.
POSTURE: inclination of the bipupillaris, shoulder and pelvis axis; evaluation of paravertebral muscles, trapezius and sterno-cleido mastoiedeus; convergence and Bascule phenonmenon; de Cyon test.

TREATMENT

In a pt we use one more of the following therapies:
Drugs for pt with signes of the central vestibular system involvement: flunarizine; ASA; TRH; citicholin. In a lot of cases miorelaxants and low dosage diazepam are usufull at the beginnig of physical rehabilitation.

VESTIBULAR REHABILITATION

Since the papers of Cowthorme and CooKsey a lot of protocols have been prposed. It is useful to divede in protocols for the treatment of typical PV (Semont, Brandt-Daoroff) and protocols for atypical PV (Norrè, Five) that are based on habituation and plurisensorial integrations.

POSTURAL CORRECTION

It is usually performed in cooperation with a phisia trist in pt with postural abnormalities. We have observed thaitin a lot of pt wich complorined atypical PV there are pelvis malities.

- SPES (superficial paravertebral electrical stimulation) it has been adopted in pt with unilateral vestibular prevalence such as in directional preponderance or in canal paresis. It has been used in pt with atypical PV but with ny always in the same direction.

The SPES has been used with a biphasic like TENS wave at 80 Hz and 100 usec on the neck paravertebral muscles of a site and the trapezins of the offsite site.

CHOICE OF THE TREATMENT

We divide PV in three groups:

A) typical PV (BPPV) the treatment of choice is Semont manouvre. It is not affective the pt has not a typical PV

B) PV as a sequela of vestibular neuritis the treatment of choice is SPES because the PV is the expression of a central vestibular imbalance. In aged pt neutotrophics may be usefull.

C) atypical PV vertigo in Rose or supime position; from sitting to recumbent position or vice-versa; without habituation,....

APY must be divided in two sub-groups:

- unipositional APY

- pluripositional APY

In booths cases SPES in employed if the direction of ny is costant.

In pluripositional APY postural abnomalities corrections must be performed.

Drugs may be associated.

If we don't reveable a VOR prevalence we prefer physical rehabilitation, postural correction and drugs.

If we retain for a pt necessary a combined treatment we prefare at begining to associate only two therapies: SPES and drugs ; rehabilitation and drugs; SPES and postural corrections......

A continuos re-evaluation of the case (at least 1/10 days) isindispensable in these pt.

CONCLUSIONS

- for the treatment of PV functional diagnosis is more important than ethio-pathogenetic diagnosis
- the evaluation of the pt must be as complete as possible
- interspecilaistic cooperation in often indispensable
- the major part of PV may be treated with success and not only BPPV.

POSITIONAL VERTIGO

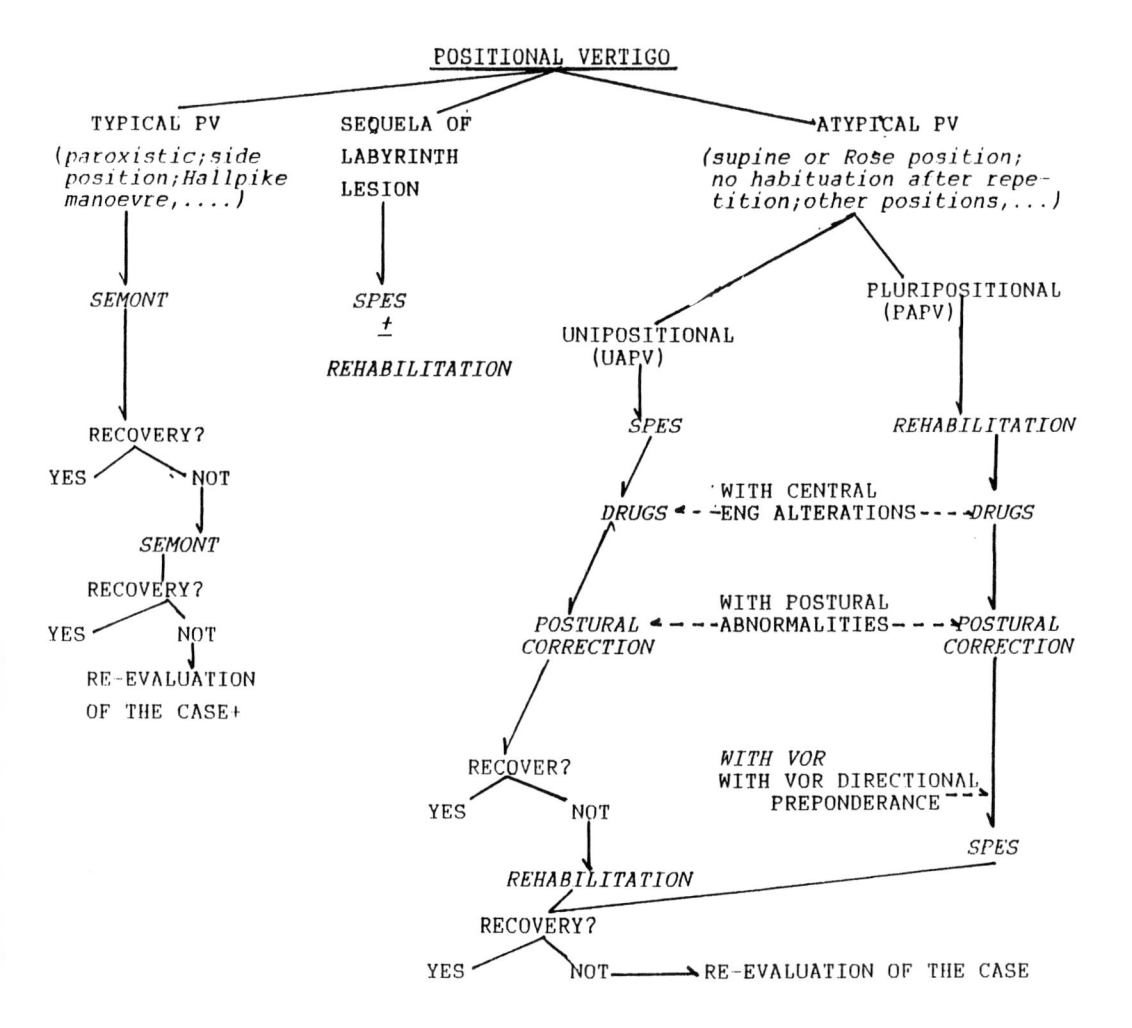

```
                          POSITIONAL VERTIGO
         ┌──────────────────────┼──────────────────────┐
   TYPICAL PV              SEQUELA OF              ATYPICAL PV
 (paroxistic;side          LABYRINTH          (supine or Rose position;
  position;Hallpike          LESION            no habituation after repe-
  manoevre,....)                               tition;other positions,...)
         │                      │                      │
         ▼                      ▼           ┌──────────┴──────────┐
      SEMONT                   SPES                          PLURIPOSITIONAL
                                ±                                (PAPV)
                          REHABILITATION   UNIPOSITIONAL
                                              (UAPV)                │
      RECOVERY?                                 │                   ▼
   YES ╱    ╲ NOT                              SPES            REHABILITATION
                                                │                   │
        SEMONT                                  │   WITH CENTRAL    │
                                             DRUGS ◄- -ENG ALTERATIONS- - - ►DRUGS
      RECOVERY?
   YES ╱    ╲ NOT                                    WITH POSTURAL
                                         POSTURAL ◄ - - -ABNORMALITIES- - - ►POSTURAL
     RE-EVALUATION                       CORRECTION                  CORRECTION
     OF THE CASE+
                                         RECOVER?           WITH VOR
                                      YES ╱    ╲ NOT    WITH VOR DIRECTIONAL
                                                          PREPONDERANCE - - ►
                                                                            SPES
                                      REHABILITATION
                                      RECOVERY?
                                   YES ╱    ╲ NOT ──────► RE-EVALUATION OF THE CASE
```

REFERENCES

1. Brandt T;, Daroff R.B.: Phisical Therapy for bening paroxysmal positional vertigo. Arch of Otolaryngol., 106, 484, 485, 1980.

2. Brandt T.: Medicamentoseund physikalische therapie des schwidels und der ataxie. Fortschr Neurol. Psychiat. 49, 88, 1981.

3. Cathorne T.: The physiological basis of head exsercises. J.Chart.Soc. Physiother ., 106, 1944

4. Cesarani A., Pertoni T., Alpini D.: L'electrostimulation cervicale posterieure dans les handicaps sensoriels vestibulaires. XXII Reunion dela societe d'otoneurologie da lange francaise. May 1988

5. Cooksey F.S.: Rehabilitation in vestibualr INJURIES. Proc. Roy. Soc. Med. 39, 273, 1946.

6. Dix M.R.: The rationale and technique of head exercises in the treatment of vertigo. Acta Otorhino-laryng Bel., 34, 370-384, 1979.

7. Hamann K.F., Bockmeyer M.: Behandling vestibularer funktionsstuorungen durch ein Ubungsprogramm. Laryng. Rhinol. Otol., 62, 474, 1983.
8. Norrè M.E.: Rationale of rehabilitation treatment for vertigo Am J. Otolaryngol, 8, 31-35, 1987
9. Semont A., Sterkers J.M.: Reducation vestibulaire. Les Chaiers d'ORL, 15, 305 1980
10. Sterkers J.M.: La methode du point de mire pou la reducation anti-vertigineuse. Revue Laryng 535, 1977.

CENTRAL MECHANISMS OF VESTIBULAR FUNCTION COMPENSATION, FOLLOWING AN EXPERIMENTAL UNILATERAL DELABYRINTHIZATION

V.CHALMANOV, H.HARALANOV, CHR.KOLCHEV.
Neurology Clinik, Medical Academy, Sofia (Bulgaria).

INTRODUCTION

In the clinical practice are not incommon the cases with unilateral vestibular function lose (VFL) due to traumatic, inflammatory or operative causes. It is impressive that the draumatic signs of vestibular disorders (vertigo, nausea and vomiting, nystagnus, ataxia, disturbances of movement, gait and posture) appearing at the early post-VFL stages reveal a well expressed tendency to restoration and diseppear within 3-5 days up to 1-2 weeks (1, 5, 8, 9, 11).

The nature and the mechanisms of this vestibular function compensation are subject of intensive exploration, however still yet there exist a lot of questions, especialy concerning the problem of participation of various brain structures-primary vestibular nuclei and pathways, cerebral and cerebellar hemispheres, visual an auditory analyzers, spinal corbs and others, in this compensation (6, 7, 10).

The aim of the present study is to create a "model" of unilateral VFL in experimental antimals (cats) and to study the dynamics of the behavioral and electrophysiological changes, in order to clarificate the neurophysiological mechanisms of the compensatory processes.

MATERIAL AND METHODS

On 7 chronicaly implanted cats were carried out 35 polygraphic (EEG, ENG, ECG, AER, VER) registraions and observations. They were performed immediately after Delabyrinthization (D) and repeated periodicaly up to the 45-th day.

Histopathological control on material from the middle and inner ear, as well as from the labyrinth-abjacent brain tisnue was made.
Delabyrinthization was performed by a modification of the combined cestructive-chemical method of Emyilianov-Alexin, 1975; eardrum was perforated unilateraly (right side) and 1,5 % solutio of mono-jodine acetic acid was applied over the verti-

cally oriented right ear by means of head fixation in a stereotaxic equipment.

EEG and evoked potential registrations were made from Gyrus Suprasyltius, Ectosylvius and Occipitalis, bilateraly. The eye's movements were registered by means of chronicaly implanted electrodes. The next parameters were used for AER-registration: Free sound field stimylation or monoaural stimulation with tone 1000 Hz, 60 dB SPL, ISI 2 sec. VER were elicited by Repetitive Light Flashes with intensity of 0,5 J, ISI 2 sec.

RESULTS

The behavioral changes begin 5 - 35 minutes after D. Head tremor arpeared, sometimes localized convulsions can be seen. Highly characteristic was the body turning to the side of damaged labyrinth, associated with a flexion of the ipsilateral limbs, while the contralateral ones were streched. There was rotation of the whole body arround the vertical axis (manege movements) in an attempt to move. The hepavioral changes showed progressive reduction in intensity and used to disappear within 4-5 days.

Well expressed electrophysiological changes were established during the varios post-D stages. ENG-registration showed the onset of a Nystagmus between 28-38 th minute after D. At the begining it was nonregular, low voltage, after 45-50 th minute in became regular, high voltage (Fig. 1). The Fast/Slow component ratio was 1:2 up to 1:4, angular velocity was 60-62°/sec with its maximum between 65-120 th minute. Progressive reduction within 2-3 days appear. (Fig. 2).

Auditory evoked potentials showed a well axpressed interhemispherec asymmetry on amplitude. The AER-amplitude was higher over the right hemisphere, following left eaer stimulation as well as the right ear stimulation (Fig.3). It can be emphized on the phase-like effect of this changes. They are most expressed between 45-120 th minute after, D. and showed a tendency

FOR NORMALIZATION or even though inversion after 2-3 days.

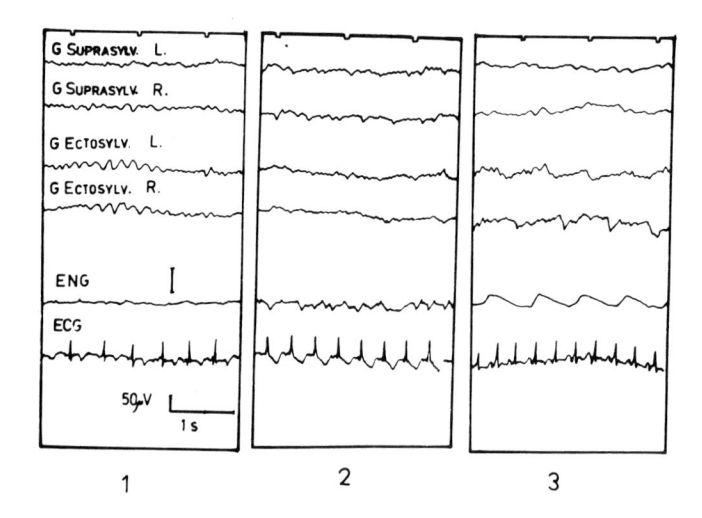

Fig.1. Polyphysiographic records made before (1), on 10 th
minute (2) and 45 th minute (3) after unilateral
(right seded) delabyrinthization in cat.

Visial Evoked potentials revealed discrete interhemispheric asymmetry in amplitude. Their latency was delayed in both hemispheres, however more expressed on the left side.

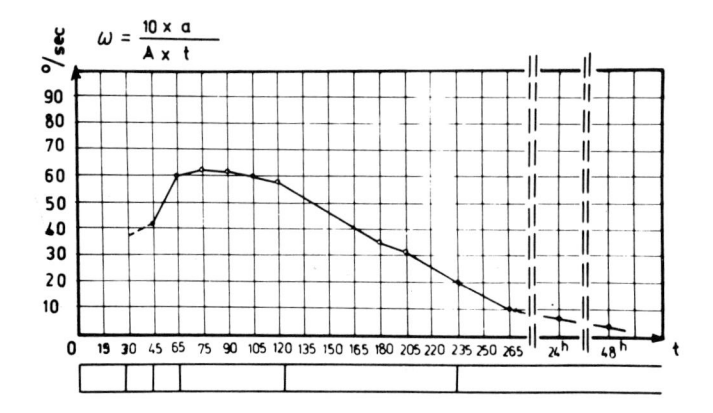

Fig.2. Graphic of the angular velocity of the Nystagmus,
following unilateral delabyrinthization of cat
(Dynamics of its average values).

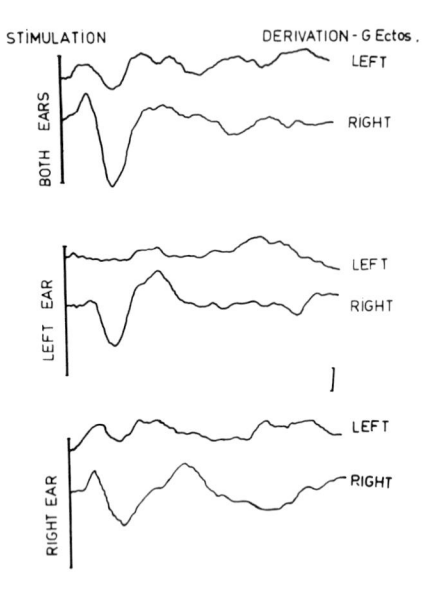

Fig.3. Auditory evoked potentials of cat, registered on 24 th hour after experimental unilateral Delabyrinthization. (See the text).

The augmentation of the VEP-amplitude occurs between the 150 ht minute and lasted up to 24 th hour, followed by progressive reduction and normalization within 2-3 days.

DISCUSSION

Despite the fact that in the present "model" of unilateral VFL the destruction concerns the peripheral part (end-organ) of the vestibular analyzer, we consider that in the compresation of disturbanced function, the central (brainstem) structures may play a leading role.

Most likely this compensatory effect is realized at the level of the primary vestibular nuclei in the brainsmet. Our electrophysiological data suggest an axcitative and reversible of the postdestructive functional changes in brainstem. A facilitation of the associative internuclear connection between ipsi- and contralateral vestibular nuclei may take place.

Most likely the basic mechanisms of vestibular compencation following an unilateral VFL can be connected with the spontaneous activation of the Ist type vestibular neurons (see 6) in the chronic post-D. stages, due to the increased sensibility of their postsynaptic membranes, because of the degeneration of the ipsilateral afferent fibres as a result of the destruction of the endogran (3, 4, 7).

REFERENCES

1. Aislan M, Rodriques-Adracos E, Inrante I. (1975). Experimental disharmonic labyrinthine syndrome. J. "Nuovo Arch. Ital.Otol., 3:110-121.
2. Bertholz A, Jones M. (Eds). Adaptive mechanism in gaze conrol. Rewiews in oculomotor research, vol.I, Elsevier, Amsterdam, 1985.
3. Haralanov H, Sachanska T, Shmarov A, Petkova K, Kolchev Chr. (1980). Complex clinical, electrophysiological, biochemical and morphological investigations in delabyrinthization. XXVIII th Int. Congress of Physiological Sciences, Budapest, Abstr. 2997, p.675.
4. Kolchev Chr. (1981). On the central mechanism of vestibular function compensation in a model of delbyrinthization. Electroencerpal.clin.Neurolophysiol., Elsevier, Amsterdam, 52, p.77 (Abstr), Soc.Proceedings.
5. Pfaltz C, Kamath R. (1971). The problem of Central Compensation in peripheral vestibular dystunctino. Acta Otolaryngol., 71, 266-272.
6. Precht W. (1974). Characteristics of Vestibular Neurons after Acute and Chronic Labyrinthine Destruction. In: Handbook of sensory Physiology (H.H.Kornhuber, Ed.), vol. VI/1, Vestibular system, part 1, Basic Mechanisms, Springer-Verlag, Berlin-Heidelberg-New York.
7. Smidt R, Thews G., Eds.(1983). Human Phusiology, Springer-Verlag, Berlin-Hejdelberg-New York, vol.1, Nervous syst.
8. Kornhuber H.(1974). Handbook of sensory physiology, vol. VI/1, Vestibular function, part 1, Basic Mechanisms, Springer-Verlag, Berlin-Heidelberg-New York.
9. Norre M, Forrez G, Beckers A.(1988). Functional Recovery of Posture in Peripheral Vestibular Disorders. In: Posture and Gait (Development, adaptation and modulation, (B.Amblard, A.Bertholz and F.Clarac, Eds), Elsevier, p, 291-299.
10. Victor M, Adams R. (1985). Common Disturbances of Vision, Osular Movements and Hearing. In: Harrison's Principles of Internal Medicine, Tenth Ed., Petersdorf-Adams-Braunwald-Isselbacher-Martin-Wilsen, Eds, Int.Student Ed.pp. 113-118.
11. Walton L.(1985). Brain's Diseases of the Nervous System, Ninth Ed, Oxford Medical Publications.

CLAMEDEX - DIAGNOSTIC NEUROOTOLOGICAL EXPERT SYSTEM WITH A NETWORK STRUCTURE

CLAUS - FRENZ CLAUSSEN, ERIKA CLAUSSEN
Neurootological Research Center, Kurhaustr. 12, 8730 Bad Kissingen, Germany

The medical diagnosis is a process of identifying a disease in a particular person and also the conclusions reached. This holds for internal medicine as well as otolaryngology as well as neurootology. Usually, after all the neurootological tests have been performed, the neurootologist is requested to find a final diagnosis which is the last stage of mental process leading to the labelling of a diseased state. After the neurootologist has collected his data, he reviews the facts he has obtained and suggested solutions. The monaural vestibular loss for example would lead to the diagnosis of a peripheral canal paresis. Then he considers the implications of the evidence. Thus, a vestibular loss patient in addition to having a caloric inhibition on that ear, should have an abnormal audiogram on the same side giving the neurootologist a history of combined vertigo and unilateral hearing loss. The neurootologist next compares the functional data with ideas that have ocurred to him to see if certain solutions for the patients condition match the data gained in the examinations. If a further study shows the presence of all of the above symtoms, for example the data would agree with the suggested solution and additionally he would find a maskable tinnitus and a history of scattered intense vertigo attacks. The diagnosis would be Meniere´s disease.

This is the method persued by the neurootologists in making a diagnosis. While the task of collecting data on the patient like history, ORL inspection, special neurootological examinations like equilibriometry, audiometry, olfactometry and gustometry, requires accurate observation, the process of correct reasoning is in the last analysis more important. False diagnoses often result not from false data, but from faulty interpretation. To assemble the data, to make use of the relevant and to discard the irrelevant information and to pass final judgement, all of which are important steps in making the diagnosis, often requires a mental ability of the highest order.

Like in other medical disciplines, we are now using the help of a modern instrumentation of our facilities. These are modern amplifiers, recorders, stimulus set-ups and during the past decade more and more modern computers. Thus, we have introduced since about 4 years CLAMEDEX, a diagnostic neurootological expert system with a network structure, which allows using this additional tool for his diagnostic work a jumping reasoning in a human manner, which we also call an associative way of thinking.

Now, expert systems have taken artificial intelligence out of research and development laboratories and are easily available in programs for personal computers, like MacSmarts from cognition technology. An expert system is a computer program for communicating knowledge or expertise. Expert systems are part of the artificial intelligence field, which includes natural language processing, robotics and medical diagnostics. Expert systems differ from conventional programs by performing symbolic, logical operations instead of numeric computations, just as you work on statistically planning a physiological experiment versus simply adding up series of measurements of blood pressure or blood sugar, for example. If you can describe it in an algorithm, which is an explicit procedure in a computer program much like a cook-book recipe, you probably do not yet need an expert system. Expert systems are dealing with problems, which are even much too complicated for algorithms.

By expert systems you can now create programs to analyse problems and make recommendations that previously required input from human experts. Even more important is that some expert systems techniques now allow a rather easy way to develop powerful programs.

3 key ideas from artificial intelligence being applied in expert systems are new ways to represent knowledge, heuristic search and the separation of knowledge from inference and control. A basic difference between conventional software and that developed by artificial intelligence programmers is that artificial intelligence focuses on verbal and graphic aspects of knowledge rather than mathematical aspects.

Basically an expert system consists of 3 components:
1. a knowledge base which contains the knowledge that is specific to the domaine of the field of expertise of your medical expert.
2. a knowledge base includes facts like normal ranges for various measurements, as well as the data of the individual neurootological measurements.
3. an expert system is acting through rules, such as if the warm and cold response of the right side of a caloric butterfly scheme are inhibited, whereas the warm and cold responses of the left side are still in normality. This demonstrates a right peripheral vestibular inhibition. The rules can also be much more complex like: The butterfly calorigram might show a right ear warm and cold response inhibition with a left ear warm and cold normal response and simultaneous left and right sided normally beating perrotatory nystagmus and a spontaneous nystagmus of slight intensity as well as direction changing. In this case we know from various interactions and rules that this is typical for a right ear peripheral vestibular degeneration, however, now under the influence of a remarkable central compensation due to the neuronal plasticity.

Rules can be explicit, so that they always work, or more complicated that they only work most of the time, but are not guaranteed. These are also called heuristics. Often, experts may not be able to articulate the rules they are using until the knowledge engineer decodes them and converts them into an explicit knowledge base. Another important constituent of an expert system is an inference engine, which is a program that forms logical operation, such as called inferencing, to reach conclusions. This program is domain independent. It remains the same, regardless of what knowledge you want to communicate. As the third important column a user interface to the person, who extracts the knowledge from the expert and transforms into a knowledge base, and to the user has to be established on a computer screen. Therefore we are using a Macintosh SE or Macintosh II computer as the front end.

The knowledge base of CLAMEDEX is comprising from our neurootological publications and handbooks, which we have been published throughout the past 20 years. The front end is displaying 6 HyperCARD screens, of which each contains buttons to navigate from one screen to another. Other buttons are specific to call for operations or informations. The CLAMEDEX opening screen contains interactive fields for the introduction of the patient, his identification, weight etc., as well as for the addresses of the corresponding medical doctors who are going to receive a case report letter. Special buttons on this field allow to call up at any stage the development of the expertise, a report upon the diagnosis, the therapy or a conclusion and prognosis. The second card contains the interactive dialogue with respect to the history as well as to the ORL inspection. All the informations and conclusions are regularly reported in a special window area on the screen with a scroll bar. An unlimited amount of verbal information can be written down there by means of preformed sentences as a result of the user dialogue with the knowledge base or after direct introduction of type written comments or remarks. The information is already transformed into a partial subdiagnosis.

The third card contains fields and buttons for evaluating the qualitative aspects of the various spontaneous and experimental nystagmus, the electrocardiogram and the cranio-corpo-gram, as well as for the quantitative evaluation of the butterfly calorigram, the perrotatory and postrotatory tests, the stepping cranio-corpo-gram and the standing cranio-corpo-gram. Also several optokinetic tests are evaluated. The result of the evalutation again is written down in verbal comments. A partial diagnosis is preformed. On a fourth screen, which can be brought to the front by clicking on the adequate button, the pure tone audiometry, the speech audiometry, tinnitus masking, impedance, facial nerve reflexes, acoustic dynamics etc. are evaluated. A fifth screen contains the evaluation of the various evoked potentials, like acoustic brainstem evoked (ABEP), acoustic late evoked (ALEP) and visually evoked potentials. As the derivation of all the evoked potentials is taking place in a bilateral manner, we can compare always homolateral and contralateral responses with responses to one receptor stimulation compared with those to the other receptor stimulation.

The sixth screen has been built up for the evaluation of olfactometry and gustometry, including rhinomanometry, the 12-component-target-olfactogram, the incremented impulse electrogustogram and the 5-component-chemogustometry.

After having run through the patient's files forward and backward and after having discussed all the interesting matters with the expert system, the initial menu is called up. From there the program jumps to a seventh screen for rolling over the final diagnosis and therapy. CLAMEDEX proposes a whole report including the descriptions of the various lesions, which have been found. Then continuing to a computer infered diagnosis the subsequent proposal for a therapy and estimating of the prognosis is performed.

The medical doctor now can correct each of the diagnostical, therapeutical or prognostical conclusions by erasing the results of the computer and/or by inserting new items by handwriting or through their selection from pop-up-menus. CLAMADEX has been revised to version 1.4 already. It is guiding the investigator through the evaluation of very complex and complicated material, such as the neurootological network evaluation. Now that the IBM-compatible world recognizes the Macintosh human interface style as a main stream idea and a desirable idea, the Apple computer of the type Macintosh SE or Macintosh II has proved that together with modern expert systems under the help of various programs which are bound into each other. It can be easily handled and is an optimal tool for every day diagnostic work. The main aspects of neurootological diagnostic and therapeutical work can as well be taken into consideration as rather rare clinical findings. It can also be used for follow-ups.

REFERENCES

1. Harmon B, Maus R (1988) Expert Systems, Tools and Applications. John Wiley & Sons. Inc., New York, Chechester, Brisbane, Toronto, Singapore

2. Goodman D (1987) The Complete HyerCard Handbook. Bantam Books, Toronto, New York, London, Sydney, Auckland

3. Mac Smarts® (1988) Instruction Manual, Version 3.2. Cognition Technology (TM), Cognition Technology Corp., Cambridge, Massachusetts

4. Fischler MA , Firschein O (1987) Intelligence, the Eye, the Brain and the Computer. Eddison Wesley Publishing Cie., Reading, Manlow Park, Don Mills, Workingham, Amsterdam, Sydney, Singapore, Tokyo, Madrid, Bogotá, Santiago, San Juan

5. Crandall RA, Colgrove MM (1986) Scientific Programming with Macintosh Pascal. John Wiley & Sons Inc., New York, Chichester, Brisbane, Toronto, Singapore
Turbo Pascal Numerical Methods Tool Box. Borland International Inc., Scott's Valley

6. Claussen C-F (1970): Über die Aufzeichnung und Auswertung ausgewählter quantitativer Gleichgewichtsfunktionsprüfungen. Fachbereich klinische Medizin, FU Berlin, Habilschrift

7. Henriksson NG, Rubin W, Jahnicke J, Claussen C-F (1970) A Synopsis of the Vestibular System. Sandoz AB, Schweden, 1970.

8. Claussen C-F, Tato JM (1971) Equilibriometria Practica. Edition Hasenclever & Cia., Buenos Aires

9. Claussen C-F, Aust G, Hortmann G, Müller-Kortkamp M (1975) Praktikum der Elektronystagmographie. Verhandlungen der GNA, Bd. II, Edition medicin & pharmacie, Hamburg und Neu-Isenburg

10. Claussen C-F, v Lühmann M (1976) Das Elektronystagmogramm und die neurootologische Kennliniendiagnostik. Edition medicin & pharmacie, Hamburg und Neu-Isenburg

11. Claussen C-F, Fort (1976) Der Schwindelkranke und seine neurootologische Begutachtung. Edition medicin & pharmacie, Hamburg und Neu-Isenburg

12. Claussen C-F, De Sa J (1978) Clinical Study of Human Equilibrium by Electronystagmography and Allied Tests. Popular Prakashan, Bombay

13. Aust G, Claussen C-F, Fort E, v. Lühmann M (1979) Ausgewählte Kapitel zum Thema Schwindel. Edition medicin & pharmacie, Hamburg und Neu-Isenburg, 1979.

14. Claussen C-F (1981) Schwindel - Ein Leitfaden für Klinik und Praxis. Edition medicin & pharmacie

15. Claussen C-F (1985) Presbyvertigo, Presbyataxie, Presbytinnitus - Gleichgewichts- und Sinnesstörungen im Alter. Springer-Verlag, Berlin, Heidelberg, New York, Tokio

16. Claussen C-F, Aust G, Schäfer WD, v. Schlachta I (1986) Atlas der Elektronystagmographie. Edition medicin & pharmacie, Hamburg

17. Claussen C-F, Claussen E (1986) Forschungsbericht Cranio-Corpo-Graphie (CCG) - Ein einfacher objektiver und quantitativer Gleichgewichtstest für die Praxis. Schriftenreihe des Hauptverbandes der gewerblichen Berufsgenossenschaften eV, D 5205 St. Augustin

18. Claussen C-F (1988) Homotoxicology - The Core of a Probiotic and Holistic Approach to Medicine. Aurelia-Verlag, Baden-Baden

19. Claussen C-F, Bergmann de Bertora JM, Bertora GO (1988) Otoneurooftalmología. Springer- Verlag, Berlin, Heidelberg, New York, London, Paris, Tokio

20. Claussen C-F, Bergmann de Bertora JM, Bertora GO (1988) Nistagmografía computerisada (CNG) - Nuevos métodos objectivos de análisis. Neurofisiología otooftalmogía. Buenos Aires

21. Claussen C-F, Kirtane MV, Schlitter K (1988) Vertigo, Nausea, Tinnitus and Hearing Loss in Metabolic Disorders. Excerpta Medica, Elsevier Science Publishers BV, Amsterdam, New York, Oxford

22. Claussen C-F, Kirtane MV (1986) Vertigo, Nausea, Tinnitus and Hearing Loss in Cardiovascular Diseases. Excerpta Medica, Elsevier Science Publishers BV, Amsterdam, New York, Oxford

23. Mira E, Buizza A, Magenes G, Manfrin M, Schmid R (1990) Expert Systems as a Diagnostic Aid in Otoneurology ORL, 52, 96-103

POSTTRAUMATIC DISTURBANCES
IN TASTE AND SMELL

ON EVENTUAL CHANGES OF LIVING HABITS DUE TO POSTTRAUMATIC DYSOSMIAS

HILMAR GUDZIOL, EGGERT BELEITES
ENT-department, Friedrich-Schiller-University, Lessingstr. 2,
Jena DDR-6900

INTRODUCTION

Physicians often assume that smell disorders result in food related problems. Food flavor is a composite sensation of taste, smell, texture, temperature and pain. If smell is missing the full flavor of food could not be enjoyed and thus appetite and body weight might be decreased.
In former textbooks chemosensory deficits are asserted to change the living habits. The patients could not eat, drink or smoke with the same enjoyment as before the smell disorder. Thus the physicians could differentiate easily between a true anosmia and aggravation or simulation. When a patient develops sudden anosmia by head injury the question arises whether the patient can adjust his behaviour to compensate for the missing olfactory information or is he at risk?

MATERIAL AND METHODS

30 patients with posttraumatic smell disorders have participated in an interview about changes in eating, drinking, smoking, sanitary and sexual behaviour since the onset of the smell deficit after their head injury. A sudden loss of sense of smell because of head trauma may be very disturbing although it is often obfuscated by dizziness, headache, vision and hearing problems. All patients were treated in ENT-department. The interviews took place between one month and seventeen years after the accident. One third of the patients were examined less than two years after the head trauma. The youngest patient was seventeen and the oldest was fifty eigth. Sixty five percent were male. Two thirds had total anosmia and one third had additional parosmia.

RESULTS

No patient has a loss of body weight. Generally the appetite is unchanged. Two patients have an increased appetite and seven pa-

tients had decreased appetite transitorily in particular immediately after the onset of their smell disorder.
Twenty five patients taste wellknown food in the same way as before the accident. Five patients complain of an altered or a decreased flavor perception or they complain that it takes longer time to the full flavor impression. That is an interesting fact. Most of the patients have no eating problems although they are no anosmics for lifetime. They may enjoy their meals by memory. The view, the taste, the texture of the food recalls olfactory engrams and elicits a constancy of flavor even if the smell perception is absent. Different stimuli may be perceived to be equivalent. They may elicit the same flavor by association. The perception of a peach may be the same whether the perception is activated by its view, its taste or its odour. For patients with smell disorders the view, the aspect of the food is especially important. The vision is combined with eating.
Many of the patients have no eating problems. A few prefer very hot, very cold or spicy foods for instance flavored with pepper, mustard, paprika etc..One patient is a so called frustrated eater. She is a fifty-two-year-old married woman with normal body weight. Again and again she eats some chocolate in an attempt to recapture the pleasure she used to get from food. This alteration did not put the patient at nutritional risk. In my research there was no patient who had lost interest in eating with eventual anorexia. Two patients enjoy cooking as a job. They have no problems related to their inability to smell. They flavor the meals by experience. Only in exceptional cases they are supported by a colleague, secretly.
Great difficulties exist in noticing spoilt food. The quality of food is controlled more carefully by the eyes or by a different person with intact sense of smell.
Coffee drinking behaviour remained the same in twenty two patients. They like to drink coffee further more. Only eight patients dislike coffee now because it tastes rather bitter or it is not tolerated. Only seven patients became antialcoholics after their head injury but nobody as a consequence of his smell deficit. Only one patient changed his smoking habit. That was independent of his anosmia. He became a non-smoker during his long hospital stay.

All patients feel uncertain in the use of city-gas. They often control or let control the gas cookers or the gas firings to detect escaping gas.

The individual body odour is not detected by all patients themselfes. Each patient needs and has a familiar person who checks his odour. During a long lasting theater performance a few patients feel handicapped because it is impossible for them to refresh.

The sanitary habits of all patients were not modified.

The sexual activity of most patients did not alter. Six patients reported they were now less active however due to older age.

Several patients have some restrictions with regard to their occupations. Special jobs as gas -workers, cookers and chemists can be practised only by the assistance of a colleague.

SUMMARY

Most patients have no problems related to their smell disorder. Established living habits are usually stable. Nevertheless a few patients develop some difficulties.

Do not be too hasty to conclude that a patient aggravates or simulates his smell disorder, if he tells us he likes eating, drinking or smoking with the same enjoyment as before the accident.

POSTTRAUMATIC DYSOSMIAS

UWE E. FRAASS, CLAUS-FRENZ CLAUSSEN

Department of Neurootology, ENT - Clinic, Head - Center, University of Würzburg, Josef-Schneider-Str. 11, 8700 Würzburg, West-Germany

INTRODUCTION

The sense of olfaction detects and identifies airborne chemicals. The olfactory sensorial epithelium in the upper choanal airways serves for chemoreception. The sense of smell may be lost, when the nerve filaments of the nose have been torn in trauma to the head or when the nerve has been damaged. In many cases vascular disturbances of the anterior cerebral artery lead to distorsions of smell or partial anosmias. The normal state of the sense of smell is called "euosmia". The absence of the sense of smell is called "anosmia". However, olfactory anesthesia must not be mixed with nasal anesthesia, where; besides, the loss of the sense of smell also the trigeminal sensations are lost. The term "preferential anosmia" expresses the lack of ability to sense certain odors only. In this respect we also use the expression "partial anosmia".

Amongst 10.335 neurootological patients of our neurootological data bank NODEC IV we had 3 % anosmias, 2,8 % hyposmias and 0,4 % parosmias. On purpose to unveil characteristic olfactory dysfunctions due to head and neck trauma in comparison with other chemosensoric affecting illnesses we investigated neurootologic patients suffering from olfactory dysfunctions. To figure out the degree of dysosmia and loss of chemosensibility we applied rhinomanometry and psychophysical chemosensoric investigation by means of the target olfactogram.

MATERIAL AND METHODS
The Target Olfaktogram

For clinical purposes we have designed the *Target Olfactogram*, a supraliminal monorhinal sniffle test using representative, chemical substances for the 9 groups of basic odors of Zwaardemaker and three trigeminal stimuli. The resulting chart is built of a polarcoordinate net of the type of a target shape. Each of the 12 partial smell tests is related to a 30 ° segment of the olfactogram. After each sniffle the patient is requested to grade his sensation according to a scale with 6 scores from descriptive identification (1) over an emotional scheme with good (2), indifferent (3), unpleasant (4) to unspecific borderline (5) and no response (6). Their statistical relation of olfactometric charts to typical underlying diseases and degenerative states are described.

Each of these 4 major classes are subdivided into 3 special qualities.These substances have been chosen according to the question that they should be typical representatives of the test groups. Also the substances should be pure, chemically stable and present in the gas above the cristals or the liquid inside the test bottle. They must have a sufficiently high rate of vaporization and should be not toxic. Further, should the typical fragrant or odor of the substance be known to most of the test persons.

Applied chemosensoric testing stimuli:
With these criteria we have chosen the following substances :

1. Odores suave olentes
    a) amylacetate
    b) nitrobenzene
    c) piperonal

2. Odores medii
    a) keton musk
    b) diallylsulfide
    c) benzene

3. Phoetores
    a) n-valeric acid
    b) pyridine
    c) scatole

4. Trigeminal stimuli
    a) formaldehyde
    b) acetic acid
    c) 25% ammonia solution.

In series after a posttraumatic state or other follow-ups, the test chart allows to differentiate between the various groups of the above mentioned smell defficiencies, especially the the degree of stimuli-corresponding smelling disturbances.

RESULTS

Data from NODEC IV

As mentioned above we firstly had a view on anamnestic data. We investigated 505 patients (mean age: 38,4 ys. , SD ±16 , 61,1 % male, 38,9 % female) . 45,1 % of the patients suffered from chemosensoric disorders, 44,2 % of the patients suffered from rhinomanometric evaluated nasal obstructions. Furthermore we noticed 2,1% patients with trigeminal dysfunctions.

Psychophysic s of chemosensoric scoring

Applying the target olfaktogram we used a psychophysic scoring scale[3] to detect chemosensoric disorders. Using the R-Factor, the ratio of odorant-specific detection within a specific patholocic entity in comparison to the whole sample we were able to measure the degree of precision in odarant sensibility. This method was established relating to a seperated view on olfactory stimuli, trigeminal-olfactory combined stimuli and trigeminal stimuli[3].

On the other hand we scored the summated mean range of unspecific gnostic judgement as like „unspecific detection" or „no sensation" refering on all odorant stimuli used[6]. This score range enables the investigator to quantify the level of missing detection in olfaction.

Whereas the R-Factor operates as a stimuli-related criterion the „unspecific gnostic judgement" expresses failure of sensibility at all.

The results of the ratio in gnostic specifity as a degree of chemosensoric detecting ability and the so called unspecific gnostic evaluation are shown in Figure 1:

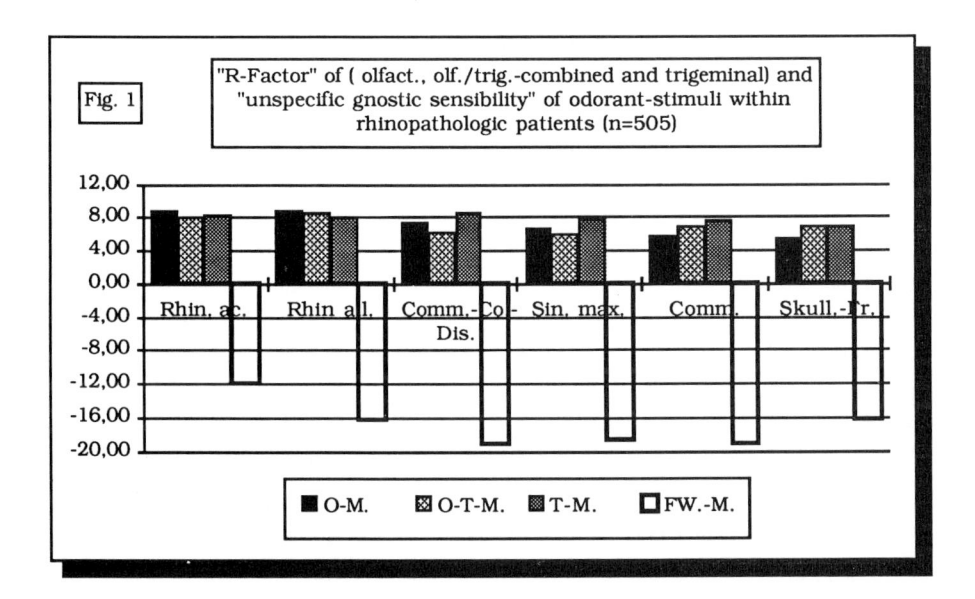

Fig. 1

"R-Factor" of (olfact., olf./trig.-combined and trigeminal) and "unspecific gnostic sensibility" of odorant-stimuli within rhinopathologic patients (n=505)

■ O-M.   ▨ O-T-M.   ▧ T-M.   ☐ FW.-M.

The R-Factor[2] expresses the degree of specific stimulus-detection. A higher level of the R-Factor as we found in non-traumatic disorders such as *Rhinitis acuta* (Olfc. 8,84) and *Rhinitis allergica* (Olfc. 8,70) indicates no severely distorted sensibility as we found in post-traumatic dysosmias (R-Factor lower than 5,50). Especially the group of patients, who suffered from a skull-fracture had the lowest level of gnostic specifity corresponding to the reference group. (Olf. 5,43). There is evidence for less disturbing trigeminal components of sensibility within the recognition of olfactorious-trigeminal stimuli as being shown by the depicted range .

Additionally the sensibility of the entire olfactory stimuli is decreased more impressive ly after head and neck trauma in comparison to a nearly equal range of all stimuli within non-traumatic patients. The level of unspecific gnostic judgement, depicted as negatively aligned columns indicates no higher scored dysfunctions within traumatic patients in relation to non-traumatic clinical features.

DISCUSSION

Posttraumatic dysosmias may arise from severe damages of the *Filae olfactoriae* or from lesions due to brain concussion or compression. Several anatomical parts of the olfactory centres may be altered by a traumatic event. Therefore it is reasonable that different specific abilities of olfaction such as gnostic evaluation of stimuli on a psychophysic scale may be lost, however with remaining unspecific sensivity to detect an odorant. Even a post-commotional state without patho-morpholgical findings may lead to disturbances of the sense of smell. Our results provide evidence for the hypothesis of temporo-spatial-coding[4,7] of chemosensoric information. In comparison to trigeminal stimuli and combined stimuli the original olfactory sensibility is altered at a significant higher level than the combined one. Traumatic lesions are subsequently causing more intensive rhinopathological disorders like *rhinitis* and *sinusitis*, as measured by scoring the stimulus-specifity-range.

As we noticed in prior investigations pleasant classes of odours seem to be affected at higher degree than unpleasant or trigeminal stimuli. Relating to results from single cell measurements in the *Limbic system* and in the area of the *Nuclei habenulae* and the *Periamygdalary region* there provides strong evidence for topologic-anatomical quality-congruence[5] in the deciphering of olfactory-sensory-input. Various types of dysosmias as depicted in the target olfactogram are corresponding to specific lesions in circumscript centres of the *rhinencephalon*. Further investigations are aiming on correlating distinct classified smell disorders with special neuropathologic and pathognomonic aspects.

REFERENCES

1. Claussen, CF (1976) Das klinische Scheibenolfaktogramm. HNO 24 (6), p 209

2. Doty, RL (1975) An Examination of Relationships between the Pleasantness, Intensity and Concentration of 10 Odorous Stimuli. Perc. & Psychophysics 17 (5) p 492-496

3. Fraaß, UE (1989) Die Repräsentation der brenzlichen Gerüche im Scheibenolfaktogram. Inauguraldissertation, Würzburg

4. Jones-Gotman M, Zattore RJ (1988) Olfactory Identification Deficits in Patients. Neuropsychologica, 26 (3) p 387-400

5. Mc Leod, P(1971) Structure and Function of Higher Olfactory Centers. In : Handbook of Sensory Physiology, L. M. Beidler Vol. IV., Olfaction, Berlin, Heidelberg, New York , Springer Verlag

6. Schiffmann S (1974) Psychophysical Correlates of Olfactory Quality. Science, Vol 185 4146 p 112-117

7. Shipley MT, Geinisman Y (1984) Anatomical Evidence for Convergence of Olfac-tory, Gustatory and Visceral Afferent Pathways in Mouse Cerebral Cortex. Brain Res Bull, 12 (3) p 221-6

Index of Authors

AANTAA, Eero — 359,
ALPINI, D. — 67, 193, 409.
ALUND, M. — 265,
AMEDEE, Ronald G. — 395,
ANADAO, Carlos Augusto — 155, 185,
AUST, Gotfried — 247, 327,

BARETTI, F. — 255,
BAROZZI, S. — 409,
BECKER, Regina — 259,
BELEITIS, Eggert — 427,
BERGMANN, Julia Matilde — 5,
BERTORA, Guilermo Oscar — 5,
BLACK, Owen F. — 167,
BODO, George — 159,
BOSSNEV, W. — 343,
BRANTBERG, Krister — 75,
BÜKI, Bela — 45, 273.

CAOVILLA, Heloisa Helena — 155, 185, 381.
CAPUTO, D. — 67, 193,
CARDENAS, Jose Luis — 201,
CASANI, Augusto — 133,
CEDIN, Antonio Carlos — 197,
CERNY, Ervin — 49,
CERNY, Rudolf — 137,
CESARANI, A. — 67, 193, 409
CHALMANOV, V. — 413,
CHERNIUK, V.I. — 171,
CHRIST, P. — 123,
CHROMEJ, Ivan — 373,
CLAUSSEN, Claus-Frenz — 5, 45, 89, 189, 419, 431.
CLAUSSEN, Erika — 5, 89, 419.
CZIGNER, Jeno — 161,

DASCALOV, M. — 343,
DEBLEN, J. — 25,
DECKER, I. — 333,
DEIKE, H. — 175,
DIEROFF, H.G. — 119,
DIMOV, D. — 269,
DOKIANAKIS, G. — 399,

EUBE, Hans — 291,

FARKAS, Zsolt — 295,
FATTORI, Bruno — 133,
FELIPE, Ricardo Galvani — 381,
FERNANDES, Jose Carlos Ramos — 197,
FIRSCHING, Raimund P. — 103,
FISCHER, B. — 339,
FRAASS, Uwe — 45, 431.
FRACHET, Bruno — 37,
FUTSCHIK, Dieter — 405,

GABERSEK, Victor — 31, 37, 63,
GANANCA, Fernando Freitas — 185,
GANANCA, Mauricio Malavasi — 155, 185, 381.
GAVALAS, G. — 301, 399.
GESTEWITZ, B. — 13, 17,
GESTEWITZ, H.R. — 21,

GHEZZI, A.	193,
GHIKOVA, S.	343,
GHILARDI, Pierluigi	133,
GITTER, Alfred H.	79, 83,
GOERTZEN, W.	123,
GOSPODINOV, Manol	221,
GRIMM, R.	167,
GUDZIOL, Hilmar	427,
GUIMARAES, Vera Helena	197,
HADJ-DJILANI, Andre M.T.	217,
HAHN, Ales	45,
HAID, C.T.	123,
HAMANN, Karin	283,
HARALANOV, Haralan	323, 413.
HARALANOV, Lyubomir	323, 363, 377,
HARALANOV, Svetlozar	363, 377,
HEDBRANT, J.	241,
HEID, Lorant	159,
HEMENWAY, W.G.	167,
HIRANANDANI, L.H.	71,
HUBER, G.	333,
INGLE, M.V.	391,
ITO, Yasuko Imasato	185, 381
JÄGER, H.	333,
JANSSON, E.	367,
JAVORKOVA, Jana	373,
JERABEK, Jaroslav	137,
JUNG, Friedrich	387,
KARIMI-NEJAD, Abbas	103,
KATONA, Gabor	295,
KESSLER, Lutz	113,
KIESEWETTER, Holger	387,
KIRTANE, M.V.	391,
KLUBA, J.	175,
KOLCHEV, Christo	141, 413.
KREJCOVA, Nana	137,
KROPF, S.	175,
LANG, Judith	307,
LARSSON, S-E.	265,
LASTOVCHENCO, V.B.	171,
LEDIN, T.	25, 229, 233, 241, 265, 367,
MAGNUSSON, Mans	75,
MANGABEIRA ALBERNAZ, Pedro Luiz	155,
MEICHELBÖCK, M.	123,
MESHCHERIAKOV, G.V.	171,
MEYER, Erhard D.	259,
MINI, M.	67, 193, 409
MÖLLER, C.	229, 265, 367
MÖLLER, M.	229,
MUKHERJEE, Kakoli	9,
NAKOVA, L.	355,
NAYAK, S.R.	391,
NETO, Teotonio T. Costa	185, 381.
NIKOLENKO, V.Y.	171,
NIKOLOVA, N.	343,
NOAKSSON, L.	25,
NORRE, Marcel E.	129, 213,

NORRIS, Charles H.	395,
ÖDKVIST, L.M.	25, 229, 233, 241, 265, 367
OLEINIK, V.S.	171,
OMLOR, A.	333,
PAPAMICHALOPOULOS, M.	399,
PASTIDIS, L.	301,
PATRIZI, M.	255,
PAVLOPOULOS, A.	399,
PESZNECKER, R.N.	167,
PETROVA, Julia	347,
PILGRAMM, M.	311,
PLINKERT, Peter K.	79, 83,
POLLASTRINI, L.	255,
POPIVANOVA, Cvetana	355,
POPOVA, Nevena	347,
POPTODOROV, Georgi	347,
RAICHEVA, Vanja	347,
RIBARI, Oto	273,
RUBIN, Wallace	3, 107, 251,
SAGNELLI, M.	255,
SCHÄFER, W.D.	189,
SCHIEFFER, Hermann-Josef	387,
SCHIMRIGK, K.	333,
SCHNEIDER, Dieter	45, 279,
SCHOLTZ, A.W.	41, 181,
SCHOLTZ, H.J.	41, 181,
SCHUHMANN, G.	119,
SCHWARTZE, Hannelore	319,
SCHWARTZE, Peter	9,
SCHWARTZE, Thomas	319,
SCHWETSCHKE, Olaf	279,
SEJNA, Ivan	287,
SFETSOS, S.	301,
SHOTECOV, Penko	323, 347,
SIEVERT, U.	41, 181,
SILVONIEMI, Pekka	359,
SPELLENBERG, Sandos	307,
SPIRIDONOVA, I.	269,
SPITZER, Stefan	387,
STAMATOVA, L.	53,
STOYNEVA, Zl.	343,
SUZUKI, Fabio Akira	185, 381
SZABADOS Eva	161,
TAKAHASHI, Sachiko	57,
TEGETMEYER, Helmut	319,
THOSS, Franz	9,
TIMAR, Tibor,	295,
TISSON, Pierre	37,
TOMAS, Jaroslav	137,
TRINUS, K.F.	171,
UZUNOV, Nicola	141,
UZUNOVA, M.	53,
VAN DEN ABBEELE, Thierry	37,
VANNUCCHI, Roberta	133,
VATHILAKIS, J.	301,
VON EINSIEDEL, Helga Gräfin	97,
VON SPECHT, H.	339,

WENNMO, Carsten 149, 205,
WILHELM, Hans-Jurgen 387,
WOLF, S. 123,

ZAFFARONI, M. 193,
ZENNER, Hans-Peter 79, 83,

Subject Index

α-bungarotoxin	83
accomodation paresis	191
acetylcholine receptor	84
acousma	364
Acoustically Evoked Potentials (AEP)	104, 177
acoustic admittance	291
acoustic alloesthesia	325
acoustic immittance	291
acoustic reflex threshold	280
acoustic trauma	311
AER (40 Hz)	104
aging	229
air-embolism	327
allergy	71
alternobaric vertigo	329
amphetaminil	406
ampullofugal	61
ampullopetal	61
anorexia	428
anosmia	427, 431
anti-vertigigenous drugs	73
artificial intelligence (AI)	419
ASHNER - DANINI reflex	355
atypical provoked dizziness	129
atypical spontaneous dizziness	129
audio-vestibular disturbances	323
auditory blink reflex	53
auditory pathway	105, 177
automatic nystagmus analysator	5, 21
BABINSKI - WEIL test	355
balance training	229
barochamber exposion	141
barotrauma	160, 327
basal skull fracture	108
BEAM (Brain Electrical Activity Mapping)	45
benign paroxistic positional vertigo	409
Berufsgenossenschaften	89
bilateral hearing loss	283

bimastoid rheoencephalography	344
binaural stereo click stimulus	377
bioelectrical analogical signals	5
biological calibration	5
biomicroscopy	343
blink reflex	53
blood flow velocity (BFV)	347
blunt brain injury	97
blurred vision	191
bodily illusions	50
Brainstem Acoustic Evoked Potentials (BAEP)	104, 269, 287, 295, 373, 377, 381
Brain Electrical Activity Mapping (BEAM)	45
brainstem	189
brain commotional syndrome	347
brain death	104
brain edema	100
brainstem lesion	53
brain stem reflexes	279
butterfly calorigram	93
calibration, biological	5
caloric test	5, 25, 59, 63, 67, 77, 130, 134, 186, 195, 205, 255, 307, 355, 359
canal paresis	134, 195
carbachol	86
CARHART-test	175
carotid	324
car accidents	255
carotid-cavernosus sinus fistulas	100
case report	63, 67
CCG (Cranio-Corpo-Gram)	93, 247
cell potential	80
central auditory transmission	375
central vertigo	133, 307
central vestibular disorders	17, 307
central vestibular system	61
centrophenoxin	406

cerebral concussion	90, 99, 124, 383
cerebral contusion	90, 99, 124
cerebral palsy	53
cerebrovascular reactivity (CVR)	347
cervical nystagmus	134, 257, 259
cervical syndrome	259
cervical vertigo	265, 333
chain incongruence	150
children	31, 53, 295
cholesteatoma	401
chronic otitis	273
CLAMEDEX - expert system	419
clonus-type eye movements	32
CNG (Computernystagmography)	5
CO_2 - test	347
cochlear hearing disorders	175
cochlear implant	37
coherence function	26
commotio labyrinthi	387
complex cranial fracture	217
computed tomography (CT)	97
computer-aided evaluation	21, 195, 205
Computernystagmography (CNG)	5
contusio labyrinthi	121
convergence paresis	191
convergent nystagmus	67
Coriolis acceleration	172
counter diffusion syndrome	328
coup- and contre-coup-focus	189
cranial injury	123
Cranio-Corpo-Gram (CCG)	93, 247
cranium-cerebral trauma (CCT)	355
CT (computed tomography)	97
cupula	61
cupula deviation	10
cupula time constant	61
dark field	13
deafness	269

decompression sickness	327
delabyrinthization	413
depolarization	80
diabetes mellitus	343, 373
diabetic autonomic neuropathy	343
diabetogenic encaphalopathy	373
dichotic speech discrimination test	119
direction-alternating phases	49
directional preponderance	43, 57, 76, 109, 133, 195, 198
disbarism	141
distorsion quotient	120
distorted speech audiometry	119
divergent nystagmus	67
divers	141
dizziness	107, 116, 129, 150, 185, 348
Doppler sonography	343, 347
dynamic posturography	229, 251, 265, 367
ear fullness	156
ear protection	314
electrical vestibular stimulation	37, 78
electromyography (EMG)	319
electronystagmography (ENG)	5, 25, 31, 57, 63, 67, 109, 134, 141, 150, 197, 217, 255
electrooculography (EOG)	25, 31
elementary auditory hallucination	364
elicitability	56
encephalic cervical syndrome of DECHER	259
endolymphatic flow	61
endolymph hydrodynamics	9
endolymphatic hydrops, post-traumatic	169
endolymphatic sac decompression	395
EOG (electrooculography)	25, 31
epidural hematoma	97, 103
epileptic nystagmoid equivalent	63
epileptic nystagmus	63

Eustachian tube function	292, 401
expert system	419
extracochlear electrode	39
extravessel compression	323
eye movements	5, 9, 13, 17, 21, 25, 31, 41, 47, 63, 75, 181
eye tracking test	46, 182
Fast Auditory Evoked Potentials (FAEP)	341
fast phase of nystagmus	6
finger-finger test	13
finger-nose test	13
flavour perception	428
fluidity of blood	387
free fall	319
fronto-basal skull fractures	119
GABA (gamma-aminobutyric acid)	79
GABA$_A$ rezeptors	81
gain	26, 75
galvanic responses	39
galvanic vestibular stimulation	37, 75, 257
gamma-aminobutyric acid (GABA)	79
Glasgow Coma Scale	103
gravitation	41
habituation	56
hair cells	9
hallucination	363
hazy vision	191
head and neck injury	185, 197, 259, 323, 333
head injuries and traumata	97, 103, 107, 133, 161, 197, 217, 221, 259, 279, 301, 323, 363, 381, 387, 391, 427, 431
head shaking nystagmus (HSN)	57, 134
heel-knee test	13
hemotympanum	303
High Pressure Nervous Syndrome (HPNS)	141
high-risk neonates	295
home accidents	91

horizontal semicircular canal	396
hormone disturbances	71
hospitalisation	137
HSN (head shaking nystagmus)	57
hydrops of the membranous labyrinth	71, 161
hydroxyethyl starch	388
Hyperbaric-associated Neurosensorial Deafness Syndrome (HaNSeDS)	141
hyperventilation	348
hypervolaemic haemodilution	388
hypoacusia	273
hyporeflexia	198
hyposmia	431
iatrogenic labyrinthine trauma	399
iatrogenic traumata	273, 399
impedance audiometry	119, 279, 287, 291
informational loading	172
infusion therapy	387
injuries of the temporal region	103
inner ear injuries	167
insulin independent diabetes	343
insurance competences	91
intracranial bleeding	113
intracranial extracerebral hemorrhage	97
intraoperative acoustic trauma	274
K^+ conductanes	80
kinesiologic disorders	138
kinetic posturography	213
labyrinthine concussion	133, 217
labyrinthine preponderance	13398
labyrinthitis	402
latex thimble	207
learning to read	31
LERMOYEZ' syndrome	325
leucodystrophy	271
linear discriminant analysis	321
living habits	427
loading experiments	171

MACHINTOSH computer	421
Magnetic Resonance Imaging (MRI)	63
Mangabeira Albernaz, Pedro Luiz	3
membrane hyperpolarization	80
Meniérè's Syndrome	71, 155, 161, 325, 395
mentally ill patients	363
microprocessors	5
mild head injury	90, 133
minor head trauma	90, 133
mono-jodine acetic acid	413
motor control	221
movement coordination	252, 367
movement coordination test (MC)	229, 265, 367
MRI (Magnetic Resonance Imaging)	63
MS (Multiple Sclerosis)	67, 193
myringotomy	401
nausea	185, 273, 283, 343
nervus vagus	343
network structure	419
neural muscular atrophy	175
neurotransmitter	79, 83
nicotinic receptor	86
NODEC - neurootological data bank	90, 431
non-nystagmic saccadic ocular movements	14
nootropics	405
nuclear paresis	191
nystagmic saccadic ocular movements	15, 17
nystagmoids	7
nystagmus	5, 25, 37, 41, 47, 57, 63, 67, 75, 109, 123, 133, 137, 150, 167, 259, 355, 359, 415
nystagmus alternans	51
nystagmus criteria	6
nystagmus recognition	6
oblique eye movements	31
oblique pursuit eye movements	181
oblique saccades	181

occupational hazards	91, 150
ocular apraxia, transitory ideomotor	35
ocular dysmetria	308
ocular epileptic equivalent	63
ocular grasping reflex	33
oculocorporal associated eye movements	32
oculoglottic occurence	33
Oculomotor Reaction Time (OMRT)	31
oculomotor crisis	63
oculomotor disturbances	31
oculomotor stimulation	63
oculopalpebral associated eye movements	32
OKAN (optokinetic afternystagmus)	41, 57, 70, 75, 156, 186
OKN (optokinetic nystagmus)	41, 75, 156, 186, 201, 255, 307
olfactory engrams	428
olivo-cochlear efferents	83
OMRT (Oculomotor Reaction Time)	31
open head injury	97
optic nerve	391
opto-vestibulo-spinal system	182
optokinetic afternystagmus (OKAN)	41, 57, 70, 75, 156, 186
optokinetic nystagmus (OKN)	41, 75, 156, 186, 201, 255, 307
optokinetic striped pattern	41
organic hallucination	363
ossicular chain discontinuity	303
oto-baro traumatism	141
otobasal fractures	89, 97, 107, 113
ototoxic aminoglycoside antibiotics	269
outer hair cells	79, 83
parasympathicotonic manifestations	356
parosmia	431
paroxysmal positional vertigo	134
patch-clamp experiment	80
pedaudiology	295
pendular sinusoidal Greiner stimulation	193

PENG method (photoelectronystagmography)	13, 17, 21, 38, 42, 182, 339, 405
perilymph fistule	159, 167, 276, 304
perilymph leakage	159, 167
perinatally hypoxic rabbits	319
peripheral facial paresis	117
peripheral vertigo	133
peripheral vestibular disorders	17
perturbation	233, 241
perturbed posturography	233, 241
petrous bone fracture	124, 217
photoelectronystagmography (PENG)	13, 17, 21, 38, 42, 182, 339, 405
piracetam	406
polyneuropathia	175
polytrauma	113
positional nystagmus	108, 186
positional oculocephalic ass. eye movements	32
positional vertigo	124, 134, 167, 259, 308, 409
positioning vertigo	124, 134, 259
post-concussion neurosis	307
post-galvanic nystagmus	39, 75
post-operative vertigo	399
post-traumatic blindness	391
postconcussion syndrome	189, 201
postcontusional ocular disturbances	189
postoperative infection	273
postrotatory nystagmus (PRN)	57
postsynaptic receptor	83
posttraumatic brain lesions	97
posttraumatic cerebrasthenic syndrome	347
posttraumatic disorders of balance	387
posttraumatic dysequilibrium	89, 129, 133, 405
posttraumatic dysosmia	427, 431
posttraumatic hearing defects	387, 405
posttraumatic vertigo	89, 129, 133, 405

posturography	130, 213, 217, 229, 233, 241, 247, 251, 367
pressure of spraying	160
PRN (postratatory nystagmus)	57
Prostaglandin E 1	388
psyco-organic syndrome (POS)	367
pulsating tinnitus	333
pure tone audiometry	120, 141, 150, 162, 175, 186
pursuit eye movement	31
pyramidal longitudinal fractures	113
pyramidal transvers fractures	113
pyritinol	406
radical mastoid cavity	205
reading glasses	191
removal of ear packing	402
retrocochlear hearing disorders	175
rhinobasal fractures	113
rhinomanometry	431
RIDT (Rotatory Intensity Damping Test)	93
ROMBERG coefficient	221
ROMBERG test	247, 355
Rotatory Intensity Damping Test (RIDT)	93
rotatory test	5, 25, 47, 57, 130, 195, 359
rotatory vertigo	360
saccadic test	134
SAK (Somato-autokinesis)	49
scull base fracture	103, 113
selective chemical vestibulectomy	395
semicircular canal	61
SEMONT manouvre	410
sensation of swaying	360
sensorineural hearing loss	107, 149, 156, 185, 269, 287, 304, 311
sensory organization	252
sensory organization test (SO)	229, 265, 367
serological findings	138

slow phase velocity (SPV)	6, 26, 42, 59, 76, 208
smooth pursuit	308
Somato-autokinesis (SAK)	49
Somatosensory Evoked Potentials (SEP)	104
speech analysis	119
speech audiometry	141, 150, 175
speech intelligibility score	186
spontaneous nystagmus	107, 134, 150, 186, 307, 339, 359
sports accidents	91
SPV (slow phase velocity)	26, 42, 59, 76
square waves	17
stabilometry	221
stapedectomy	273, 275
stapedius reflex	292
static posturography	213, 369
streptomycin	395
subdural hematoma	97, 103, 377
substantia reticularis	51
sudden hearing loss (SHL)	287
supranuclear paresis	191
surgical treatment	395
symmetrical sensor coordinatometry	221
sympathicotonic manifestations	356
target olfactogram	431
temporal bone fracture	107, 149, 185, 301
thermistor thermography	343
thrombosis	324
tinnitus	152, 156, 159, 167, 186, 311, 329, 333
topodiagnostics	17, 48, 177, 273, 363
tractor drivers	173
traffic accidents	91, 113, 150
tramping test	217
trans-ethmoid decompression	391
transfer function	26
transient vertigo attacks	348
transitory ideomotor ocular apraxia	35

traumatic carotid dissection	333
trauma classification	91
treatment	73, 405, 409
tremorometry	222
triffling trauma	283
tripelenamine	406
tympanic membrane defect	205
tympanic membrane rupture	303
tympanotomy	159, 168
undulations	7
unilateral sensorineural hearing loss	107, 186
unilateral subdural hematom	377
unilateral vestibular function loss	413
UNTERBERGER-FUKUDA stepping test	248
VALSALVA test	348
vascular pathology	71
vasodilators	73
vectornystagmography (VENG)	155, 197
vegetative responses	355
velocity storage mechanism	41, 61
venesection	388
VEP (Visual Evoked Potentials)	45
vergence nystagmus	67
vertebro-basiliar insufficiency (VBI)	138, 339
vertigo	63, 92, 107, 116, 123, 129, 133, 137, 149, 156, 159, 167, 186, 255, 259, 273, 283, 333, 343, 359, 363
vestibular afferents, thick	9
vestibular afferents, thin	9
vestibular asymmetry	57, 75, 413
vestibular compensation	107, 117, 123, 131, 252, 413
vestibular evoked potentials (VestEP)	171
vestibular loss	283
vestibular neuronitis	359
vestibular physical therapy	168

vestibular rehabilitation	252
vestibular stimulation	9
vestibular system	9
vestibulo-motor reflexes	319
vestibulo-ocular reflex (VOR)	11, 25, 41, 75, 130, 193
vestibulo-spinal reflex (VSR)	130, 247
vibration	172
viral labyrinthitis	71
viral neuronitis	71
virus intoxication	269
Visual Evoked Potentials (VEP)	45, 104, 415
visual disturbances	189
visual hallucinations	63
visual-vestibular interaction	201
visual suppression (VS)	25
visual suppression test	193
visuomotor coordination	32
vomitus	185
VOR (vestibulo-ocular reflex)	11, 25, 41, 75, 130
VS (visual suppression)	25
VS quotient	25
WARDENBURG's syndrome	271
whiplash injury	110, 133, 255, 259, 333
whole-body vibration	171